Global Exosome Trials

Jeffrey N. Weiss

Global Exosome Trials

Springer

Jeffrey N. Weiss
American College of Regenerative Medicine
Parkland, FL, USA

ISBN 978-3-031-96419-0 ISBN 978-3-031-96420-6 (eBook)
https://doi.org/10.1007/978-3-031-96420-6

This Springer imprint is published by the registered company Springer Nature Switzerland AG
The registered company address is: Gewerbestrasse 11, 6330 Cham, Switzerland

For the patients that have allowed us the privilege to serve.

Preface

This book is a compendium of Active global exosome trials that are registered with clinicaltrials.gov. Clinicaltrials.gov, the website of the United States National Institutes of Health, is the largest listing of research studies in the world. The information is accurate as of January 2025.

I have corrected the mischaracterization of studies, to only include those that truly belong within each category, and to correct spelling and grammar, without changing the spirit or intentions of the submitters, in order to produce a consistent and easy to read format. The studies are listed according to the treated diagnosis.

I hope that by providing this reference, the field of exosome therapy research will be advanced.

Parkland, FL, USA   Jeffrey N. Weiss

Contents

1 What Are Exosomes? 1

2 Cancer Exosome Trials 3

3 Cardiac Exosome Trials 133

4 Renal Exosome Trials 143

5 Diabetes Exosome Trials 149

6 Miscellaneous Exosome Trials 175

7 Ophthalmology Exosome Trials 247

8 Orthopedic Exosome Trials 271

9 Pulmonary Exosome Trials 289

10 Rectum/Anus Exosome Trials 321

11 Skin Exosome Trials 329

12 Stroke Exosome Trials 349

Index 369

Chapter 1
What Are Exosomes?

Exosomes are extracellular vesicles, 30–150 nm in diameter, enclosed by a lipid membrane, that are secreted by cells. They contain mRNA, miRNA, non-coding RNA, DNA, lipids, and proteins and provide intercellular communication, maintain cellular homeostasis, and remove cellular debris. They are primarily found in saliva, urine, cerebrospinal fluid, and serum and travel in all body fluids. Their contents reflect that of the originating cell.

Exosome properties include low immunogenicity, stability, biomembrane penetration, and biocompatibility making them a potential innovation for drug delivery and for diagnostics. Encapsulating drugs in exosomes avoids the possibility of inactivation and dilution by blood. Exosomes have been demonstrated to control apoptosis, offer cytoprotection, and promote angiogenesis. They have the ability to cross the blood-brain barrier.

Exosomes may be isolated from blood and urine, and since they contain proteins reflective of many diseases and cancer, the hope is that they can be biomarkers of these conditions as a new diagnostic test.

The United States and China lead in both the number of published journal articles and the number of patents. Most exosome manufacturers are located in the United States, followed by Europe, and then Asia.

Naturally occurring exosomes may be modified to improve their targeting ability, improve their drug loading capacity and efficiency, and resist clearance from the body.

J. N. Weiss, *Global Exosome Trials*, https://doi.org/10.1007/978-3-031-96420-6_1

Bibliography

1. Krylova SV, Feng D. The machinery of exosomes: biogenesis, release, and uptake. Int J Mol Sci. 2023;24(2):1337. https://doi.org/10.3390/ijms24021337. PMID: 36674857; PMCID: PMC9865891.
2. Tenchov R, Sasso JM, Wang X, Liaw WS, Chen CA, Zhou QA. Exosomes—Nature's lipid nanoparticles, a rising star in drug delivery and diagnostics. ACS Nano. 2022;16(11):17802–46. https://doi.org/10.1021/acsnano.2c08774. Epub 2022 Nov 10. PMID: 36354238; PMCID: PMC9706680.
3. Rajput A, Varshney A, Bajaj R, Pokharkar V. Exosomes as new generation vehicles for drug delivery: biomedical applications and future perspectives. Molecules. 2022;27(21):7289. https://doi.org/10.3390/molecules27217289. PMID: 36364116; PMCID: PMC9658823.
4. Tian J, Han Z, Song D, Peng Y, Xiong M, Chen Z, Duan S, Zhang L. Engineered exosome for drug delivery: recent development and clinical applications. Int J Nanomedicine. 2023;18:7923–40. https://doi.org/10.2147/IJN.S444582. PMID: 38152837; PMCID: PMC10752020.
5. Wang B, Xing D, Zhu Y, Dong S, Zhao B. The state of exosomes research: a global visualized analysis. Biomed Res Int. 2019;2019:1495130. https://doi.org/10.1155/2019/1495130. PMID: 31073519; PMCID: PMC6470441.

Chapter 2
Cancer Exosome Trials

Cancer

Recruiting

Non-small Cell Lung Cancer with Central Nervous System Metastasis

ClinicalTrials.gov ID NCT06026735

Sponsor: National Taiwan University Hospital

Information provided by National Taiwan University Hospital (responsible party)

Last update posted: 2023-09-07

Study Overview

Brief Summary

Cerebrospinal fluid was obtained from the cerebrospinal cavity of non-small cell lung cancer patients with central nervous system metastasis, blood was obtained from veins, and metastatic lung cancer tumor tissue was obtained from surgically resected brain tumors or meningeal tumors. Then, comprehensively analyze the exosomes contained in the aforementioned samples and compare and analyze the clinical data of the patients, so as to explore whether the cancer cell-related substances contained in the cerebrospinal fluid, blood, and tumor tissue can be used to predict lung cancer metastasis and bioindicators of treatment effect.

Official Title

Comprehensive Profiling of Promising Biomarkers in Exosomes from Non-small Cell Lung Cancer with Central Nervous System Metastasis

Conditions

Lung cancer with central nervous system metastasis

Intervention/Treatment

J. N. Weiss, *Global Exosome Trials*, https://doi.org/10.1007/978-3-031-96420-6_2

- Other: lung cancer with brain/leptomeningeal metastasis

Other Study ID Numbers

- 202209032RINB

Study Start (Actual)
2023-01-13
Primary Completion (Estimated)
2027-12
Study Completion (Estimated)
2027-12
Enrollment (Estimated)
30
Study Type
Observational
Study Contact
Name: Abel Huang, MD
Phone Number: +8860223123456 ext 265913
Email: how.how0622@gmail.com
Study Contact Backup
Name: Abel Huang
Phone Number: +8860223123456 ext 265913
Email: how.how0622@gmail.com
This study has one location.
Taiwan
Taipei, Taiwan, 100
Recruiting
National Taiwan University Hospital
Contact:
Abel Huang
023123456 ext 265913 how.how0622@gmail.com
Eligibility Criteria
Description
Inclusion criteria:

A. Non-small cell lung cancer patients diagnosed with brain metastases or meningeal metastases on brain computed tomography (CT) or magnetic resonance (MRI) images
B. Patients with non-small cell lung cancer who are about to undergo surgical brain surgery, such as brain tumor resection, lumbar abdominal drainage, Euclidean storage, or ventriculoperitoneal drainage

Exclusion criteria:

A. Non-small cell lung cancer patients without brain metastases or meningeal metastases
B. Physical condition does not allow surgical removal of the tumor

Study population

Non-small cell lung cancer patients with brain metastases or meningeal metastases

Ages Eligible for Study

20 to 90 years (adult, older adult)

Sexes Eligible for Study

All

Accepts Healthy Volunteers

No

Sampling Method

Probability sample

Design Details

Observational model: case-only

Time perspective: prospective

Groups and Interventions

Groups/cohorts	Intervention/treatment
Lung cancer with brain metastasis	Other: lung cancer with brain/leptomeningeal metastasis Cerebrospinal fluid was obtained from the cerebrospinal cavity of non-small cell lung cancer patients with central nervous system metastasis, blood was obtained from veins, and metastatic lung cancer tumor tissue was obtained from surgically resected brain tumors or meningeal tumors. Then, comprehensively analyze the exosomes contained in the aforementioned samples, and compare and analyze the clinical data of the patients, so as to explore whether the cancer cell-related substances contained in the cerebrospinal fluid, blood, and tumor tissue can be used to predict lung cancer metastasis and bioindicators of treatment effect.
Lung cancer with leptomeningeal metastasis	Other: lung cancer with brain/leptomeningeal metastasis Cerebrospinal fluid was obtained from the cerebrospinal cavity of non-small cell lung cancer patients with central nervous system metastasis, blood was obtained from veins, and metastatic lung cancer tumor tissue was obtained from surgically resected brain tumors or meningeal tumors. Then, comprehensively analyze the exosomes contained in the aforementioned samples, and compare and analyze the clinical data of the patients, so as to explore whether the cancer cell-related substances contained in the cerebrospinal fluid, blood and tumor tissue can be used to predict lung cancer metastasis and bioindicators of treatment effect.

Primary Outcome Measures

Outcome measure	Measure description	Time frame
Predict lung cancer metastasis and bioindicators of treatment effect	Cerebrospinal fluid was obtained from the cerebrospinal cavity of non-small cell lung cancer patients with central nervous system metastasis, blood was obtained from veins, and metastatic lung cancer tumor tissue was obtained from surgically resected brain tumors or meningeal tumors. Then, comprehensively analyze the exosomes contained in the aforementioned samples, and compare and analyze the clinical data of the patients, so as to explore whether the cancer cell-related substances contained in the cerebrospinal fluid, blood, and tumor tissue can be used to predict lung cancer metastasis and bioindicators of treatment effect.	Follow 3 years

Sponsor: National Taiwan University Hospital

Active, Not Recruiting

Exosome as the Prognostic and Predictive Biomarker in EBC Patients

ClinicalTrials.gov ID NCT05955521

Sponsor: Samsung Medical Center

Information provided by JI-YEON, KIM, Samsung Medical Center (responsible party)

Last update posted: 2023-07-21

Study Overview

Brief Summary

This study is the experimental study for serial ctDNA and exosome evaluation in EBC patients

Official Title

Development of a Prognostic and Predictive Biomarker for Locally Advanced Breast Cancer Patients Treated with Neoadjuvant Chemotherapy Using Exosome

Conditions

Triple-negative breast cancer

HER2-positive breast cancer

Intervention/treatment

- Procedure: exosome and ctDNA evaluation

Other Study ID Numbers

- EXO_Breast

Study Start (Actual)
2021-05-01

Primary Completion (Actual)
2023-07-01
Study Completion (Estimated)
2028-07-01
Enrollment (Actual)
200
Study Type
Interventional
Phase
Not applicable
This study has one location.
Republic of Korea
Seoul, Republic of Korea, 06351
Ji-Yeon Kim
Eligibility Criteria
Description
Inclusion criteria:

- Early breast cancer
- Planned neoadjuvant chemotherapy
- Triple negative breast cancer or HER2-positive breast cancer

Exclusion criteria:

- Stage IV breast cancer
- Hormone receptor positive breast cancer

Ages Eligible for Study
Child, adult, older adult
Sexes Eligible for Study
Female
Accepts Healthy Volunteers
Yes
Design Details
Primary purpose: screening
Allocation: N/A
Interventional model: single group assignment
Masking: none (open label)

Arms and Interventions

Participant group/arm	Intervention/treatment
Experimental: CtDNA/exosome evaluation	Procedure: exosome and ctDNA evaluation Serial exosome and ctDNA evaluation during follow-up period between neoadjuvant chemotherapy and surveillance after curative surgery

Primary Outcome Measures

Outcome measure	Measure description	Time frame
Prognostic biomarker for EBC	Positive predictive value of ctDNA/exosome for BC recurrence	60 months

Sponsor: Samsung Medical Center

Not Yet Recruiting

Effects of Exosome Administration in Preventing Early Leakage in Rectal Cancer Patients Undergoing Low Anterior Resection

ClinicalTrials.gov ID NCT06536712

Sponsor: Tehran University of Medical Sciences

Information provided by Ahmadi Tafti, Tehran University of Medical Sciences (responsible party)

Last update posted: 2024-08-05

Study Overview

Brief Summary

The goal of this clinical trial is to assess the safety and efficacy of human placenta mesenchymal stem cell-derived exosomes in preventing early anastomosis leak in patients undergoing low anterior resection for rectal cancer. The main question it aims to answer is as follows:

Do mesenchymal stem cell-derived exosomes prevent early anastomosis leak in patients undergoing low anterior resection for rectal cancer?

If there is a comparison group: researchers will compare mesenchymal stem cell-derived exosomes to placebo to see if it can prevent early anastomotic leakage.

Participants will receive intraperitoneal mesenchymal stem cell-derived exosomes at the end of their surgery.

Detailed Description

Anastomotic leakage remains one of the most severe complications following colorectal surgery, leading to increased morbidity, prolonged hospitalization, and reduced quality of life. Despite advances in surgical techniques and perioperative care, the incidence of early anastomotic leaks persists. Practical strategies to reduce this risk are crucial for improving patient outcomes.

Recent studies have highlighted the potential role of mesenchymal stem cell-derived exosomes in enhancing tissue repair and modulating inflammation. These extracellular vesicles, derived from human placenta mesenchymal stem cells (hPMSC), contain bioactive molecules such as proteins, lipids, and RNA that facilitate cellular communication and promote healing processes. Preclinical research suggests that exosomes can support anastomotic healing by reducing local inflammation.

This study aims to evaluate the safety and efficacy of intraperitoneal administration of hPMSC-derived exosomes in preventing early anastomotic leakage in patients undergoing low anterior resection (LAR) for rectal cancer. We hypothesize that the exosome treatment will significantly reduce the incidence of anastomotic leaks compared to placebo, thereby improving postoperative recovery and reducing hospital stay.

Official Title

Investigating the Effect of Intraperitoneal Administration of Exosome in Preventing Early Anastomotic Leakage in Rectal Cancer Patients Who Undergo Low Anterior Resection

Conditions

Rectal cancer

Intervention/treatment

- Biological: mesenchymal stem cell-derived exosomes
- Other: placebo

Other Study ID Numbers

- IR.TUMS.IKHC.REC.1403.114

Study Start (Estimated)

2024-08

Primary Completion (Estimated)

2024-10

Study Completion (Estimated)

2024-12

Enrollment (Estimated)

20

Study Type

Interventional

Phase

Phase 1

Study Contact

Name: Seyed Mohsen Ahmadi Tafti, MD

Phone Number: +98(912)2109773

Email: smahmadit@sina.tums.ac.ir

This study has one location.

Islamic Republic of Iran

Tehran, Iran, Islamic Republic of, 1419733141

Division of Colorectal Surgery, Department of Surgery, Tehran University of Medical Sciences, Tehran, Iran

Eligibility Criteria

Description

Inclusion criteria:

Patients with stage II–III rectal cancer who underwent neoadjuvant chemoradiation therapy and are candidates for low anterior resection surgery

Exclusion criteria:

- Patients who need emergency surgery (presenting with peritonitis or signs of obstruction)
- Patients with apparent malnutrition or patients who have serum albumin levels of less than 3 g/dl
- Patients who receive corticosteroids (an equivalent dose of prednisolone 5 mg/day or more)
- Patients with chronic pulmonary disease
- Patients who need more than two units of blood transfusion perioperatively

Ages Eligible for Study
18 to 75 years (adult, older adult)
Sexes Eligible for Study
All
Accepts Healthy Volunteers
No
Design Details
Primary purpose: prevention
Allocation: non-randomized
Interventional model: parallel assignment
Masking: quadruple (participant, care provider, investigator, outcomes assessor)

Arms and Interventions

Participant group/arm	Intervention/treatment
Experimental: mesenchymal stem cell-derived exosomes 10 patients in this arm will receive mesenchymal stem cell-derived exosomes at the end of their low anterior resection surgery.	Biological: mesenchymal stem cell-derived exosomes Mesenchymal stem cell-derived exosomes will be administered intraperitoneally to patients at the end of their surgery.
Placebo comparator: placebo 10 patients in this arm will receive placebo at the end of their low anterior resection surgery.	Other: placebo 10 patients will receive intraperitoneal placebo at the end of their surgery.

Primary Outcome Measures

Outcome measure	Measure description	Time frame
Number of patients with early anastomotic leakage	Failed surgical anastomosis after surgery measured with interview and physical examinations in follow-up sessions in clinic	1 month

Secondary Outcome Measures

Outcome measure	Measure description	Time frame
Mean serum and peritoneal interleukin-6 and tumor necrosis factor-alpha levels in participants	The level of serum and peritoneal inflammatory markers in postoperative days measured with laboratory tests	1 month
Anastomosis integrity in colonoscopy exam	A colonoscopy will be conducted one month after surgery to assess the integrity of the colorectal anastomosis, detect early signs of local recurrence, identify polyps, and monitor for any postoperative complications such as strictures or inflammatory changes. Baseline colonoscopies will be compared with post-surgical colonoscopy at one month. This outcome will help determine the efficacy of surgical intervention and guide future surveillance strategies in rectal cancer management.	1 month
Hospitalization length of stay	The number of days that the patient in hospitalized postoperatively	1 month

Sponsor: Tehran University of Medical Sciences

Investigators

- Study director: Seyed Mohsen Ahmadi Tafti, MD, Colorectal Research Center, Imam Khomeini Hospital, Tehran University of Medical Sciences

Publications

- Platell C, Barwood N, Dorfmann G, Makin G. The incidence of anastomotic leaks in patients undergoing colorectal surgery. Colorectal Dis. 2007;9(1):71–9. https://doi.org/10.1111/j.1463-1318.2006.01002.x.
- Lipska MA, Bissett IP, Parry BR, Merrie AE. Anastomotic leakage after lower gastrointestinal anastomosis: men are at a higher risk. ANZ J Surg. 2006;76(7):579–85. https://doi.org/10.1111/j.1445-2197.2006.03780.x.
- Choi HK, Law WL, Ho JW. Leakage after resection and intraperitoneal anastomosis for colorectal malignancy: analysis of risk factors. Dis Colon Rectum. 2006;49(11):1719–25. https://doi.org/10.1007/s10350-006-0703-2.
- Barnhoorn MC, Wasser MNJM, Roelofs H, Maljaars PWJ, Molendijk I, Bonsing BA, Oosten LEM, Dijkstra G, van der Woude CJ, Roelen DL, Zwaginga JJ, Verspaget HW, Fibbe WE, Hommes DW, Peeters KCMJ, van der Meulen-de Jong AE. Long-term Evaluation of Allogeneic Bone Marrow-derived Mesenchymal Stromal Cell Therapy for Crohn's Disease Perianal Fistulas. J Crohns Colitis. 2020;14(1):64–70. https://doi.org/10.1093/ecco-jcc/jjz116.

- Tashak Golroudbari H, Banikarimi SP, Ayati A, Hadizadeh A, Khorasani Zavareh Z, Hajikhani K, Heirani-Tabasi A, Ahmadi Tafti M, Davoodi S, Ahmadi Tafti H. Advanced micro-/nanotechnologies for exosome encapsulation and targeting in regenerative medicine. Clin Exp Med. 2023;23(6):1845–66. https://doi.org/10.1007/s10238-023-00993-7. Epub 2023 Jan 27.

Recruiting

Study Investigating the Ability of Plant Exosomes to Deliver Curcumin to Normal and Colon Cancer Tissue

ClinicalTrials.gov ID NCT01294072

Sponsor: University of Louisville

Information provided by Gerald W. Dryden, Jr., University of Louisville (responsible party)

Last update posted: 2023-12-20

Study Overview

Brief Summary

This clinical trial will investigate the ability of plant exosomes to more effectively deliver curcumin to normal colon tissue and colon tumors. Curcumin is the yellow pigment of turmeric, a natural product with diverse biological activities. Exosomes are small endosome-derived vesicles (50–100 nm in size). Previous clinical trials conducted with oral curcumin have demonstrated only limited bioavailability even at very high doses of 8–12 grams per day. This trial plans to address this problem of curcumin delivery by using plant exosomes to deliver the drug to colon tumors and normal colon tissue.

Detailed Description

Curcumin is a constituent of the spice turmeric, which is one of the primary ingredients of curry powder. Curcumin has been shown to interfere with colon carcinogenesis in a variety of chemical and genetic rodent models. It has also been shown to have a strong inhibitory effect on the growth of colon cancer cell lines. There is considerable evidence that the effects of curcumin are mediated by changes in signal transduction. There is an extensive body of work showing effects on several signaling pathways, including the beta-catenin and NF-κB pathways. Although curcumin has been viewed as an ideal chemopreventative agent in colon cancer for many years, its application has been impeded by important issues with drug delivery and bioavailability in the reported clinical trials of this compound.

Work from the James Graham Brown Cancer Center published recently suggests that using exosomes as a delivery vehicle leads to overcoming all the major obstacles of using curcumin as an anti-inflammatory agent, including increased stability, solubility, and bioavailability of curcumin. The work was further extended to define the resource that can supply a large quantity of exosomes with a maximum binding capacity of curcumin. Emerging data indicate that exosomes derived from many fruits release exosome-like particles strongly bind to many hydrophobic drugs including curcumin and are taken up by the intestine cells as well as the immune cells in the intestine. These results suggest that these fruit-derived exosomes are potentially used as a delivery vehicle to treatment of intestinal diseases. Moreover, both fruit exosomes and curcumin should not generate any side-effects since they are consumed by humans daily.

In this clinical trial, the effect of exosomally delivered curcumin on the immune modulation, cellular metabolism, and phospholipid profile of normal and malignant colon cells in subjects who are undergoing surgery for newly diagnosed colon cancer will be characterized. In selected subjects, the effect of exosomally delivered curcumin on the production of cytokines, the changes of immune cells, and glucose metabolism by administration of 13C-glucose prior to surgical resection will also be characterized.

Official Title

Phase I Clinical Trial Investigating the Ability of Plant Exosomes to Deliver Curcumin to Normal and Malignant Colon Tissue

Conditions

Colon cancer

Intervention/Treatment

- Dietary supplement: curcumin
- Dietary supplement: curcumin conjugated with plant exosomes
- Other: no intervention

Other Study ID Numbers

- BCC-GI-10 curcumin

Study Start

2011-01

Primary Completion (Estimated)

2024-11

Study Completion (Estimated)

2024-11

Enrollment (Estimated)

35

Study Type

Interventional

Phase

Not applicable

Study Contact

Name: Gerald W Dryden Jr, MD, PhD

Phone number: 502-852-6991

Email: gerald.dryden@louisville.edu

This study has one location.

United States

Kentucky locations

Louisville, Kentucky, United States, 40202
Recruiting
University of Louisville Hospital
Principal investigator: Gerald W Dryden, MD, PhD
Eligibility Criteria
Description
Inclusion criteria:

- Subjects must have definitive diagnosis of colon cancer.
- Surgical resection of the primary tumor must be an option for the newly diagnosed cancer.
- No history of diabetes.
- Subjects must be informed of the investigational nature of this study and sign and give written informed consent in accordance with institutional and federal guidelines.
- Absence of life-limiting medical conditions.
- Ability to understand and willingness to sign a written informed consent document.
- Eastern Cooperative Oncology Group (ECOG) performance status 0, 1, or 2 (Karnofsky > 60%; see Appendix A).
- Subjects must have adequate bone marrow function. ANC > 1000/microliters (microL) and platelet count >100,000/microL.
- Age >20 years

Exclusion criteria:

- Known familial colon cancer syndrome
- Pregnancy
- Known human immunodeficiency virus (HIV)
- Patients receiving immunosuppressive drugs
- Inflammatory bowel disease
- Active second malignancy in the last 5 years
- Patients receiving any other investigational agent(s)
- Patients who have received any prior chemotherapy or radiation therapy to the primary colon cancer
- Intolerance to grapes, grapefruit, or curcumin
- History of diabetes mellitus

Ages Eligible for Study
20 Years and older (adult, older adult)
Sexes Eligible for Study
All
Accepts Healthy Volunteers
No
Design Details
Primary purpose: basic science
Allocation: randomized
Interventional model: parallel assignment

Interventional model description: curcumin alone in capsule form (Arm 1), curcumin combined with plant exosomes (Arm 2), and will not take curcumin or plant exosomes (Arm 3)

Masking: none (open label)

Arms and Interventions

Participant group/arm	Intervention/treatment
Experimental: Arm 1: curcumin alone Subjects take curcumin orally.	Dietary supplement: curcumin Tablets: 3.6 gram (gm) taken daily for 7 days—15 subjects
Experimental: Arm 2: curcumin with plant exosomes Subjects take curcumin conjugated with plant exosomes.	Dietary supplement: curcumin conjugated with plant exosomes Tablets: taken daily for 7 days—15 subjects
Experimental: Arm 3: no treatment Subjects will not take curcumin or plant exosomes	Other: no intervention No treatment

Primary Outcome Measures

Outcome measure	Measure description	Time frame
Concentration of curcumin in normal and cancerous tissue	Concentration of curcumin delivered with curcumin alone or curcumin conjugated with plant exosomes to normal and cancerous colon cells will be compared. This exploratory trial is designed to estimate the effect of a fixed concentration of curcumin when delivered by plant exosomes compared to oral tablets of curcumin alone.	7 days after start of curcumin ingestion

Secondary Outcome Measures

Outcome measure	Measure description	Time frame
Safety and tolerability of curcumin alone as determined by adverse events	Curcumin will be taken orally.	7 days after study enrollment
Effects of curcumin on normal and cancerous colon cells by measuring the biomarkers using histochemical staining		7 days after patient enrollment
The immune system response to curcumin, measured by serum cytokine levels		7 days after patient enrollment in study
Immune response in ex vivo cell cultures of colon cancer cells treated with curcumin and Exo-cur, to be evaluated by using histochemical staining		7 days after patient enrollment in study
Measurement of curcumin alone on metabolic characteristics of normal colon mucosa and colon tumors		7 days after patient enrollment
Safety and tolerability of curcumin with plant exosomes as determined by adverse events	Curcumin and plant exosomes will be taken orally.	7 days after study enrollment
Measurement of curcumin mixed with plant exosomes on metabolic characteristics of normal colon mucosa and colon tumors		7 days after patient enrollment on study

Sponsor: University of Louisville

Investigators

- Principal investigator: Gerald W Dryden Jr, MD, PhD, University of Louisville

Publications

- Wu K, Xing F, Wu SY, Watabe K. Extracellular vesicles as emerging targets in cancer: Recent development from bench to bedside. Biochim Biophys Acta Rev Cancer. 2017;1868(2):538–63. https://doi.org/10.1016/j.bbcan.2017.10.001. Epub 2017 Oct 18.

Recruiting

Pancreatic Cancer Detection Consortium (PCDC)

ClinicalTrials.gov ID NCT06388967

Sponsor: City of Hope Medical Center

Information provided by City of Hope Medical Center (responsible party)

Last update posted: 2024-04-29

Study Overview

Brief Summary

This study aims to prospective validate an exosome-based miRNA signature for noninvasive and early detection of pancreatic ductal adenocarcinoma.

Detailed Description

Pancreatic ductal adenocarcinoma (PDAC) is one of the deadliest forms of cancer. It often goes undetected until it is at an advanced stage, making it challenging to treat. Currently, only a small percentage of patients are diagnosed early enough for effective treatment. While a blood marker exists, called serum carbohydrate antigen 19-9 (CA19-9), it is used primarily to track the disease and it is unreliable for early detection.

To address this problem, the researchers have developed a new method to analyze circulating vesicles (called exosomes), which contain specific genetic material called microRNAs (miRNAs). In a previous study, by analyzing both the miRNAs that circulate freely in serum and the miRNAs that are inside the exosomes, the researchers have already identified a combination of 13 miRNAs that could accurately detect early-stage PDAC.

In this study, the researchers will test this method in a larger international cohort study. This study aims to confirm the effectiveness of this approach in accurately identifying PDAC at its earliest stages.

Official Title

Early Detection of Pancreatic Cancer: Prospective Study

Conditions

Pancreatic cancer

Pancreatic carcinoma

Pancreatic adenocarcinoma

Pancreatic ductal adenocarcinoma
Intervention/Treatment

- Diagnostic test: PANcreatic cancer Exosome Early detectiON (PANXEON)

Other Study ID Numbers

- 19288/PCDC

Study Start (Actual)
2023-03-15
Primary Completion (Estimated)
2025-11-21
Study Completion (Estimated)
2025-11-21
Enrollment (Estimated)
2000
Study Type
Observational
Study Contact
Name: Ajay Goel, PhD
Phone Number: 6262183452
Email: AJGOEL@COH.ORG
This study has 11 locations.
United States
Arizona locations
Phoenix, Arizona, United States, 85004
Recruiting
Translational Genomics Research Institute
Contact:
Daniel Von Hoff
dvh@tgen.org
Principal investigator: Daniel Von Hoff
Scottsdale, Arizona, United States, 85258
Recruiting
Honorhealth
Contact:
Erkut Borazanci
erkut.borazanci@honorhealth.com
Sub-investigator:
Erkut Borazanci
California locations
Monrovia, California, United States, 91016
Recruiting
City of Hope Medical Center
Contact:
Ajay Goel, PhD

626-218-3452 AJGOEL@COH.ORG
Principal investigator: Ajay Goel
Newport Beach, California, United States, 92663
Recruiting
Hoag Center
Contact:
Michael Demeure
michael.demeure@hoag.org
Sub-investigator:
Michael Demeure
Illinois locations
Peoria, Illinois, United States, 61637
Recruiting
OSF HealthCare
Contact:
Chandler Wilfong
chandler.d.wilfong@osfhealthcare.org
Sub-investigator:
Chandler Wilfong
Louisiana locations
Jefferson, Louisiana, United States, 70121
Recruiting
Ochsner Medical Center
Contact:
John Bolton
jbolton@ochsner.org
Sub-investigator:
John Bolton
New Jersey locations
Morristown, New Jersey, United States, 07960
Recruiting
Atlantic Health System
Contact:
Angela Alistar
angela.alistar@atlantichealth.org
Sub-investigator:
Angela Alistar
South Carolina locations
Rock Hill, South Carolina, United States, 29732
Recruiting
Piedmont Medical Center
Contact:
Andrew Page
Andrew.Page@piedmont.org
Sub-investigator:
Andrew Page

Wisconsin locations
Milwaukee, Wisconsin, United States, 53226
Recruiting
Medical College of Wisconsin
Contact:
Douglas Evans
devans@mcw.edu
Sub-investigator:
Douglas Evans
Japan
Nagoya, Japan
Recruiting
Nagoya University
Contact:
Yasuhiro Kodera
ykodera@med.nagoya-u.ac.jp
Sub-investigator:
Yasuhiro Kodera
Republic of Korea
Seoul, Republic of Korea
Recruiting
Asan Medical Center
Contact:
Song Cheol Kim
drksc@amc.seoul.kr
Sub-investigator:
Song Cheol Kim
Eligibility Criteria
Description
Inclusion criteria:

- Histological diagnosis of pancreatic ductal adenocarcinoma, stages I–IV (TNM classification, 8th edition)
- Received standard diagnostic and staging procedures as per local guidelines, and at least one sample was drawn before receiving any curative-intent treatment
- Imaging- or endoscopy-based proof of lack of pancreatic ductal adenocarcinoma at the time of sampling (non-disease controls)

Exclusion criteria:

- Lack of written informed consent

Study Population
Independent cohorts of individuals with and without pancreatic cancer (cases and controls, respectively)
Ages Eligible for Study
18 Years and older (adult, older adult)

Sexes Eligible for Study
All
Accepts Healthy Volunteers
Yes
Sampling Method
Non-probability sample
Design Details
Observational model: case-control
Time perspective: prospective
Biospecimen retention: samples without DNA
Biospecimen description: serum

Groups and Interventions

Groups/cohorts	Intervention/treatment
Patients with pancreatic cancer ductal adenocarcinoma (training) Individuals diagnosed with pancreatic ductal adenocarcinoma	Diagnostic test: PANcreatic cancer Exosome Early detectiON (PANXEON) This test will utilize quantitative reverse transcriptase polymerase chain reaction (qRT-PCR) to quantify the expression levels of 5 cell-free and 8 exosome-miRNAs in plasma samples obtained from patients with pancreatic ductal adenocarcinoma and from individuals without it Other names: PANXEON (PANcreatic cancer Exosome Early detectiON)
Individuals without pancreatic cancer ductal adenocarcinoma (training) Individuals without pancreatic ductal adenocarcinoma	Diagnostic test: PANcreatic cancer Exosome Early detectiON (PANXEON) This test will utilize quantitative reverse transcriptase polymerase chain reaction (qRT-PCR) to quantify the expression levels of 5 cell-free and 8 exosome-miRNAs in plasma samples obtained from patients with pancreatic ductal adenocarcinoma and from individuals without it Other names: PANXEON (PANcreatic cancer Exosome Early detectiON)
Patients with pancreatic cancer ductal adenocarcinoma (validation) Individuals diagnosed with pancreatic ductal adenocarcinoma	Diagnostic Test: PANcreatic cancer Exosome Early detectiON (PANXEON) This test will utilize quantitative reverse transcriptase polymerase chain reaction (qRT-PCR) to quantify the expression levels of 5 cell-free and 8 exosome-miRNAs in plasma samples obtained from patients with pancreatic ductal adenocarcinoma and from individuals without it Other names: PANXEON (PANcreatic cancer Exosome Early detectiON)
Individuals without pancreatic cancer ductal adenocarcinoma (validation) Individuals without pancreatic ductal adenocarcinoma	Diagnostic test: PANcreatic cancer Exosome Early detectiON (PANXEON) This test will utilize quantitative reverse transcriptase polymerase chain reaction (qRT-PCR) to quantify the expression levels of 5 cell-free and 8 exosome-miRNAs in plasma samples obtained from patients with pancreatic ductal adenocarcinoma and from individuals without it Other names: PANXEON (PANcreatic cancer Exosome Early detectiON)

Primary Outcome Measures

Outcome measure	Measure description	Time frame
Sensitivity	True positive rate: the probability of a positive test result, conditioned on the individual truly being positive	Through study completion, an average of 1 year

Secondary Outcome Measures

Outcome measure	Measure description	Time frame
Specificity	True negative rate: the probability of a negative test result, conditioned on the individual truly being negative	Through study completion, an average of 1 year
Accuracy	A measure of trueness: proportion of correct predictions (both true positives and true negatives) among the total number of cases examined	Through study completion, an average of 1 year

Sponsor: City of Hope Medical Center

Investigators

- Principal investigator: Ajay Goel, PhD, City of Hope Medical Center

Publications

- Ryan DP, Hong TS, Bardeesy N. Pancreatic adenocarcinoma. N Engl J Med. 2014;371(11):1039–49. https://doi.org/10.1056/NEJMra1404198. No abstract available.
- Kleeff J, Korc M, Apte M, La Vecchia C, Johnson CD, Biankin AV, Neale RE, Tempero M, Tuveson DA, Hruban RH, Neoptolemos JP. Pancreatic cancer. Nat Rev Dis Primers. 2016;2:16022. https://doi.org/10.1038/nrdp.2016.22.
- Mizrahi JD, Surana R, Valle JW, Shroff RT. Pancreatic cancer. Lancet. 2020;395(10242):2008–2020. https://doi.org/10.1016/S0140-6736(20)30974-0.
- Sung H, Ferlay J, Siegel RL, Laversanne M, Soerjomataram I, Jemal A, Bray F. Global Cancer Statistics 2020: GLOBOCAN Estimates of Incidence and Mortality Worldwide for 36 Cancers in 185 Countries. CA Cancer J Clin. 2021;71(3):209–249. https://doi.org/10.3322/caac.21660. Epub 2021 Feb 4.
- Rahib L, Smith BD, Aizenberg R, Rosenzweig AB, Fleshman JM, Matrisian LM. Projecting cancer incidence and deaths to 2030: the unexpected burden of thyroid, liver, and pancreas cancers in the United States. Cancer Res. 2014;74(11):2913–21. https://doi.org/10.1158/0008-5472.CAN-14-0155. Erratum In: Cancer Res. 2014 Jul 15;74(14):4006.
- Vincent A, Herman J, Schulick R, Hruban RH, Goggins M. Pancreatic cancer. Lancet. 2011;378(9791):607–20. https://doi.org/10.1016/S0140-6736(10)62307-0. Epub 2011 May 26.
- Uesaka K, Boku N, Fukutomi A, Okamura Y, Konishi M, Matsumoto I, Kaneoka Y, Shimizu Y, Nakamori S, Sakamoto H, Morinaga S, Kainuma O, Imai K, Sata

N, Hishinuma S, Ojima H, Yamaguchi R, Hirano S, Sudo T, Ohashi Y; JASPAC 01 Study Group. Adjuvant chemotherapy of S-1 versus gemcitabine for resected pancreatic cancer: a phase 3, open-label, randomised, non-inferiority trial (JASPAC 01). Lancet. 2016 Jul 16;388(10041):248–57. https://doi.org/10.1016/S0140-6736(16)30583-9. Epub 2016 Jun 2.

- Conroy T, Hammel P, Hebbar M, Ben Abdelghani M, Wei AC, Raoul JL, Chone L, Francois E, Artru P, Biagi JJ, Lecomte T, Assenat E, Faroux R, Ychou M, Volet J, Sauvanet A, Breysacher G, Di Fiore F, Cripps C, Kavan P, Texereau P, Bouhier-Leporrier K, Khemissa-Akouz F, Legoux JL, Juzyna B, Gourgou S, O'Callaghan CJ, Jouffroy-Zeller C, Rat P, Malka D, Castan F, Bachet JB; Canadian Cancer Trials Group and the Unicancer-GI-PRODIGE Group. FOLFIRINOX or Gemcitabine as Adjuvant Therapy for Pancreatic Cancer. N Engl J Med. 2018;379(25):2395–2406. https://doi.org/10.1056/NEJMoa1809775.
- Conroy T, Desseigne F, Ychou M, Bouche O, Guimbaud R, Becouarn Y, Adenis A, Raoul JL, Gourgou-Bourgade S, de la Fouchardiere C, Bennouna J, Bachet JB, Khemissa-Akouz F, Pere-Verge D, Delbaldo C, Assenat E, Chauffert B, Michel P, Montoto-Grillot C, Ducreux M; Groupe Tumeurs Digestives of Unicancer; PRODIGE Intergroup. FOLFIRINOX versus gemcitabine for metastatic pancreatic cancer. N Engl J Med. 2011;364(19):1817–25. https://doi.org/10.1056/NEJMoa1011923.
- Von Hoff DD, Ervin T, Arena FP, Chiorean EG, Infante J, Moore M, Seay T, Tjulandin SA, Ma WW, Saleh MN, Harris M, Reni M, Dowden S, Laheru D, Bahary N, Ramanathan RK, Tabernero J, Hidalgo M, Goldstein D, Van Cutsem E, Wei X, Iglesias J, Renschler MF. Increased survival in pancreatic cancer with nab-paclitaxel plus gemcitabine. N Engl J Med. 2013;369(18):1691–703. https://doi.org/10.1056/NEJMoa1304369. Epub 2013 Oct 16.
- Golan T, Hammel P, Reni M, Van Cutsem E, Macarulla T, Hall MJ, Park JO, Hochhauser D, Arnold D, Oh DY, Reinacher-Schick A, Tortora G, Algul H, O'Reilly EM, McGuinness D, Cui KY, Schlienger K, Locker GY, Kindler HL. Maintenance Olaparib for Germline BRCA-Mutated Metastatic Pancreatic Cancer. N Engl J Med. 2019;381(4):317–327. https://doi.org/10.1056/NEJMoa1903387. Epub 2019 Jun 2.
- Fahrmann JF, Schmidt CM, Mao X, Irajizad E, Loftus M, Zhang J, Patel N, Vykoukal J, Dennison JB, Long JP, Do KA, Zhang J, Chabot JA, Kluger MD, Kastrinos F, Brais L, Babic A, Jajoo K, Lee LS, Clancy TE, Ng K, Bullock A, Genkinger J, Yip-Schneider MT, Maitra A, Wolpin BM, Hanash S. Lead-Time Trajectory of CA19-9 as an Anchor Marker for Pancreatic Cancer Early Detection. Gastroenterology. 2021;160(4):1373–1383.e6. https://doi.org/10.1053/j.gastro.2020.11.052. Epub 2020 Dec 14.
- Majumder S, Taylor WR, Foote PH, Berger CK, Wu CW, Mahoney DW, Bamlet WR, Burger KN, Postier N, de la Fuente J, Doering KA, Lidgard GP, Allawi HT, Petersen GM, Chari ST, Ahlquist DA, Kisiel JB. High Detection Rates of Pancreatic Cancer Across Stages by Plasma Assay of Novel Methylated DNA Markers and CA19-9. Clin Cancer Res. 2021;27(9):2523–2532. https://doi.org/10.1158/1078-0432.CCR-20-0235. Epub 2021 Feb 16.

- Gui JC, Yan WL, Liu XD. CA19-9 and CA242 as tumor markers for the diagnosis of pancreatic cancer: a meta-analysis. Clin Exp Med. 2014;14(2):225–33. https://doi.org/10.1007/s10238-013-0234-9. Epub 2013 Mar 3.
- Tempero MA, Uchida E, Takasaki H, Burnett DA, Steplewski Z, Pour PM. Relationship of carbohydrate antigen 19-9 and Lewis antigens in pancreatic cancer. Cancer Res. 1987;47(20):5501–3.
- Martin LK, Wei L, Trolli E, Bekaii-Saab T. Elevated baseline CA19-9 levels correlate with adverse prognosis in patients with early- or advanced-stage pancreas cancer. Med Oncol. 2012;29(5):3101–7. https://doi.org/10.1007/s12032-012-0278-9. Epub 2012 Jun 24.
- Luo G, Liu C, Guo M, Cheng H, Lu Y, Jin K, Liu L, Long J, Xu J, Lu R, Ni Q, Yu X. Potential Biomarkers in Lewis Negative Patients With Pancreatic Cancer. Ann Surg. 2017;265(4):800–805. https://doi.org/10.1097/SLA.0000000000001741.
- Cescon DW, Bratman SV, Chan SM, Siu LL. Circulating tumor DNA and liquid biopsy in oncology. Nat Cancer. 2020;1(3):276–90. https://doi.org/10.1038/s43018-020-0043-5. Epub 2020 Mar 20.
- Pantel K, Alix-Panabieres C. Liquid biopsy and minimal residual disease – latest advances and implications for cure. Nat Rev Clin Oncol. 2019;16(7):409–24. https://doi.org/10.1038/s41571-019-0187-3.
- Crowley E, Di Nicolantonio F, Loupakis F, Bardelli A. Liquid biopsy: monitoring cancer-genetics in the blood. Nat Rev Clin Oncol. 2013;10(8):472–84. https://doi.org/10.1038/nrclinonc.2013.110. Epub 2013 Jul 9.
- Kilgour E, Rothwell DG, Brady G, Dive C. Liquid Biopsy-Based Biomarkers of Treatment Response and Resistance. Cancer Cell. 2020;37(4):485–95. https://doi.org/10.1016/j.ccell.2020.03.012.
- Bloomston M, Frankel WL, Petrocca F, Volinia S, Alder H, Hagan JP, Liu CG, Bhatt D, Taccioli C, Croce CM. MicroRNA expression patterns to differentiate pancreatic adenocarcinoma from normal pancreas and chronic pancreatitis. JAMA. 2007;297(17):1901–8. https://doi.org/10.1001/jama.297.17.1901.
- Jin X, Chen Y, Chen H, Fei S, Chen D, Cai X, Liu L, Lin B, Su H, Zhao L, Su M, Pan H, Shen L, Xie D, Xie C. Evaluation of Tumor-Derived Exosomal miRNA as Potential Diagnostic Biomarkers for Early-Stage Non-Small Cell Lung Cancer Using Next-Generation Sequencing. Clin Cancer Res. 2017;23(17):5311–9. https://doi.org/10.1158/1078-0432.CCR-17-0577. Epub 2017 Jun 12.
- Yu W, Hurley J, Roberts D, Chakrabortty SK, Enderle D, Noerholm M, Breakefield XO, Skog JK. Exosome-based liquid biopsies in cancer: opportunities and challenges. Ann Oncol. 2021;32(4):466–77. https://doi.org/10.1016/j.annonc.2021.01.074. Epub 2021 Feb 4.
- Krug AK, Enderle D, Karlovich C, Priewasser T, Bentink S, Spiel A, Brinkmann K, Emenegger J, Grimm DG, Castellanos-Rizaldos E, Goldman JW, Sequist LV, Soria JC, Camidge DR, Gadgeel SM, Wakelee HA, Raponi M, Noerholm M, Skog J. Improved EGFR mutation detection using combined exosomal RNA and circulating tumor DNA in NSCLC patient plasma. Ann Oncol. 2018 Mar 1;29(3):700–6. https://doi.org/10.1093/annonc/mdx765.

- San Lucas FA, Allenson K, Bernard V, Castillo J, Kim DU, Ellis K, Ehli EA, Davies GE, Petersen JL, Li D, Wolff R, Katz M, Varadhachary G, Wistuba I, Maitra A, Alvarez H. Minimally invasive genomic and transcriptomic profiling of visceral cancers by next-generation sequencing of circulating exosomes. Ann Oncol. 2016;27(4):635–41. https://doi.org/10.1093/annonc/mdv604. Epub 2015 Dec 17.
- Ingenito F, Roscigno G, Affinito A, Nuzzo S, Scognamiglio I, Quintavalle C, Condorelli G. The Role of Exo-miRNAs in Cancer: A Focus on Therapeutic and Diagnostic Applications. Int J Mol Sci. 2019;20(19):4687. https://doi.org/10.3390/ijms20194687.
- Toiyama Y, Okugawa Y, Fleshman J, Richard Boland C, Goel A. MicroRNAs as potential liquid biopsy biomarkers in colorectal cancer: A systematic review. Biochim Biophys Acta Rev Cancer. 2018;1870(2):274–82. https://doi.org/10.1016/j.bbcan.2018.05.006. Epub 2018 May 29.
- Shigeyasu K, Toden S, Zumwalt TJ, Okugawa Y, Goel A. Emerging Role of MicroRNAs as Liquid Biopsy Biomarkers in Gastrointestinal Cancers. Clin Cancer Res. 2017;23(10):2391–9. https://doi.org/10.1158/1078-0432.CCR-16-1676. Epub 2017 Jan 31.
- Nishiwada S, Cui Y, Sho M, Jun E, Akahori T, Nakamura K, Sonohara F, Yamada S, Fujii T, Han IW, Tsai S, Kodera Y, Park JO, Von Hoff D, Kim SC, Li W, Goel A. Transcriptomic Profiling Identifies an Exosomal microRNA Signature for Predicting Recurrence Following Surgery in Patients With Pancreatic Ductal Adenocarcinoma. Ann Surg. 2022 Dec 1;276(6):e876–85. https://doi.org/10.1097/SLA.0000000000004993. Epub 2021 Jun 16.
- Nakamura K, Zhu Z, Roy S, Jun E, Han H, Munoz RM, Nishiwada S, Sharma G, Cridebring D, Zenhausern F, Kim S, Roe DJ, Darabi S, Han IW, Evans DB, Yamada S, Demeure MJ, Becerra C, Celinski SA, Borazanci E, Tsai S, Kodera Y, Park JO, Bolton JS, Wang X, Kim SC, Von Hoff D, Goel A. An Exosome-based Transcriptomic Signature for Noninvasive, Early Detection of Patients With Pancreatic Ductal Adenocarcinoma: A Multicenter Cohort Study. Gastroenterology. 2022;163(5):1252–66.e2. https://doi.org/10.1053/j.gastro.2022.06.090. Epub 2022 Jul 16.

Recruiting

Exosomes in Rectal Cancer

ClinicalTrials.gov ID NCT03874559

Sponsor: University of Kansas Medical Center

Information provided by Andrew Hoover, University of Kansas Medical Center (responsible party)

Last update posted: 2024-10-16

Study Overview

Brief Summary

The primary aims of this study is to characterize exosomal biomarker levels in patients with locally advanced rectal cancer undergoing neoadjuvant chemoradiation therapy. Compare rates of exosomal expression before during and after chemoradiation therapy with pathologic response rates at the time of APR or LAR. The researchers will also examine the functionality of these exosomes in malignant colonic organoids and mouse models of colorectal cancer.

Detailed Description

All male and female patients, aged 18 and older with a histologically proven diagnosis of rectal adenocarcinoma, treated in this study will receive neo adjuvant chemotherapy (consisting of 5 FU or capecitabine) given concurrently with external beam radiation therapy to a dose of 50.4 Gy in 28 fractions. Radiation treatments will be administered daily, Monday through Friday. Within 1 week prior to beginning chemotherapy and radiation treatments, a serum sample will be obtained from each patient. Patients will also have serum samples collected every two weeks during radiation, and on the last day of radiation therapy, as well as at their 1 month follow-up visit after completion of radiation and prior to planned surgery. A final serum sample will be collected within one month after definitive surgery. Each serum sample collected will be less than 50 mL.

The study will involve obtaining serum samples from patients before during and after chemoradiation therapy. These serum samples will be analyzed to determine exosomal biomarker levels, which will be correlated with clinical, imaging, laboratory, and pathologic data obtained from the medical record.

Additional data from the patients' medical records will be collected, including demographic data, clinical information from notes in the medical record, radiology images and reports, results of diagnostic tests, and information from procedure notes and pathology reports.

Official Title

Exosomes As Correlative Biomarker in Clinical Outcomes in Patients Undergoing Neoadjuvant Chemoradiation Therapy for Rectal Cancer

Conditions

Rectal cancer

Intervention/Treatment

- Diagnostic test: blood draw

Other Study ID Numbers

- Protocol IIT-RE-0

Study Start (Actual)

2018-02-13

Primary Completion (Estimated)

2025-02-01

Study Completion (Estimated)

2026-02-01

Enrollment (Estimated)

30
Study Type
Observational (patient registry)
Study Contact
Name: Leah K Miller, MS
Phone Number: 913-588-3670
Email: lmiller25@kumc.edu
Study Contact Backup
Name: Michelle Faucheux, RN
Phone Number: 913-588-9927
Email: mfaucheux@kumc.edu
This study has one location.
United States
Kansas locations
Eligibility Criteria
Description
Inclusion criteria:

- Male and female patients aged 18 and older
- Histologically proven diagnosis of rectal adenocarcinoma
- Will be receiving neoadjuvant chemoradiation therapy prior to a planned definitive surgical resection

Exclusion criteria:

- Age less than 18
- Patients who are unable or unwilling to undergo definitive surgery
- Patients with a prior history of pelvic external beam radiation, brachytherapy, or chemotherapy
- Patients with a prior history of cancer (excluding non-melanoma skin cancers)
- Patients who are immunocompromised

Study Population

All patients seen in the Department of Radiation Oncology at The University of Kansas Health System that are over the age of 18 and have a histologically proven diagnosis of rectal adenocarcinoma and will be receiving neoadjuvant chemoradiation therapy before a planned, definitive surgical resection has been performed.

Ages Eligible for Study
18 Years and older (adult, older adult)
Sexes Eligible for Study
All
Accepts Healthy Volunteers
No
Sampling Method
Probability sample
Design Details
Observational model: cohort

Time perspective: prospective

Target follow-up duration: 1 month

Biospecimen retention: samples with DNA

Biospecimen description: Blood serum samples will be collected from patients before, during, and after chemoradiation therapy. These samples will be analyzed and stored for 10 years.

Groups and Interventions

Groups/cohorts	Intervention/treatment
Arm A All patients enrolled will be placed in Arm A. Serum blood draw samples will be collected as well as additional data from medical records will be collected. This data includes demographic data, clinical information from notes, radiology images and reports, diagnostic test results, and procedure and pathology reports.	Diagnostic test: blood draw Serum samples will be obtained from each patient enrolled.

Primary Outcome Measures

Outcome measure	Measure description	Time frame
Exosomal Biomarkers Assessment	Characterize exosomal biomarker levels in patients with locally advanced rectal cancer undergoing neoadjuvant chemoradiation therapy.	Up to 10 years after treatment completion

Secondary Outcome Measures

Outcome measure	Measure description	Time frame
Exosomal expression	Compare rates of exosomal expression before during and after chemoradiation therapy with pathologic response rates at the time of APR or LAR. Response rates will be graded based on College of American Pathologists Guidelines on neoadjuvant treatment effect, which consists of a 4-tiered grading system categorizing response to neoadjuvant chemoradiation as "complete," "moderate," "minimal," or "poor." These grades are routinely documented in pathology reports for patients undergoing neoadjuvant chemoradiation for rectal cancer and will be obtained from review of pathology reports in the patient medical records.	Up to 10 years after treatment completion
Exosomal functionality assessment	Examine the functionality of these exosomes in malignant colonic organoids and mouse models of colorectal cancer	Up to 10 years after treatment completion

Sponsor: University of Kansas Medical Center

Investigators

- Principal investigator: Andrew Hoover, MD, The University of Kansas Medical Center

Recruiting

Study of Exosomes in Monitoring Patients with Sarcoma (EXOSARC) (EXOSARC)

ClinicalTrials.gov ID NCT03800121

Sponsor: Centre Georges Francois Leclerc

Information provided by Centre Georges Francois Leclerc (responsible party)

Last update posted: 2023-12-15

Study Overview

Brief Summary

Sarcomas are rare cancers with a high risk of metastatic progression and a major pejorative factor with respect to patient survival. The estimation of the metastatic risk of sarcomas is very complex given the histological heterogeneity of this entity. It is therefore essential that, at diagnosis, a reliable evaluation of this metastatic potential be made, in order to adapt the therapeutic strategy as well as possible.

It has recently been discovered that sarcomas secrete many exosomes that appear to play an important role in tumorgenesis, growth, tumor progression, and the onset of metastases. They contain many proteins and nucleic acids (DNA, RNA, microRNA), reflecting the characteristics of the tumor. It has been shown that the amount of exosomes can be correlated with the grade of malignancy of the tumor. Present in the blood, exosomes offer the possibility of non-invasively analyzing the molecular information of the cancer cell. As a result, the study of serum exosomes derived from sarcomas has a high potential as a liquid biopsy to evaluate cancer pathogenesis, progression, and treatment efficacy.

The purpose of this study is to demonstrate in patients with sarcomas that exosomes can be used to monitor their disease and be used as a predictor of the risk of recurrence.

Detailed Description

The main objective of this pilot study is to quantify exosomes and analyze their protein and RNA content in patients with sarcoma with disease:

- Localized before and after treatment with surgery
- Localized for which neoadjuvant chemotherapy is being considered
- Metastatic or locally advanced cancer before and after treatment with first-line chemotherapy which may include neoadjuvant therapy

The secondary objectives are as follows:

1. Determine whether the initial exosome concentration and the protein and RNA profile they contain vary with the localized or metastatic stage of the disease
2. Determine if the exosome concentration as well as the protein and RNA profile they contain varies after treatment
3. Determine if the initial exosome concentration (at T0) is associated with a response to treatment
4. Determine whether the change in exosome concentration before and after treatment is associated with a response to treatment

5. Identify a protein marker or RNA associated with a treatment response (marker present at T0 or occurring during follow-up)

Official Title
Study of Exosomes in Monitoring Patients with Sarcoma (EXOSARC)
Conditions
Sarcoma
Intervention/Treatment

- Biological: blood samples

Other Study ID Numbers

- 2018-A01393-52

Study Start (Actual)
2018-11-19
Primary Completion (Estimated)
2024-11-19
Study Completion (Estimated)
2025-11-19
Enrollment (Estimated)
34
Study Type
Observational
Study Contact
Name: Alice HERVIEU
Phone Number: 03 80 73 75 00
Email: ahervieu@cgfl.fr
Study Contact Backup
Name: Emilie REDERSTORFF
Phone Number: 03 80 73 75 00
Email: erederstorff@cgfl.fr
This study has three locations.
France
Besançon, France, 25000
Recruiting
CHU de Besançon
Contact:
Loic Chaigneau
Contact:
echaigneau@chu-besancon.fr
Sub-investigator:
Elsa Kalbacher
Dijon, France, 21000
Recruiting
Centre Georges François Leclerc

Contact:
Alice Hervieu
03 80 73 75 00 ahervieu@cgfl.fr
Sub-investigator:
Sylvain Causeret
Poitiers, France, 86000
Recruiting
CHU de Poitiers
Contact:
Nicolas Isambert, PU-PH
05 49 44 45 38 nicolas.isambert@chu-poitiers.fr
Sub-investigator:
Sheik Emambux
Eligibility Criteria
Description
Inclusion criteria:

1. Men and women newly diagnosed with localized, metastatic, or locally advanced soft tissue sarcoma.
2. Previous treatment of the disease with chemotherapy, radiotherapy, or surgery is allowed if it has been completed for more than 12 months at the time of inclusion.
3. For metastatic or locally advanced (inoperable) sarcoma, patients for whom first-line metastatic chemotherapy is indicated.
4. Age ≥18 years.
5. Affiliation to a social security scheme.
6. Patients who signed informed consent to participate in the study.

Exclusion criteria:
Patients who meet at least one of the following criteria will not be eligible:

1. Patient with another synchronous tumor
2. Patient with sarcoma in irradiated territory
3. Patient with a history of cancer other than sarcoma in the 5 years preceding the diagnosis of sarcoma
4. Patient unable to undergo medical follow-up for geographical, social or psychological reasons
5. Person benefiting from a protection system for adults (including guardianship and trusteeship)
6. Serology HIV and / or HBV and / or HCV positive.
7. Pregnant or lactating woman
8. Patients unable to understand, read, and/or sign informed consent

Study Population
Patients with soft tissue sarcoma
Ages Eligible for Study
18 Years and older (adult, older adult)
Sexes Eligible for Study

All
Accepts Healthy Volunteers
No
Sampling Method
Probability sample
Design Details
Observational model: cohort
Time perspective: prospective

Groups and Interventions

Groups/cohorts	Intervention/treatment
Localized sarcoma with neoadjuvant chemotherapy In total, several blood tests specific to the EXOSARC study will be necessary: A first blood test of 7 mL during the initial assessment (inclusion) Then, four blood samples of 32mL distributed over 6 months	Biological: blood samples Localized sarcoma group: 1 blood sample during inclusion (7 ml) + 1 blood sample before surgery (32 ml) + 1 blood sample 1 month after surgery (32 ml) + 1 blood sample 3 month after surgery (32 ml) + 1 blood sample 6 month after surgery (32 ml) Metastatic sarcoma group: 1 blood sample during inclusion (7 ml) + 1 blood sample during chemotherapy cure 1 (32 ml) + 1 blood sample during chemotherapy cure 3 (32 ml) + 1 blood sample during chemotherapy cure 6 (32 ml) Other names: Localized sarcoma Metastatic sarcoma
Metastatic or locally advanced sarcoma In total, several blood tests specific to the EXOSARC study will be necessary: A first blood of 7 mL during the initial assessment (inclusion) Then, three blood samples of 32 mL distributed over 3 months	Biological: blood samples Localized sarcoma group: 1 blood sample during inclusion (7 ml) + 1 blood sample before surgery (32 ml) + 1 blood sample 1 month after surgery (32 ml) + 1 blood sample 3 month after surgery (32 ml) + 1 blood sample 6 month after surgery (32 ml) Metastatic sarcoma group: 1 blood sample during inclusion (7 ml) + 1 blood sample during chemotherapy cure 1 (32 ml) + 1 blood sample during chemotherapy cure 3 (32 ml) + 1 blood sample during chemotherapy cure 6 (32 ml) Other names: Localized sarcoma Metastatic sarcoma

Primary Outcome Measures

Outcome measure	Measure description	Time frame
Concentration of exosomes in blood	Blood samples	Up to 6 months after inclusion

Sponsor: Centre Georges Francois Leclerc

Not Yet Recruiting

UCMSC-Exo for Chemotherapy-induced Myelosuppression in Acute Myeloid Leukemia

ClinicalTrials.gov ID NCT06245746

Sponsor: Wuhan Union Hospital, China

Information provided by Qiubai Li, Wuhan Union Hospital, China (responsible party)

Last update posted: 2024-02-09

Study Overview

Brief Summary

The purpose of the study is to explore the safety and efficacy of UCMSC-Exo in consolidation chemotherapy-induced myelosuppression in patients with acute myeloid leukemia after achieving complete remission.

Detailed Description

Despite the improved prognosis of patients with acute myeloid leukemia, almost all patients will experience severe myelosuppression induced by chemotherapy, leading to a series of complications such as infection due to neutropenia, bleeding due to thrombocytopenia and/or impaired major organ function such as cardiac function due to anemia, which are the main reasons for dose reduction, dose interruptions of chemotherapy, and also treatment-related death. It is of significant clinical importance and an urgent need to promote early recovery of myelosuppression and reduce risks of related complications as well as medical burdens. Umbilical cord-derived mesenchymal stem cells exosomes (UCMSC-Exo), as the key effector of the stem cells with multipotential, can widely act on the functional cell units of bone marrow microenvironment and promote the repairment and regeneration of key cells such as hematopoietic stem cells, mesenchymal stem cells and endothelial cells, thus making it an ideal means for effectively promoting recovery of myelosuppression. Patients with acute myeloid leukemia who have achieved complete remission (CR) and are going to receive consolidation chemotherapy will be invited to participate in the study, to receive UCMSC-Exo intravenous infusion and follow-up visits of up to 1 year after enrollment.

Official Title

A Single-center, Prospective Trial of the Safety and Efficacy of UCMSC-Exo in Consolidation Chemotherapy-induced Myelosuppression in Patients with Acute Myeloid Leukemia After Achieving Complete Remission

Conditions

Acute myeloid leukemia

Neutropenia

Anemia

Thrombocytopenia

Intervention/Treatment

- Biological: umbilical cord-derived mesenchymal stem cells exosomes (UCMSC-Exo)

Other Study ID Numbers

- UHCT231013

  Study Start (Estimated)
  2024-03
  Primary Completion (Estimated)
  2024-12
  Study Completion (Estimated)
  2025-12
  Enrollment (Estimated)
  9
  Study Type
  Interventional
  Phase
  Phase 1
  Study Contact
  Name: Qiubai Li, Professor
  Phone Number: 85726808 ext 027
  Email: qiubaili@hust.edu.cn
  Study Contact Backup
  Name: Di Wu
  Phone Number: 18790696175 ext 86
  Email: 373181302@qq.com
  No location data
  Eligibility Criteria
  Description
  Inclusion criteria:

1. Aged between 18 and 60 years old
2. Acute myeloid leukemia (AML, AML subtype M3 excluded) diagnosed according to the 2016 revision to the World Health Organization classification of myeloid neoplasms and acute leukemia, who have achieved complete remission (CR) by cytarabine and daunorubicin/cytarabine and idarubicin induction chemotherapy and are going to receive consolidation chemotherapy by cytarabine
3. The participant or his/her legal guardian is adequately informed of the nature and risks of the study, voluntarily participates in the study with signed informed consent
4. Male or female
5. Weight between 55 and 75kg
6. Eastern Cooperative Oncology Group (ECOG) performance status (PS) of 0 to 2 (by the day chemotherapy is initiated)
7. Estimated survival of at least 3 months
8. Adequate major organ function:

   1. Respiratory function: indoor oxygen saturation of at least 95%
   2. Cardiac function: ejection fraction of left ventricular of at least 45%

3. Hepatic function: alanine aminotransferase/aspartate aminotransferase of at most 2.5 times/upper limit of normal value and serum total bilirubin of at most 1.5 times/upper limit of normal value
4. Renal function: Serum creatinine of at most 1.5 times/upper limit of normal value

9. Participants who do not receive any type of anti-cancer therapy within 2 weeks before enrollment (radiation therapy, chemotherapy, and/or immune therapy, et al.), and treatment-associated toxicities induced by previous therapy has recovered to Grade 1 or below (except for low grade toxicities such as alopecia)
10. For female participants, they should be surgical sterilized or postmenopausal, or agree to utilize a medically recognized method of contraception (such as intrauterine device, condom) during treatment period of the study and within 6 months after the end of treatment period of the study. For male participants, they should be surgical sterilized or agree to utilize a medically recognized method of contraception (such as intrauterine device, condom) during treatment period of the study and within 6 months after the end of treatment period of the study

Exclusion criteria:

1. Central nervous system manifestations of acute myeloid leukemia at diagnosis
2. Secondary acute myeloid leukemia
3. Myelosuppression induced by conditions other than anti-cancer therapy
4. Previous radiation therapy performed on sternum or pelvis
5. Specifically diagnosed and uncontrolled infection at enrollment (uncontrolled is defined as exhibiting ongoing signs and symptoms of infection without improvement despite anti-infective agents)
6. Uncontrolled active bleeding at enrollment
7. Severe underlying comorbidities affecting survival, including cachexia, severe malnutrition, etc.
8. Estimated survival of at most 48 hours
9. Active hepatitis B virus (HBV) or hepatitis C virus (HCV) infection
10. History of or current human immunodeficiency virus (HIV) infection
11. Syphilis infection
12. Continuous usage of immunosuppressants or received organ transplantation in the last 6 months
13. Participation in clinical trials of other drugs within 6 weeks before enrollment
14. Previous participation in clinical stem cell or exosome research
15. Receive any agent concurrently with UCMSC-Exo infusion which inhibits cell division (hydroxyurea, low-dose cytarabine or methotrexate, etc.)
16. Severe allergic constitution, or known or suspected allergy to the study drug and its components
17. Known contraindication to receiving hematopoietic growth factors, transfusion of blood components, anti-infective agents
18. Female participants who are pregnant or breast feeding

19. Participants suffering from mental illness
20. Presence of drug abuse/addiction
21. History of other malignancies other than hematological malignancies within 3 years
22. Participants without signed informed consent
23. Participants with poor compliance and are unable to complete the whole course of the study
24. Participants with circumstances that, in the opinion of the investigator, may increase the risk of the participants or interfere with conduct of the clinical trial and the judgment of results (excessive tension, sensitivity or cognitive impairment, etc.)
25. Participants with other circumstances that are ineligible for enrollment in this study, in the opinion of the investigator

Ages Eligible for Study
18 to 60 years (adult)
Sexes Eligible for Study
All
Accepts Healthy Volunteers
No
Design Details
Primary purpose: treatment
Allocation: N/A
Interventional model: single group assignment
Masking: none (open label)

Arms and Interventions

Participant group/arm	Intervention/treatment
Experimental: UCMSC-Exo intervention UCMSC-Exo will be preset with 3 escalation dose levels in single time infusion.	Biological: umbilical cord-derived mesenchymal stem cells exosomes (UCMSC-Exo) UCMSC-Exo will be infused intravenously.

Primary Outcome Measures

Outcome measure	Measure description	Time frame
Incidence of adverse events (AEs) and serious adverse events (SAEs)	To investigate the safety characteristics, percentages will be calculated and grade will be evaluated.	From the day that UCMSC-Exo is infused to up to 28 days (short-term safety follow-up) and 1 year (long-term safety follow-up)

(continued)

Outcome measure	Measure description	Time frame
Dose-limiting toxicities (DLT)	During the DLT observation period, the subject has an adverse event that is reasonably related to UCMSC-Exo infusion (possibly, likely, or definitely related).	From the day that UCMSC-Exo is infused to up to 14 days
Maximum tolerated dose (MTD)	During the dose-escalation, the highest dose of dose-limiting toxicity for subjects no more than 1/6 in the dose group of at least 6 evaluable subjects of the study drug.	From the day that UCMSC-Exo is infused to up to 14 days

Secondary Outcome Measures

Outcome measure	Measure description	Time frame
Time to absolute neutrophil count recovery	To investigate the efficacy characteristics, time will be measured in days.	From the start of chemotherapy to up to 42 days
Incidence of febrile neutropenia	To investigate the efficacy characteristics, percentages will be calculated.	From the start of chemotherapy to up to 42 days
Duration of febrile neutropenia	To investigate the efficacy characteristics, the duration will be measured in days.	From the start of chemotherapy to up to 42 days
Incidence of severe thrombocytopenia	To investigate the efficacy characteristics, percentages will be calculated.	From the start of chemotherapy to up to 42 days
Time to severe thrombocytopenia recovery	To investigate the efficacy characteristics, time will be measured in days.	From the start of chemotherapy to up to 42 days
Incidence of severe anemia	To investigate the efficacy characteristics, percentages will be calculated.	From the start of chemotherapy to up to 42 days
Time to severe anemia recovery	To investigate the efficacy characteristics, time will be measured in days.	From the start of chemotherapy to up to 42 days
Incidence of infection	To investigate the efficacy characteristics, percentages will be calculated.	From the start of chemotherapy to up to 42 days
Duration of infection	To investigate the efficacy characteristics, the duration will be measured in days.	From the start of chemotherapy to up to 42 days
Incidence of bleeding	To investigate the efficacy characteristics, percentages will be calculated.	From the start of chemotherapy to up to 42 days
Duration of bleeding	To investigate the efficacy characteristics, the duration will be measured in days.	From the start of chemotherapy to up to 42 days

(continued)

Outcome measure	Measure description	Time frame
Application rate of blood transfusion	To investigate the efficacy characteristics, percentages will be calculated.	From the start of chemotherapy to up to 42 days
Application rate of anti-infective agents	To investigate the efficacy characteristics, percentages will be calculated.	From the start of chemotherapy to up to 42 days

Sponsor: Wuhan Union Hospital, China

Investigators

- Principal investigator: Qiubai Li, Professor, Wuhan Union Hospital, China

Active, Not Recruiting

Analysis of Circulating Exosomes in Melanoma Patients (EXOMEL1)

ClinicalTrials.gov ID NCT05744076

Sponsor: Centre Hospitalier Universitaire de Besancon

Information provided by Centre Hospitalier Universitaire de Besancon (responsible party)

Last update posted: 2023-02-24

Study Overview

Brief Summary

The hypothesis is that PD-L1 (programmed death-ligand 1) labeling in exosomes could be a biomarker of disease progression in melanoma. The rate of circulating exosomes, their size, and the exosomal expression of PD-L1 could be correlated with the stage of the disease, the response to treatment, and/or the prognosis of patients. In this study, blood samples (EDTA tubes taken as part of routine care at Besançon University Hospital) and associated clinical data are reused.

Official Title

Analysis of Circulating Exosomes in Melanoma Patients

Conditions

Melanoma

Other Study ID Numbers

- P/2018/401

Study Start (Actual)

2019-03-01

Primary Completion (Estimated)

2024-03

Study Completion (Estimated)

2024-03

Enrollment (Estimated)
150
Study Type
Observational
This study has one location.
France
Besançon, France
CHU de Besançon
Eligibility Criteria
Description
Inclusion criteria:

- Melanoma patients admitted in Besançon University Hospital
- eligible for immunotherapy such as anti PD-L1/PD-1
- Age ≥18 years
- Affiliation to a social security system

Exclusion criteria:

- Minor patients
- Patients who have expressed their opposition to the reuse of their data and biological samples

Study Population
Melanoma patients admitted in Besançon University Hospital
Ages Eligible for Study
18 Years and older (adult, older adult)
Sexes Eligible for Study
All
Accepts Healthy Volunteers
No
Sampling Method
Non-probability sample
Design Details
Observational model: cohort
Time perspective: other

Primary Outcome Measures

Outcome measure	Measure description	Time frame
Quantification of circulating exosomes	Dosage of protein biomarkers in circulating exosomes, plasma and tumor tissues. Blood samples were taken in standard care, before initiation of immunotherapy and then during disease follow-up until progression and tumor evaluation	Day 1

Secondary Outcome Measures

Outcome measure	Measure description	Time frame
PDL1 marking	Compare PD-L1 labeling in exosomes to PD-L1 labeling in plasma and in tumor tissue. Blood samples were taken in standard care, before initiation of immunotherapy and then during disease follow-up until progression and tumor evaluation	Day 1
Other protein detection	Identify other proteins of interest in circulating exosomes. Blood samples were taken in standard care, before initiation of immunotherapy and then during disease follow-up until progression and tumor evaluation.	Day 1
Determine whether the initial exosome concentration (at T0) is Associated with a response to treatment.	Dosage of PD-L1 in circulating exosomes. Blood samples were taken in standard care, before initiation of immunotherapy and then during disease follow-up until progression and tumor evaluation	Day 1

Sponsor: Centre Hospitalier Universitaire de Besancon

Collaborators

- Centre Georges Francois Leclerc

Recruiting

Clinical Relevance of Detecting Molecular Abnormalities in Glial Tumor Exosomes (ExoGLIE)

ClinicalTrials.gov ID NCT06116903

Sponsor: University Hospital, Limoges

Information provided by University Hospital, Limoges (responsible party)

Last update posted: 2024-12-13

Study Overview

Brief Summary

The purpose of this pilot study is that exosomes constitute a more interesting support for analyzes allowing a broader screening of molecular alterations to be carried out with more reliable, more sensitive, and more efficient results than the reference Foundation One Liquid CDx test.

Detailed Description

Gliomas are the most common primary brain tumors in adults. The heterogeneity of tumors and the lack of reliable criteria for identifying different subtypes make their histopathological diagnosis and their management complex. The molecular profiling from circulating exosomes is one of the most promising approaches to better characterize gliomas.

We will demonstrate the superiority of detection by NGS of molecular abnormalities present in exosomes from glioblastomas, compared to detection by the Foundation One Liquid CDx test on ctDNA.

Official Title

Clinical Relevance of Detecting Molecular Abnormalities in Glial Tumor Exosomes

Conditions

Glioma

Intervention/Treatment

- Genetic: blood sampling

Other Study ID Numbers

- 87RI22_0011-ExoGLIE

Study Start (Actual)

2024-04-11

Primary Completion (Estimated)

2025-05-15

Study Completion (Estimated)

2025-12-15

Enrollment (Estimated)

60

Study Type

Interventional

Phase

Not applicable

This study has one location.

France

Limoges, France, 87042

Recruiting

CHU de Limoges

Contact:

Deluche Elise, MD

+33505556309 elise.deluche@chu-limoges.fr

Eligibility Criteria

Description

Inclusion criteria:

- Subject of both sexes at least 18 years of age with glioblastoma
- Patient for whom an FMI test is indicated, progressing after a first line following the chemotherapy and radiotherapy protocol (STUPP protocol)
- Patient affiliated to French social security

Exclusion criteria:

- Patient included in another research protocol using an experimental molecule
- Any medical or psychiatric condition which, in the investigator's opinion, would preclude the patient from adhering to the protocol or completing the study per protocol
- Patient under legal protection, guardianship, or curatorship
- Patient with active malignancy or a previous malignancy within the past 5 years, except for patient with resected basocarcinoma and resected carcinoma in-situ of the cervix

Ages Eligible for Study
18 Years and older (adult, older adult)
Sexes Eligible for Study
All
Accepts Healthy Volunteers
No
Design Details
Primary purpose: diagnostic
Allocation: N/A
Interventional model: single group assignment
Masking: none (open label)

Arms and Interventions

Participant group/arm	Intervention/treatment
Experimental: detection of molecular abnormalities Blood samples will be taken from 2 + 3 cell-free DNA collection tubes (Roche): for the comparative performance of the two methods (main objective) 3 cell-free DNA collection tubes will be collected at 3 months (post chemotherapy) to evaluate the clinical relevance of a new analysis of molecular alterations on exosomes	Genetic: blood sampling Blood sampling for testing of the detection of molecular abnormalities in exosomes of glial tumors

Primary Outcome Measures

Outcome measure	Measure description	Time frame
Analyze next-generation sequencing (NGS)	Higher proportion of contributory samples identified by NGS analysis (via exosomes) compared to that of FMI (Foundation Medicine International) test (at inclusion)	3 months

Secondary Outcome Measures

Outcome measure	Measure description	Time frame
Expression of biomarkers	Level of expression of biomarkers, for the same patient, by molecular analysis of exosomes and blood sampling according to the FMI test protocol	3 months
Molecular alterations	Modification or not modification of the profile of the molecular alterations	3 months
Carbon footprint	Evaluation of the carbon footprint for each of the 2 techniques (NGS via exosomes and FMI test)	3 months

Sponsor: University Hospital, Limoges

Recruiting

Evaluation of Urinary Exosomes Presence from Clear Cell Renal Cell Carcinoma (PEP-C)

ClinicalTrials.gov ID NCT04053855

Sponsor: Centre Hospitalier Universitaire de Saint Etienne

Information provided by Centre Hospitalier Universitaire de Saint Etienne (responsible party)

Last update posted: 2024-10-26

Study Overview

Brief Summary

Clear cell renal cell carcinoma is diagnosed by imaging, sometimes associated with biopsy. This diagnosis is expensive, invasive, and sometimes late. The development of a simple biological test for diagnosis is essential. Exosomes are 30- to 150-nm membrane vesicles secreted into the extracellular space by various living cells. These exosomes can be isolated from biological fluids, including urine. The recent study of urinary exosomes is a promising topic for analyzing tumor markers in urine. The investigator's goal is to develop a reliable technique for detecting tumor exosomes in urine in patients with clear cell renal cell carcinoma. The analysis of urinary exosomes could provide a new liquid biopsy tool for the early diagnosis of clear cell renal cell carcinoma.

Detailed Description

The primary objective is to detect urinary exosomes, by electron microscopy technique, from clear cell renal cell carcinoma due to exosome markers (CD9) and clear cell kidney cancer (CA9).

Official Title

Evaluation of Urinary Exosomes Presence from Clear Cell Renal Cell Carcinoma

Conditions

Clear cell renal cell carcinoma

Intervention/Treatment

- Biological: urinary sample

Other Study ID Numbers

- 19CH048
- 2019-A01408-49 (other identifier) (OTHER: ANSM)

Study Start (Actual)
2020-01-29
Primary Completion (Estimated)
2026-08-01
Study Completion (Estimated)
2026-08-01
Enrollment (Estimated)
100
Study Type
Observational
Study Contact
Name: Nicolas Mottet, MD PhD
Phone Number: (0)477828331 ext +33
Email: nicolas.mottet@chu-st-etienne.fr
Study Contact Backup
Name: Arnauld Garcin, CRA
Phone Number: (0)477120286 ext +33
Email: Arnauld.Garcin@chu-st-etienne.fr
This study has one location.
France
Saint-Étienne, France
Recruiting
Chu Saint-Etienne
Principal investigator: Nicolas Mottet, MD PhD
Eligibility Criteria
Description
Inclusion criteria:
Patients:

- All patients with renal mass requiring surgery (partial or total nephrectomy)
- Social security affiliation
- Signed informed consent

Control:

- Unscheduled nephrectomy
- Social security affiliation
- Signed informed consent

Exclusion criteria:

- Insufficient volume of urine sample (< 100 ml)

- Patients with a urinary catheter
- Patients under court-ordered guardianship or curators

Study Population
60 patients and 40 controls will be included.
Ages Eligible for Study
18 Years and older (adult, older adult)
Sexes Eligible for Study
All
Accepts Healthy Volunteers
No
Sampling Method
Non-probability sample
Design Details
Observational model: cohort
Time perspective: prospective
Biospecimen retention: samples without DNA
Biospecimen description: urinary sample

Groups and Interventions

Groups/cohorts	Intervention/treatment
Renal mass patients Patients with renal mass requiring surgery (partial or total nephrectomy) will be included. They will have a urinary sample.	Biological: urinary sample Urinary sample (100 ml) will be collected in the urology department to analysis urinary exosomes.
Control patients Control patients (without renal mass) will be included. They will have a urinary sample.	Biological: urinary sample Urinary sample (100 ml) will be collected in the urology department to analysis urinary exosomes.

Primary Outcome Measures

Outcome measure	Measure description	Time frame
Number of patients (with clear cell kidney cancer) with CD9+ and CA9+ exosomes by electron microscopy technique	Measured by analysis in electron microscopy technique of urinary sample	At inclusion

Secondary Outcome Measures

Outcome measure	Measure description	Time frame
Percentage of CD9+ /CA9+ exosomes by electron microscopy technique (%) for patients with clear cell kidney cancer	Measured by analysis in electron microscopy technique of urinary sample	At inclusion
Percentage of CD9+ /CA9+ exosomes by electron microscopy technique (%) for control patients	Measured by analysis in electron microscopy technique of urinary sample	At inclusion

(continued)

Outcome measure	Measure description	Time frame
Percentage of CD9+ /CA9+ exosomes by flow cytometry (%) for patients with clear cell kidney cancer	Measured by analysis in flow cytometry of urinary sample	At inclusion
Percentage of CD9+ /CA9+ exosomes by flow cytometry (%) for control patients	Measured by analysis in flow cytometry of urinary sample	At inclusion
Percentage of CD9+ /CA9+ exosomes by reverse transcription quantitative polymerase chain reaction (RT-qPCR) (%) for control patients	Measured by analysis in reverse transcription quantitative polymerase chain reaction (RT-qPCR) of urinary sample	At inclusion
Percentage of CD9+ /CA9+ exosomes by reverse transcription quantitative polymerase chain reaction (RT-qPCR) (%) for patients with clear cell kidney cancer	Measured by analysis in reverse transcription quantitative polymerase chain reaction (RT-qPCR) of urinary sample	At inclusion
Percentage of CD9+/CD63+/CD81+/CA9+ exosomes by electron microscopy technique (%) for patients with clear cell kidney cancer	Measured by analysis in electron microscopy technique of urinary sample	At inclusion
Percentage of CD9+/CD63+/CD81+/CA9+ exosomes by electron microscopy technique (%) for control patients	Measured by analysis in electron microscopy technique of urinary sample	At inclusion
Percentage of CD9+/CD63+/CD81+/CA9+ exosomes by flow cytometry (%) for patients with clear cell kidney cancer	Measured by analysis in flow cytometry of urinary sample	At inclusion
Percentage of CD9+/CD63+/CD81+/CA9+ exosomes by flow cytometry (%) for control patients	Measured by analysis in flow cytometry of urinary sample.	At inclusion
Percentage of CD9+/CD63+/CD81+/CA9+ exosomes by reverse transcription quantitative polymerase chain reaction (RT-qPCR) (%) for patients with clear cell kidney cancer	Measured by analysis in reverse transcription quantitative polymerase chain reaction (RT-qPCR) of urinary sample	Years: 2
Percentage of CD9+/CD63+/CD81+/CA9+ exosomes by reverse transcription quantitative polymerase chain reaction (RT-qPCR) (%) for control patients	Measured by analysis in reverse transcription quantitative polymerase chain reaction (RT-qPCR) of urinary sample	Years: 2
Percentage of CD9+/VGEFR2+ exosomes by electron microscopy technique (%) for patients with clear cell kidney cancer	Measured by analysis in electron microscopy technique of urinary sample	At inclusion
Percentage of CD9+/VGEFR2+ exosomes by electron microscopy technique (%) for control patients	Measured by analysis in electron microscopy technique of urinary sample	At inclusion
Percentage of CD9+/VGEFR2+ exosomes by flow cytometry (%) for patients with clear cell kidney cancer	Measured by analysis in flow cytometry of urinary sample	At inclusion

(continued)

Outcome measure	Measure description	Time frame
Percentage of CD9+/VGEFR2+ exosomes by flow cytometry (%) for control patients	Measured by analysis in flow cytometry of urinary sample	At inclusion
Percentage of CD9+/VGEFR2+ exosomes by reverse transcription quantitative polymerase chain reaction (RT-qPCR) (%) for patients with clear cell kidney cancer	Measured by analysis in reverse transcription quantitative polymerase chain reaction (RT-qPCR) of urinary sample	At inclusion
Percentage of CD9+/VGEFR2+ exosomes by reverse transcription quantitative polymerase chain reaction (RT-qPCR) (%) for control patients	Measured by analysis in reverse transcription quantitative polymerase chain reaction (RT-qPCR) of urinary sample	At inclusion

Sponsor: Centre Hospitalier Universitaire de Saint Etienne

Investigators

- Principal investigator: Nicolas Mottet, MD PhD, CHU de Saint-Etienne
- Study Chair: Nora Mallouk, PhD, University Saint-Etienne
- Study Chair: Guorong Li, PhD, CHU de Saint-Etienne

Publications

- Li G, Mallouk N, Flandrin P, Garcin A, Lambert C, Berremila SA, Habchi H, Mottet N. Presence of urinary exosomes for liquid biopsy of clear cell renal cell carcinoma: protocol for a pilot feasibility study. JMIR Res Protoc. 2021;10(7):e24423. https://doi.org/10.2196/24423.

Recruiting

Exosomes and Immunotherapy in Non-Hodgkin B-cell Lymphomas (ExoReBLy)

ClinicalTrials.gov ID NCT03985696

Sponsor: University Hospital, Limoges

Information provided by University Hospital, Limoges (responsible party)

Last update posted: 2022-07-25

Study Overview

Brief Summary

Diffuse large B cell lymphomas (DLBCL) are highly aggressive and heterogeneous B cell lymphoma that would imminently be fatal without treatment. Monoclonal anti-CD20 antibody, rituximab, in combination of CHOP chemotherapy (R-CHOP) is widely used with favorable results. Although more than half of patients achieve long-term remission, many are not cured with this immunotherapy. Suboptimal response and/or resistance to rituximab have remained a challenge in the therapy of DLBCL but also of all B-NHL. Exosomes are microvesicles released from tumor B cells that are found in plasma of patients with B-NHL. Exosomes carry therapeutic targets (as CD20, PDL-1) and could act as "decoy-receptors" for immunotherapy. Our objective is to determine, in aggressive B-NHL, the role of exosomes in immunotherapy escape.

Detailed Description

Diffuse large B cell lymphomas (DLBCL) are highly aggressive and heterogeneous B cell lymphoma that would imminently be fatal without treatment. Monoclonal anti-CD20 antibody, rituximab, in combination of CHOP chemotherapy (R-CHOP) is widely used with favourable results. Although more than half of patients achieve long-term remission, many are not cured with this immunotherapy. Decreased CD20 expression has been postulated to be one of the most important contributing to rituximab resistance. Moreover, R-CHOP therapies are sometimes ineffective, and new treatment strategies based notably on host immune responses modulation are being explored. Among them, programmed cell death ligand 1 (PD-L1) protein was identified as a potent predicting biomarker in DLBCL. Exosomes are small membrane vesicles secreted by several cell types during exocytic fusion of multivesicular bodies with the plasma membrane. Many cancer cells have been shown to secrete exosomes in greater amounts than normal cells. Exosome secretion may contribute to drug resistance. Indeed, exosome release from B cell non-Hodgkin lymphoma (B-NHL), by the expression of CD20, has been suggest to act as decoy targets upon rituximab exposure, allowing lymphoma cells to escape from humoral immunotherapy. Finally, as exosome composition seems to be cell and tissue specific, they are highly suitable to serve as diagnostic markers.

Our hypothesis is that high expression of the immunotherapeutic targets (CD20, PD-L1) on exosomes derived from aggressive or resistant B-NHL may allow tumor cells to escape therapeutic antibodies and thus contribute in vivo to therapeutic resistance. For this objective, we will use exosomes derived from DLBCL human cells and exosomes isolated from plasma of DLBCL patients. We will analyze, on these microvesicles, CD20 and PDL-1 expression in function of DLBCL subtypes and outcome of patients. Moreover, exosome capacity to interfere with immunotherapy will be also studied from in vitro and in vivo (xenografts) models.

Official Title

Exosomes and Resistance to Immunotherapy in Aggressive Non-Hodgkin B-cell Lymphomas (B-NHL)

Conditions

Lymphoma, B cell, aggressive non-Hodgkin (B-NHL)

Intervention/Treatment

- Other: blood sample

Other Study ID Numbers

- 87RI18_0025 (ExoReBLy)

Study Start (Actual)
2019-07-02

Primary Completion (Estimated)
2025-07-02
Study Completion (Estimated)
2025-07-02
Enrollment (Estimated)
90
Study Type
Interventional
Phase
Not applicable
Study Contact
Name: Julie ABRAHAM, Dr
Phone Number: +33 (0) 555 056 651
Email: julie.abraham@chu-limoges.fr
Study Contact Backup
Name: Danielle TROUTAUD, Pr
Email: danielle.troutaud@unilim.fr
This study has one location.
France
Limoges, France, 87042
Recruiting
University Hospital Limoges
Contact:
Julie Abraham, PH
julie.abraham@chu-limoges.fr
Eligibility Criteria
Description
Inclusion criteria:

- Patients over 18 years old with DLBCL at diagnostic or relapsed patients after R-CHOP therapy.
- Healthy volunteers over 18 years old

Exclusion criteria:

- Other B cell diseases

Ages Eligible for Study
18 Years and older (adult, older adult)
Sexes Eligible for Study
All
Accepts Healthy Volunteers
Yes
Design Details
Primary purpose: basic science
Allocation: non-randomized
Interventional model: parallel assignment
Masking: none (open label)

Arms and Interventions

Participant group/arm	Intervention/treatment
Experimental: patients with DLBCL	Other: blood sample 1 blood volume (5–7 ml EDTA)
Active comparator: healthy volunteers	Other: blood sample 1 blood volume (5–7 ml EDTA)

Primary Outcome Measures

Outcome measure	Measure description	Time frame
Quantification of CD20 and PDL-1 in exosomes purified from cell cultures of DLBCL human cell lines and from healthy volunteers	From D0 until the end of the inclusion period (36 months)	Month 36

Secondary Outcome Measures

Outcome measure	Measure description	Time frame
Evaluation if peripheral exosomes can be used as novel diagnostic biomarkers in DLBCL	To analyze the prognostic value of exosomal markers on therapeutic response and patient outcome, each patient included in the study at diagnostic (D0) will be followed up until 36 months after inclusion.	Month 36

Sponsor: University Hospital, Limoges

Not Yet Recruiting

Integrative Analysis of Exosome-Mediated Single-Cell Transcriptomics and Proteomics in Gastric Cardia Cancer

ClinicalTrials.gov ID NCT06702891

Sponsor: Qilu Hospital of Shandong University

Information provided by Qilu Hospital of Shandong University (responsible party)

Last update posted: 2024-11-25

Study Overview

Brief Summary

This is an observational study with a case control design. This study included patients with gastric cancer confirmed by pathological diagnosis of gastric tissue, and matched the control population according to age, gender, etc. In this study, researchers collected clinical information and multiple biological samples such as serum and tissue from the study subjects. The researchers combined exosome sequencing, proteomics, and single-cell RNA sequencing to explore the heterogeneity of cardia cancer, identify specific biomarkers and potential therapeutic targets for cardia cancer, and provide a basis for the development of new diagnostic tools and therapeutic strategies.

Official Title

Integrative Analysis of Exosome-Mediated Single-Cell Transcriptomics and Proteomics in Gastric Cardia Cancer

Conditions

Gastric cardia cancer

Intervention/Treatment

- Other: detection of biological samples based on exosome sequencing, proteomics, and single-cell RNA sequencing

Other Study ID Numbers

- 2024SDU-QILU-2

Study Start (Estimated)
2024-11
Primary Completion (Estimated)
2025-10
Study Completion (Estimated)
2027-10
Enrollment (Estimated)
20
Study Type
Observational (Patient Registry)
Study Contact
Name: Xiaoya Wang, Bachelor
Phone Number: (86)13821379210
Email: xiaoyawang99@163.com
No location data
Eligibility Criteria
Description
Inclusion criteria:

- Study population signing informed consent form
- Age: 18 years old or older
- The study population must undergo endoscopic examination and was confirmed by pathological diagnosis as gastric cancer: including high-level intraepithelial neoplasia, early gastric cancer, and advanced gastric cancer.

Exclusion criteria:

- Those who have undergone gastrointestinal surgery within the past 1 year; patients who have undergone neoadjuvant chemotherapy and have developed tumors in the residual stomach after previous partial gastrectomy.

- Those who have used proton pump inhibitors, antibiotics, probiotics, and prebiotics daily within the past month, and those who have recently received hormone therapy.
- People with infectious diseases and other digestive system diseases that interfere with the experimental results, such as inflammatory bowel disease, irritable bowel syndrome, etc.

Study Population

Case:

The population in the case group signed an informed consent form, aged 18 years old or older. All subjects underwent endoscopic examination and were confirmed by pathological diagnosis as gastric cancer, including high-grade intraepithelial neoplasia, early gastric cancer, and advanced gastric cancer.

Control:

The age and gender of the study subjects in the control group were matched to the study population in the case group. The pathological results of the stomach of all subjects showed no malignant changes, including normal gastric mucosa, superficial gastritis, non-atrophic gastritis, and gastric polyps, etc.

Ages Eligible for Study

18 Years and older (adult, older adult)

Sexes Eligible for Study

All

Accepts Healthy Volunteers

Yes

Sampling Method

Non-probability sample

Design Details

Observational model: case-control

Time perspective: cross-sectional

Target follow-up duration: 2 years

Groups and Interventions

Groups/cohorts	Intervention/treatment
Case group The case group includes high-grade intraepithelial neoplasia of the stomach, early gastric cancer, and advanced gastric cancer.	Other: detection of biological samples based on exosome sequencing, proteomics, and single-cell RNA sequencing The researchers combined exosome sequencing, proteomics, and single-cell RNA sequencing to explore the heterogeneity of cardia cancer and identify specific biomarkers and potential therapeutic targets for cardia cancer.

(continued)

Groups/cohorts	Intervention/treatment
Control group Pathological findings in the control group showed no malignant changes in the stomach, including normal gastric mucosa, superficial gastritis, non-atrophic gastritis, and gastric polyps, etc.	Other: detection of biological samples based on exosome sequencing, proteomics, and single-cell RNA sequencing The researchers combined exosome sequencing, proteomics and single-cell RNA sequencing to explore the heterogeneity of cardia cancer and identify specific biomarkers and potential therapeutic targets for cardia cancer.

Primary Outcome Measures

Outcome measure	Measure description	Time frame
Differential protein		6 months

Secondary Outcome Measures

Outcome measure	Measure description	Time frame
Key miRNA		10 months
Differential cell subsets	Differential cell subsets between cardiac cancer tissue and normal tissue	12 months

Sponsor: Qilu Hospital of Shandong University

Not Yet Recruiting

Exosome-Based OCS Scores for Predicting Ovarian Cancer Recurrence

ClinicalTrials.gov ID NCT06558019

Sponsor: Lei Li

Information provided by Lei Li, Peking Union Medical College Hospital (responsible party)

Last update posted: 2024-08-16

Study Overview

Brief Summary

Ovarian cancer is the third most common malignant tumor of the female reproductive system in China in terms of incidence rate and the first in terms of mortality. Surgery and systemic chemotherapy are the cornerstone of first-line treatment for patients with epithelial ovarian cancer. The efficacy rate of first-line platinum combined with taxus chemotherapy is more than 80%, and more than half of them reach complete remission (CR). However, even if advanced patients reach CR, 50–70% still relapse, with a median disease-free interval of 16 months. Most patients lack typical symptoms when they relapse. The sensitivity of CA125 in monitoring recurrence is poor (43–74%), which means that more than 25% of ovarian cancer patients cannot detect recurrence in a timely manner during follow-up. Therefore, more sensitive biomarkers are needed for monitoring ovarian cancer recurrence after treatment. More and more studies have explored the application value of extracellular vesicle technology in the diagnosis and treatment of ovarian cancer, including auxiliary diagnosis, prognosis, monitoring, etc. China already has an approved exosome ovarian cancer diagnostic product by the National Medical Products Administration, namely the Ovarian Cancer Diagnostic Score (OCS) product based on exosome technology, which is also the world's first exosome technology diagnostic kit for ovarian cancer. Clinical trial data shows that OCS products have demonstrated excellent performance in distinguishing between benign and malignant ovarian tumors. Under high specificity (90.2%), it has a higher sensitivity than serum CA125, reaching 95.5% (95% CI 92.7–97.3%), and has a sensitivity of 89.7% in the diagnosis of stage I ovarian cancer. OCS exhibits better sensitivity than CA125, especially in early ovarian cancer, suggesting that OCS may be a better tool for monitoring recurrence in ovarian cancer patients. The main purpose of this study is to establish an OCS scoring ovarian cancer recurrence prediction and monitoring model based on exosome technology, providing an effective tool for clinical ovarian cancer recurrence prediction and monitoring. Secondly, we hope to explore the correlation between OCS score and tumor staging, chemotherapy sensitivity, PFS, OS indicators, etc. and determine the performance of recurrence prediction models in different subgroups, such as different pathological subtypes of ovarian cancer and different treatment methods.

Detailed Description

This research subjects are patients with epithelial ovarian cancer. The training set adopts case-control analysis, using the PASS software Test for Two Related Proportions in a Matched Case Control Design module. Setting $\alpha = 0.05$, $\beta = 0.1$, assuming $P0 = 10\%$, OR = 4, and a 1:1 ratio between the case group and the control group, 101 cases need to be separately enrolled in the case group and the control group. The case group consists of patients who have achieved response to first-line treatment and experienced imaging recurrence. Therefore, 101 recurrence events need to be observed during the 18-month follow-up period. Assuming that the response rate to platinum-based chemotherapy in first-line treatment is 80% and the recurrence rate at 18 months is 50%, they need to be enrolled in group 101 / 80% / 50% = 253 cases. The control group consisted of at least 101 patients who achieved CR with first-line treatment and had no recurrence of OCS imaging during follow-up testing. Assuming a CR rate of 70% with first-line treatment, 145 patients need to be enrolled. Therefore, the inclusion of 253 cases can meet the sample size requirements for both the case group and the control group. Considering a dropout rate of 15%, a total of 298 cases need to be enrolled. Evaluate the performance of the validation set in predicting recurrence. Assuming the sensitivity of predicting recurrence increases from 75% to 90%, with $\alpha = 0.05$ and $\beta = 0.2$, 45 recurrence events are required. Assuming an 80% response rate to platinum-based chemotherapy as first-line treatment and a 50% recurrence rate within 18 months, 45 recurrence events observed during the 18-month follow-up period need to be enrolled / 80% / 50% = 113 patients. Assuming a specificity of not less than 90%, $\alpha = 0.05$, $\beta = 0.2$, 179 patients are required for enrollment. Assuming a dropout rate of 15%, a total of 211 patients needs to be included. Taking into account both sensitivity and specificity performance evaluation, a total of 211 patients were included in the validation set.

This project will announce the findings and main achievements of this research through the publication of core Chinese papers and SCI indexed articles. In addition, this project will organize experts in the field to explore consensus and write guidelines, announcing the technical routes and application directions related to this research.

Official Title

Exosome-based OCS Scores for Predicting Ovarian Cancer Recurrence: A Prospective Multicenter Observational Cohort

Conditions

Ovarian cancer

Other Study ID Numbers

- OCS-OvaRPM

Study Start (Estimated)

2024-10-01

Primary Completion (Estimated)

2026-12-31

Study Completion (Estimated)

2026-12-31

Enrollment (Estimated)

509

Study Type

Observational

Study Contact

Name: Lei Li, M.D.

Phone Number: 86-139-1198-8831

Email: lileigh@163.com

This study has one location.

China

Beijing locations

Beijing, Beijing, China

Peking Union Medical College Hospital

Eligibility Criteria

Description

Inclusion criteria:

- Women over 18 years old
- Pathological diagnosis of stage I–IV epithelial ovarian cancer
- Eastern Cooperative Oncology Group (ECOG) score ≤ 2

- Expected survival period exceeding 6 months
- Within 8 weeks between diagnosis and enrollment
- Sign informed consent form

Exclusion criteria:

- Non-epithelial ovarian tumors
- History of cancer in the past 5 years
- Received systematic treatment for ovarian cancer
- Gestation
- Previous bilateral oophorectomy

Study Population
The research subjects are patients with epithelial ovarian cancer.
Ages Eligible for Study
18 Years and older (adult, older adult)
Sexes Eligible for Study
Female
Accepts Healthy Volunteers
No
Sampling Method
Non-probability sample

Primary Outcome Measures

Outcome measure	Measure description	Time frame
Progression-free survival	Progression-free survival after diagnosis	2 years
Overall survival	Overall survival after diagnosis	2 years

Sponsor: Lei Li

Investigators

- Principal investigator: Lei Li, MD, Peking Union Medical College Hospital

Active, Not Recruiting

Molecular Profiling of Exosomes in Tumor-draining Vein of Early-staged Lung Cancer (ExOnSite-Pro)

ClinicalTrials.gov ID NCT04939324
Sponsor: University Hospital, Limoges
Information provided by University Hospital, Limoges (responsible party)
Last update posted: 2023-04-10
Study Overview
Brief Summary

This is an observational prospective single-center study of 30 patients operated for early-stage non-small cell lung cancer. The main aim is the analysis of molecular profiling of exosome with a sample in tumor-draining vein in order to identify prognostic molecular characteristics associated with cancer recurrence after surgery.

Detailed Description

Surgical resection remains the best chance for cure in patients with early-stage non-small cell lung cancer (NSCLC). Unfortunately, approximately 30–50% of patients will relapse within 5-year of curative surgery despite early TNM stage. The identification of prognostic biomarkers of relapse is a necessity. Among them, extracellular vesicles (exosomes) study seems promising in early-staged cancers and samples directly in tumor-draining vein to. The pulmonary vein is draining blood directly from the lungs and sampling at this location could provide a higher yield. The literature reports that Navarro et al. are the only team to have link exosome characteristics to oncological outcomes following surgery. The investigators propose to analyze the molecular profiling mediated by these extracellular vesicles in the tumor-draining vein of operated patients.

A peripheral blood sample is obtained before surgery (D-1 or D0). During oncological lung surgery, the pulmonary tumor-drainage vein is first exposed and punctured with a needle prior to subsequent surgical manipulation for resection (D0). A piece of resected tumor will be analyzed for the study (D0). Quantification and size distribution of exosome and molecular cargo of exosome in blood samples (peripheral and pulmonary vein) and tumor are analyzed (DNA sequencing).

Standard clinical and radiological follow-up is then performed and 2-year overall survival and 2-year disease-free survival are checked.

Official Title

Analyse du Profil moléculaire Des Exosomes de la Veine Pulmonaire Dans le Cancer Bronchique de Stade précoce

Conditions

Lung cancer

Exosomes

Non-small cell lung cancer

Intervention/Treatment

- Biological: blood samples at two sites: peripheral vein and tumor-draining vein

Other Study ID Numbers

- 87RI20-0067 (ExOnSite-Pro)

Study Start (Actual)

2021-06-21

Primary Completion (Estimated)

2023-08-21

Study Completion (Estimated)

2024-06-06

Enrollment (Actual)

30

Study Type
Interventional
Phase
Not applicable
This study has one location.
France
Limoges, France, 87042
CHU de Limoges
Eligibility Criteria
Description
Inclusion criteria:

- Surgical non-small cell lung cancer with pure solid nodule or part-solid ground glass nodule on CT-scan

Exclusion criteria:

- Pure ground glass nodule
- Neoadjuvant therapy
- Second cancer or cancer in the 5 years
- Pregnancy
- Patients <18 years old
- Tutorship

Ages Eligible for Study
18 Years and older (adult, older adult)
Sexes Eligible for Study
All
Accepts Healthy Volunteers
No
Design Details
Primary purpose: diagnostic
Allocation: N/A
Interventional model: single group assignment
Masking: none (open label)

Arms and Interventions

Participant group/arm	Intervention/treatment
Other: blood samples at 2 sites: peripheral vein and tumor-draining vein D0: surgery (inclusion): oncological lung resection Blood samples at 2 sites: peripheral vein and tumor-draining vein Resected tumor analysis: standard clinical and radiological follow-up during 2 years (medical consultation or phone call)	Biological: blood samples at 2 sites: peripheral vein and tumor-draining vein D0: surgery (inclusion): oncological lung resection Blood samples at 2 sites: peripheral vein and tumor-draining vein Resected tumor analysis: standard clinical and radiological follow-up during 2 years (medical consultation or phone call)

Primary Outcome Measures

Outcome measure	Measure description	Time frame
Evaluate size distribution, concentration and molecular profiling of pulmonary vein exosomes at inclusion	Concentration of extracellular vesicle (millions of particle/mL of blood)	36 months

Secondary Outcome Measures

Outcome measure	Measure description	Time frame
Size distribution, molecular profiling of peripheral vein exosome sat inclusion	The size distribution of extracellular vesicles harvested	36 months
Mutations and polymorphism in resected lung cancer	Analysis of the molecular profile in the resected tumor tissue	36 months
Overall survival	Overall survival	36 months
2-year disease-free survival	2-year disease-free survival	24 months

Sponsor: University Hospital, Limoges

Investigators

- Principal investigator: Jérémy Tricard, MD, University Hospital, Limoges

Recruiting

An Exosome-Based Liquid Biopsy for the Differential Diagnosis of Primary Liver Cancer (ELUCIDATE)

ClinicalTrials.gov ID NCT06342414

Sponsor: City of Hope Medical Center

Information provided by City of Hope Medical Center (responsible party)

Last update posted: 2024-04-02

Study Overview

Brief Summary

It is sometimes difficult to precisely understand whether a primary liver cancer is a hepatocellular carcinoma or a cholangiocarcinoma. The researchers will develop and validate a liquid biopsy, based on exosomal content analysis and powered by machine learning, to help clinicians differentiate these two cancers before surgery.

Detailed Description

Primary liver cancers (PLCs) encompass a diverse group of malignancies originating from the liver, collectively ranking as the third leading cause of cancer-related mortality worldwide in 2020. Among PLCs, intrahepatic cholangiocarcinoma (ICC) and hepatocellular carcinoma (HCC) represent the most predominant subtypes. Despite their collective grouping as PLCs, ICC and HCC patients exhibit distinct etiologies, pathologies, and clinical characteristics, necessitating different treatment approaches. Accurate differentiation between ICC and HCC is paramount to optimize patient outcomes and guide personalized treatment decisions. However, a definitive diagnosis is often obtained only after the pathological review of the resected neoplastic tissue, which requires invasive tumor sampling and poses risks of complications such as hemorrhage and tumor cell seeding. Consequently, there is a pressing clinical need to develop noninvasive diagnostic approaches to achieve an accurate differential diagnosis for patients with these distinct forms of PLCs.

This study involves the development and validation of a liquid biopsy, assessing circulating exosomal microRNAs (exo-miRNA) for indirect sampling of tumor tissue in the bloodstream. The researchers intend to harness machine learning and bioinformatics to create a cost-efficient, non-invasive, clinic-friendly assay with high sensitivity and specificity, aiding the differential diagnosis between ICC and HCC.

The researchers intend to do so in three phases:

1. To perform comprehensive small RNA-Seq from exo-miRNA from patients with ICC and HCC
2. To develop and train a differential diagnosis panel based on advanced machine-learning models to obtain a final differential diagnosis biomarker
3. To validate the findings in an independent cohort of ICC and HCC

In summary, this proposal promises to improve patient care and help clinicians perform a more reliable differential diagnosis between ICC and HCC in patients with primary liver cancer.

Official Title

An Exosome-Based Liquid Biopsy for the Differential Diagnosis of Primary Liver Cancer

Conditions

Hepatocellular carcinoma

Intrahepatic cholangiocarcinoma

Cholangiocarcinoma

Primary liver cancer

Intervention/Treatment

- Diagnostic test: ELUCIDATE

Other Study ID Numbers

- 23228/ELUCIDATE

Study Start (Actual)

2024-03-15

Primary Completion (Estimated)

2025-03-15

Study Completion (Estimated)

2025-03-15

Enrollment (Estimated)

400
Study Type
Observational
Study Contact
Name: Ajay Goel, PhD
Phone Number: 6262183452
Email: AJGOEL@COH.ORG
United States
California locations
Duarte, California, United States, 91010
Recruiting
City of Hope Medical Center
Contact:
Ajay Goel, PhD
626-218-3452 AJGOEL@COH.ORG
Sub-Investigator:
Caiming Xu, MD, PhD
Japan
Fukuoka, Japan
Recruiting
Graduate School of Medical Sciences, Kyushu University
Contact:
Tomoharu Yoshizumi
Sub-investigator: Tomoharu Yoshizumi
Kumamoto, Japan
Recruiting
Graduate School of Medical Sciences, Kumamoto University
Contact:
Hideo Baba
Sub-investigator: Hideo Baba
Sapporo, Japan
Recruiting
Hokkaido University Graduate School of Medicine
Contact:
Akinobu Taketomi
Principal investigator: Akinobu Taketomi
Tokushima, Japan
Recruiting
Tokushima University
Contact:
Mitsuo Shimada
Sub-investigator: Mitsuo Shimada
Eligibility Criteria
Description
Inclusion criteria:

- A histologically confirmed diagnosis of hepatocellular carcinoma
- A histologically confirmed diagnosis of intrahepatic cholangiocarcinoma
- Received standard diagnostic and staging procedures as per local guidelines
- Availability of at least one blood-derived sample, drawn before receiving any curative-intent treatment

Exclusion criteria:

- Lack of or inability to provide informed consent
- Synchronous hepatocellular carcinoma and intrahepatic cholangiocarcinoma
- Primary liver cancer other than hepatocellular carcinoma or intrahepatic cholangiocarcinoma
- Secondary liver cancer

Study Population

Individuals who were diagnosed with either intrahepatic cholangiocarcinoma or hepatocellular carcinoma (case-case design for a differential diagnosis study)

Ages Eligible for Study

18 Years and older (adult, older adult)

Sexes Eligible for Study

All

Accepts Healthy Volunteers

No

Sampling Method

Non-probability sample

Design Details

Observational model: case-only

Time perspective: retrospective

Groups and Interventions

Groups/cohorts	Intervention/treatment
Hepatocellular carcinoma (training) A cohort of patients with histologically confirmed hepatocellular carcinoma (HCC)	Diagnostic test: ELUCIDATE ELUCIDATE (Evaluation of Liver Cholangiocarcinoma Intrahepatic) Other names: ELUCIDATE (Evaluation of Liver Cholangiocarcinoma Intrahepatic)
Intrahepatic cholangiocarcinoma (training) A cohort of patients with histologically confirmed intrahepatic cholangiocarcinoma (ICC)	Diagnostic test: ELUCIDATE ELUCIDATE (Evaluation of Liver Cholangiocarcinoma Intrahepatic) Other names: ELUCIDATE (Evaluation of Liver Cholangiocarcinoma Intrahepatic)
Hepatocellular carcinoma (validation) A cohort of patients with histologically confirmed hepatocellular carcinoma (HCC)	Diagnostic test: ELUCIDATE ELUCIDATE (Evaluation of Liver Cholangiocarcinoma Intrahepatic) Other names: ELUCIDATE (Evaluation of Liver Cholangiocarcinoma Intrahepatic)

(continued)

Groups/cohorts	Intervention/treatment
Intrahepatic cholangiocarcinoma (validation) A cohort of patients with histologically confirmed intrahepatic cholangiocarcinoma (ICC)	Diagnostic test: ELUCIDATE ELUCIDATE (Evaluation of Liver Cholangiocarcinoma Intrahepatic) Other names: ELUCIDATE (Evaluation of Liver Cholangiocarcinoma Intrahepatic)

Primary Outcome Measures

Outcome measure	Measure description	Time frame
Sensitivity	True positive rate: the probability of a positive test result, conditioned on the individual truly being positive	Through study completion, an average of 1 year

Secondary Outcome Measures

Outcome measure	Measure description	Time frame
Specificity	True negative rate: the probability of a negative test result, conditioned on the individual truly being negative	Through study completion, an average of 1 year
Proportion of correct predictions (true positives and true negatives) among the total number of cases (i.e., accuracy)	A measure of trueness: proportion of correct predictions (both true positives and true negatives) among the total number of cases examined	Through study completion, an average of 1 year

Sponsor: City of Hope Medical Center

Investigators

- Principal investigator: Ajay Goel, PhD, City of Hope Medical Center

Publications

- Marrero JA, Kulik LM, Sirlin CB, Zhu AX, Finn RS, Abecassis MM, Roberts LR, Heimbach JK. Diagnosis, Staging, and Management of Hepatocellular Carcinoma: 2018 Practice Guidance by the American Association for the Study of Liver Diseases. Hepatology. 2018;68(2):723–50. https://doi.org/10.1002/hep.29913. No abstract available.
- Wu Y, Xia C, Chen J, Qin Q, Ye Z, Song B. Diagnostic performance of magnetic resonance imaging and contrast-enhanced ultrasound in differentiating intrahepatic cholangiocarcinoma from hepatocellular carcinoma: a meta-analysis. Abdom Radiol (NY). 2024;49(1):34–48. https://doi.org/10.1007/s00261-023-04064-z. Epub 2023 Oct 12.
- El-Serag HB, Marrero JA, Rudolph L, Reddy KR. Diagnosis and treatment of hepatocellular carcinoma. Gastroenterology. 2008;134(6):1752–63. https://doi.org/10.1053/j.gastro.2008.02.090.

- Vigano L, Lleo A, Muglia R, Gennaro N, Sama L, Colapietro F, Roncalli M, Aghemo A, Chiti A, Di Tommaso L, Solbiati L, Colombo M, Torzilli G. Intrahepatic cholangiocellular carcinoma with radiological enhancement patterns mimicking hepatocellular carcinoma. Updates Surg. 2020;72(2):413–21. https://doi.org/10.1007/s13304-020-00750-5. Epub 2020 Apr 22.
- Kovac JD, Jankovic A, Dikic-Rom A, Grubor N, Antic A, Dugalic V. Imaging Spectrum of Intrahepatic Mass-Forming Cholangiocarcinoma and Its Mimickers: How to Differentiate Them Using MRI. Curr Oncol. 2022;29(2):698–723. https://doi.org/10.3390/curroncol29020061.
- Arbelaiz A, Azkargorta M, Krawczyk M, Santos-Laso A, Lapitz A, Perugorria MJ, Erice O, Gonzalez E, Jimenez-Aguero R, Lacasta A, Ibarra C, Sanchez-Campos A, Jimeno JP, Lammert F, Milkiewicz P, Marzioni M, Macias RIR, Marin JJG, Patel T, Gores GJ, Martinez I, Elortza F, Falcon-Perez JM, Bujanda L, Banales JM. Serum extracellular vesicles contain protein biomarkers for primary sclerosing cholangitis and cholangiocarcinoma. Hepatology. 2017;66(4):1125–43. https://doi.org/10.1002/hep.29291. Epub 2017 Aug 26.
- Banales JM, Inarrairaegui M, Arbelaiz A, Milkiewicz P, Muntane J, Munoz-Bellvis L, La Casta A, Gonzalez LM, Arretxe E, Alonso C, Martinez-Arranz I, Lapitz A, Santos-Laso A, Avila MA, Martinez-Chantar ML, Bujanda L, Marin JJG, Sangro B, Macias RIR. Serum Metabolites as Diagnostic Biomarkers for Cholangiocarcinoma, Hepatocellular Carcinoma, and Primary Sclerosing Cholangitis. Hepatology. 2019;70(2):547–62. https://doi.org/10.1002/hep.30319. Epub 2019 Feb 14.
- Huang C, Xu X, Wang M, Xiao X, Cheng C, Ji J, Fang M, Gao C. Serum N-glycan fingerprint helps to discriminate intrahepatic cholangiocarcinoma from hepatocellular carcinoma. Electrophoresis. 2021;42(11):1187–95. https://doi.org/10.1002/elps.202000392. Epub 2021 Mar 1.
- Chen VL, Xu D, Wicha MS, Lok AS, Parikh ND. Utility of Liquid Biopsy Analysis in Detection of Hepatocellular Carcinoma, Determination of Prognosis, and Disease Monitoring: A Systematic Review. Clin Gastroenterol Hepatol. 2020;18(13):2879–902.e9. https://doi.org/10.1016/j.cgh.2020.04.019. Epub 2020 Apr 11.
- Foda ZH, Annapragada AV, Boyapati K, Bruhm DC, Vulpescu NA, Medina JE, Mathios D, Cristiano S, Niknafs N, Luu HT, Goggins MG, Anders RA, Sun J, Meta SH, Thomas DL, Kirk GD, Adleff V, Phallen J, Scharpf RB, Kim AK, Velculescu VE. Detecting Liver Cancer Using Cell-Free DNA Fragmentomes. Cancer Discov. 2023;13(3):616–31. https://doi.org/10.1158/2159-8290.CD-22-0659.
- Lapitz A, Azkargorta M, Milkiewicz P, Olaizola P, Zhuravleva E, Grimsrud MM, Schramm C, Arbelaiz A, O'Rourke CJ, La Casta A, Milkiewicz M, Pastor T, Vesterhus M, Jimenez-Aguero R, Dill MT, Lamarca A, Valle JW, Macias RIR, Izquierdo-Sanchez L, Perez Castano Y, Caballero-Camino FJ, Riano I, Krawczyk M, Ibarra C, Bustamante J, Nova-Camacho LM, Falcon-Perez JM, Elortza F, Perugorria MJ, Andersen JB, Bujanda L, Karlsen TH, Folseraas T, Rodrigues PM, Banales JM. Liquid biopsy-based protein biomarkers for risk prediction,

early diagnosis, and prognostication of cholangiocarcinoma. J Hepatol. 2023;79(1):93–108. https://doi.org/10.1016/j.jhep.2023.02.027. Epub 2023 Mar 1.

- Wang P, Song Q, Ren J, Zhang W, Wang Y, Zhou L, Wang D, Chen K, Jiang L, Zhang B, Chen W, Qu C, Zhao H, Jiao Y. Simultaneous analysis of mutations and methylations in circulating cell-free DNA for hepatocellular carcinoma detection. Sci Transl Med. 2022;14(672):eabp8704. https://doi.org/10.1126/scitranslmed.abp8704. Epub 2022 Nov 23.
- Ye Q, Ling S, Zheng S, Xu X. Liquid biopsy in hepatocellular carcinoma: circulating tumor cells and circulating tumor DNA. Mol Cancer. 2019;18(1):114. https://doi.org/10.1186/s12943-019-1043-x.
- Li S, Yao J, Xie M, Liu Y, Zheng M. Exosomal miRNAs in hepatocellular carcinoma development and clinical responses. J Hematol Oncol. 2018;11(1):54. https://doi.org/10.1186/s13045-018-0579-3.
- Sasaki R, Kanda T, Yokosuka O, Kato N, Matsuoka S, Moriyama M. Exosomes and Hepatocellular Carcinoma: From Bench to Bedside. Int J Mol Sci. 2019;20(6):1406. https://doi.org/10.3390/ijms20061406.
- Wang M, Gao Y, Feng H, Warner E, An M, Jia J, Chen S, Fang M, Ji J, Gu X, Gao C. A nomogram incorporating six easily obtained parameters to discriminate intrahepatic cholangiocarcinoma and hepatocellular carcinoma. Cancer Med. 2018;7(3):646–54. https://doi.org/10.1002/cam4.1341. Epub 2018 Feb 23.
- Si YQ, Wang XQ, Pan CC, Wang Y, Lu ZM. An Efficient Nomogram for Discriminating Intrahepatic Cholangiocarcinoma From Hepatocellular Carcinoma: A Retrospective Study. Front Oncol. 2022;12:833999. https://doi.org/10.3389/fonc.2022.833999. eCollection 2022.
- Wang Y, Zhang C, Zhang P, Guo G, Jiang T, Zhao X, Jiang J, Huang X, Tong H, Tian Y. Serum exosomal microRNAs combined with alpha-fetoprotein as diagnostic markers of hepatocellular carcinoma. Cancer Med. 2018;7(5):1670–1679. https://doi.org/10.1002/cam4.1390. Epub 2018 Mar 23.

Enrolling By Invitation

Tumor Exosome Liquid Biopsy Strategy to Diagnose Pancreatic Cancer

ClinicalTrials.gov ID NCT06108531

Sponsor: Shanghai Jiao Tong University School of Medicine

Information provided by Yingbin Liu, MD, PhD, FACS, Shanghai Jiao Tong University School of Medicine (responsible party)

Last update posted: 2023-10-31

Study Overview

Brief Summary

This is an observational study of patients diagnosed with pancreatic cancer by pathology, with a control group of patients with pathology suggestive of benign pancreatic lesions and normal subjects, and the diagnostic ability of exosomes to identify patients with pancreatic cancer was assessed through the detection of exosomes in the peripheral blood.

Official Title

Study on the Application of Tumor Exosome Liquid Biopsy in the Early Diagnosis of Pancreatic Cancer

Conditions

Pancreatic

Intervention/Treatment

- Other:

Other Study ID Numbers

- IIT-2023-0118

Study Start (Estimated)
2023-11-01
Primary Completion (Estimated)
2025-08-01
Study Completion (Estimated)
2026-08-01
Enrollment (Estimated)
400
Study Type
Observational
This study has one location.
China
Shanghai locations
Shanghai, Shanghai, China, 20092
Xinhua Hospital, Affiliated to Shanghai Jiao Tong University, School of Medicine
Eligibility Criteria
Description
Inclusion criteria:

- Diagnosis of pancreatic cancer confirmed by imaging (case)
- Diagnosis of chronic pancreatitis confirmed by imaging (hospital control)

Exclusion criteria:

- The pathology diagnosis and imaging does not match
- Patients with other malignant tumors
- Patients with other severe systemic diseases

Study Population

Cases will be patients with newly diagnosed pancreatic cancer. Controls will be selected from patients with pancreatitis in the same hospital as the cases, matched by sex, race, and age (1:1). A total of 400 patients with gallbladder cancer will be recruited.

Ages Eligible for Study
18 to 80 years (adult, older adult)
Sexes Eligible for Study
All
Accepts Healthy Volunteers
Yes
Sampling Method
Probability sample
Design Details
Observational model: case-control
Time perspective: prospective
Biospecimen retention: samples without DNA
Biospecimen description: serum

Groups and Interventions

Groups/cohorts	Intervention/treatment
Pancreatic patients Cases will be the patients with newly diagnosed pancreatic.	Other:
The controls Controls will be selected from patients with pancreatitis from the same hospital as the case, matched by gender, race, and age (1:1).	Other:

Primary Outcome Measures

Outcome measure	Measure description	Time frame
Characterization of proteins in tumor exosomes from patients with pancreatic cancer	We will select specific protein A from circulating exosomes of pancreatic cancer patients for further analysis.	Up to 2 years from start of study
The expression of protein A in the circulating exosomes from patients	By detecting the expression of protein A in circulating exosomes of patients. the ROC curve of A+ circulating exosomes will be compared to clinical standard tumor biomarkers (e.g., CA199) in pancreatic cancer patients.	Up to 2 years from start of study

Sponsor: Shanghai Jiao Tong University School of Medicine

Active, Not Recruiting

Circulating Exosome RNA in Lung Metastases of Primary High-Grade Osteosarcoma

ClinicalTrials.gov ID NCT03108677

Sponsor: Ruijin Hospital
Information provided by Yuhui Shen, Ruijin Hospital (responsible party)
Last update posted: 2023-10-03
Study Overview
Brief Summary

The purpose of this study is to learn whether the profile of RNA from circulating exosomes can be used as a biomarker for lung metastases of primary high-grade osteosarcoma. Circulating exosomes plays roles in metastases in many kinds of cancer including osteosarcoma. By RNA profiling, researchers may find lung metastases earlier than conventional work-up and predict the oncological outcomes.

Detailed Description

Investigators have performed a four-patient pilot study under the oversight of hospital's ethics committee, and the investigator found that the levels and mutations of circulating exosome RNA from patients with or without lung metastasis have significant differences. Then, investigators wish to register this study to do further research, in order to reveal the roles of circulating exosome RNA in metastases of osteosarcoma.

Official Title

A Pilot Study of Circulating Exosome RNA as Diagnostic and Prognostic Markers in Lung Metastases of Primary High-Grade Osteosarcoma

Conditions
Lung metastases
Osteosarcoma
Intervention/Treatment

- Other: blood samples

Other Study ID Numbers

- RJ2017NO13

Study Start (Actual)
2017-05-01
Primary Completion (Actual)
2023-09-19
Study Completion (Estimated)
2023-12-30
Enrollment (Actual)
90
Study Type
Observational (patient registry)
This study has one location.
China
Shanghai locations
Shanghai, Shanghai, China, 200025
Ruijin Hospital Shanghai Jiao Tong University School of medicine
Eligibility Criteria

Description
Inclusion criteria:

- Diagnosis by biopsy: primary high-grade osteosarcoma, including conventional osteosarcoma, telangiectatic osteosarcoma, small cell osteosarcoma, and high-grade surface osteosarcoma
- Tumor located in the extremities or pelvis
- Age 12–60 years
- No prior history of cancer and no prior treatment elsewhere
- No prior history of chronic diseases including autoimmune disease, chronic infection, etc. which may interfere the level of circulating exosomes

Exclusion criteria:

- Initial misdiagnosis confirmed by specimen of definitive surgery
- Applying target drugs in the period of treatment which may reduce tumor derived exosomes
- Withdraw from the study for any reason

Study Population
Patients with primary high-grade osteosarcoma aged 12–60
Ages Eligible for Study
12 to 60 years (child, adult)
Sexes Eligible for Study
All
Accepts Healthy Volunteers
No
Sampling Method
Non-probability sample
Design Details
Observational model: cohort
Time perspective: prospective
Target follow-up duration: 3 years
Biospecimen retention: samples without DNA
Biospecimen description: samples with purified exosome RNA

Groups and Interventions

Groups/cohorts	Intervention/treatment
Metastatic For osteosarcoma patients with metastasis, collecting blood samples	Other: blood samples 15 ml peripheral blood
Non-metastatic For osteosarcoma patients without metastasis, collecting blood samples	Other: blood samples 15 ml peripheral blood

Primary Outcome Measures

Outcome measure	Measure description	Time frame
Differences in the levels and mutations of circulating exosome RNA from patients with or without lung metastasis	Next-generation sequencing will be performed to the whole RNA sequencing.	Before the neo-adjuvant chemotherapy, before the definitive surgery procedure, and every 6 months after surgery, up to 3 years.

Secondary Outcome Measures

Outcome measure	Measure description	Time frame
Differences in the classic cell signal pathway mutations of circulating exosome RNA from patients with or without lung metastasis	Next-generation sequencing will be performed to the whole RNA sequencing.	Before the neo-adjuvant chemotherapy, before the definitive surgery procedure, and every 6 months after surgery, up to 3 years
Differences in the therapeutic target mutations of circulating exosome RNA from patients with or without lung metastasis	Next-generation sequencing will be performed to the whole RNA sequencing.	Before the neo-adjuvant chemotherapy, before the definitive surgery procedure, and every 6 months after surgery, up to 3 years
The correlation between circulating exosome RNA mutation levels and 3-year disease-free survival (DFS), progression-free survival (PFS), and lung metastases	Next-generation sequencing will be performed to the whole RNA sequencing.	Before the neo-adjuvant chemotherapy, before the definitive surgery procedure, and every 6 months after surgery, up to 3 years
The correlation between specific circulating exosome RNA mutations and 3-year disease-free survival (DFS), progression-free survival (PFS), and lung metastases	Next-generation sequencing will be performed to the whole RNA sequencing.	Before the neo-adjuvant chemotherapy, before the definitive surgery procedure, and every 6 months after surgery, up to 3 years
The roles of circulating exosome micro-RNA mutations on regulation of circulating exosome RNA	Next-generation sequencing will be performed to the whole RNA sequencing.	Before the neo-adjuvant chemotherapy, before the definitive surgery procedure, and every 6 months after surgery, up to 3 years
The mutations of circulating exosome RNA from patients without metastasis	Next-generation sequencing will be performed to the whole RNA sequencing.	Before the neo-adjuvant chemotherapy, before the definitive surgery procedure, and every 6 months after surgery, up to 3 years.

Sponsor: Ruijin Hospital

Investigators

- Principal investigator: Yuhui Shen, PhD, MD, Ruijin Hospital
- Principal investigator: Weibin Zhang, PhD, MD, Ruijin Hospital

Publications

- Bao Q, Gong L, Wang J, Wen J, Shen Y, Zhang W. Extracellular Vesicle RNA Sequencing Reveals Dramatic Transcriptomic Alterations Between Metastatic and Primary Osteosarcoma in a Liquid Biopsy Approach. Ann Surg Oncol. 2018;25(9):2642–51. https://doi.org/10.1245/s10434-018-6642-z. Epub 2018 Jul 6.

Enrolling By Invitation

Plasma Exosomes Reveal the Efficacy of Targeted Therapy in Patients with EGFR Mutation in Lung Adenocarcinoma

ClinicalTrials.gov ID NCT06730477

Sponsor: Wuhan Union Hospital, China

Information provided by Yang Jin, Wuhan Union Hospital, China (responsible party)

Last update posted: 2024-12-12

Study Overview

Brief Summary

The objective of this observational study is to explore the therapeutic trajectory of targeted therapy in lung adenocarcinoma patients with epidermal growth factor receptor (EGFR) mutations. The main objective is to identify potential biomarkers that can predict the efficacy of targeted therapy through plasma exosomes and to explore strategies to reverse drug resistance to targeted therapy. Biological specimens and medical imaging data will be collected from patients already receiving targeted therapy as a first-line treatment, and followed-up will be conducted to analyze prognosis based on different patterns.

Detailed Description

The medical imaging data will be collected retrospectively and prospectively, and the blood samples and tumor tissues will be collected prospectively.

Official Title

Based on Plasma Exosomes Combined with Multi-omics Analysis to Reveal the Trajectory of Targeted Therapy Resistance and Novel Target Intervention Therapy in Patients with EGFR Mutation in Lung Adenocarcinoma

Conditions

Lung adenocarcinoma

EGFR-activating mutation

Intervention/Treatment

- Other: observational study

Other Study ID Numbers

- XHJY20240912

Study Start (Actual)

2021-01-01
Primary Completion (Estimated)
2026-12-30
Study Completion (Estimated)
2027-12-30
Enrollment (Estimated)
500
Study Type
Observational
This study has one location.
China
Hubei locations
Wuhan, Hubei, China, 430022
Union hospital, Tongji Medical college, Huazhong University of Science and Technology
Eligibility Criteria
Description
Inclusion criteria:

- Pathological examination confirmed lung adenocarcinoma.
- No other type of tumor was present.
- Common sensitive EGFR (Ex19Del L858R or combined with other sites) mutations have been identified.
- Receive targeted therapy with or without chemotherapy as first-line treatment.
- ≥ 18 and ≤80 years old.

Exclusion criteria:

- History of other malignant tumors
- Irregular treatment or poor compliance
- Incomplete clinical information or lost to follow-up

Study Population
From January 2021 to December 2026, about 500 patients with EGFR-mutated lung adenocarcinoma who receive targeted therapy with or without chemotherapy as first-line treatment will be included in this cohort study.
Ages Eligible for Study
18 to 80 years (adult, older adult)
Sexes Eligible for Study
All
Accepts Healthy Volunteers
No
Sampling Method
Non-probability sample
Design Details
Observational model: cohort
Time perspective: other

Biospecimen retention: samples with DNA
Biospecimen description: Blood samples and tumor tissues will be retained.

Groups and Interventions

Groups/cohorts	Intervention/treatment
Untreated EGFR-mutated lung adenocarcinoma patients Patients diagnosed with lung adenocarcinoma with EGFR mutations for the first time	Other: observational study Efficacy of targeted therapy combined with or without chemotherapy as first-line therapy in patients with EGFR-mutated lung adenocarcinoma
Patients with EGFR-mutated lung adenocarcinoma who are responding to targeted therapy Patients with EGFR-mutated lung adenocarcinoma treated with targeted therapy combined with or without chemotherapy as first-line therapy, and the therapeutic effect was in the response stage.	Other: observational study Efficacy of targeted therapy combined with or without chemotherapy as first-line therapy in patients with EGFR-mutated lung adenocarcinoma
Patients with EGFR-mutated lung adenocarcinoma who are resistant to targeted therapy Patients with EGFR-mutated lung adenocarcinoma treated with targeted therapy combined with or without chemotherapy as first-line therapy, and the therapeutic effect was in drug resistance stage, or disease progression.	Other: observational study Efficacy of targeted therapy combined with or without chemotherapy as first-line therapy in patients with EGFR-mutated lung adenocarcinoma.

Primary Outcome Measures

Outcome measure	Measure description	Time frame
Progression-free survival	The time of disease progression is evaluated according to the Response Evaluation Criteria in Solid Tumors, version 1.1.	A 2-year period after starting treatment (regular follow-up every 3 months after receiving targeted therapy combined with or without chemotherapy as first-line treatment)

Secondary Outcome Measures

Outcome measure	Measure description	Time frame
Overall survival	The survival time after receiving targeted therapy combined with or without chemotherapy as first-line treatment	A 3-year period after starting treatment (regular follow-up every 6 months after receiving targeted therapy combined with or without chemotherapy as first-line treatment)

Sponsor: Wuhan Union Hospital, China

Collaborators

- Yichang Central People's Hospital
- Suizhou Hospital, Hubei University of Medicine

Recruiting

A Companion Diagnostic Study to Develop Circulating Exosomes as Predictive Biomarkers for the Response to Immunotherapy in Renal Cell Carcinoma

ClinicalTrials.gov ID NCT05705583

Sponsor: Zhejiang Cancer Hospital

Information provided by ZHAO An, Zhejiang Cancer Hospital (responsible party)

Last update posted: 2023-01-31

Study Overview

Brief Summary

Immune checkpoint inhibitors targeting PD-1 or PD-L1 have been developed and clinical trials showing a better response in unselected patients with metastatic renal cell carcinoma (RCC). At the moment, no clear biomarker exists to accurately predict anti-PD1/PDL1 RCC responsiveness. The objective of this study is to develop and evaluate the utility of circulating exosomes as companion diagnostic biomarker for predicting response to immunotherapy in patients with RCC.

Official Title

A Companion Diagnostic Study to Develop Circulating Exosomes as Predictive Biomarkers for the Response to Immunotherapy in Renal Cell Carcinoma

Conditions

Renal cell carcinoma

Intervention/Treatment

- Other: blood and urine collection

Other Study ID Numbers

- RCC-CDx-001

Study Start (Actual)

2023-01-01

Primary Completion (Estimated)

2025-12-31

Study Completion (Estimated)

2025-12-31

Enrollment (Estimated)

100

Study Type

Observational

This study has one location.
China
Hangzhou, China, 310022
Recruiting
An Zhao
Contact:
An Zhao, Dr
+8618258863556 zhaoan@zjcc.org.cn
Principal investigator: An Zhao, PhD
Eligibility Criteria
Description
Inclusion criteria:

- Advanced metastatic RCC
- Scheduled to initiate an immunocheckpoint inhibitors or in combination with them
- Age >= 18 years
- Able to provide informed consent

Exclusion criteria:

- Other, unrelated, concomitant active, invasive malignancy

Study Population
Adults with renal cell carcinoma
Ages Eligible for Study
18 Years and older (adult, older adult)
Sexes Eligible for Study
All
Accepts Healthy Volunteers
No
Sampling Method
Probability sample
Design Details
Observational model: cohort
Time perspective: prospective
Biospecimen retention: samples with DNA

Biospecimen description: collection of blood and urine specimens from patients receiving immunotherapy as part of their standard of care for the treatment of RCC

Groups and Interventions

Intervention/treatment
Other: blood and urine collection Blood and urine collection

Primary Outcome Measures

Outcome measure	Measure description	Time frame
The correlation between the circulating exosomes levels and the tumor responsiveness	The measurement: the concentration of circulating exosomes and the expression level of exosomal RNA The measurement tool: RT-PCR,WB, and Elisa	3 years

Sponsor: Zhejiang Cancer Hospital

Publications

- Wang H, Zhu Z, Zhang Y, Jiang T, Zhang M, Wang Z, Zhang Y, Zhao A, Su B. New insight into immune checkpoint inhibitors in the treatment of advanced renal cell carcinoma. Sci China Life Sci. 2023;66(4):875–8. https://doi.org/10.1007/s11427-022-2197-7. Epub 2022 Dec 1. No abstract available.
- Yu M, Liu X, Xu H, Shen S, Wang F, Chen D, Li G, Wang Z, Zuo Z, Zhao A. Comprehensive Evaluation of the m6A Regulator Prognostic Risk Score in the Prediction of Immunotherapy Response in Clear Cell Renal Cell Carcinoma. Front Immunol. 2022;13:818120. https://doi.org/10.3389/fimmu.2022.818120. eCollection 2022.
- Zhang W, Ni M, Su Y, Wang H, Zhu S, Zhao A, Li G. MicroRNAs in Serum Exosomes as Potential Biomarkers in Clear-cell Renal Cell Carcinoma. Eur Urol Focus. 2018;4(3):412–9. https://doi.org/10.1016/j.euf.2016.09.007. Epub 2016 Oct 14.

Recruiting

Exosome-Based Detection of Molecular Residual Disease in Stage II–III Colorectal Cancer

ClinicalTrials.gov ID NCT06654622

Sponsor: City of Hope Medical Center

Information provided by Ajay Goel, City of Hope Medical Center (responsible party)

Last update posted: 2024-10-23

Study Overview

Brief Summary

This study aims to establish an exosome-based liquid biopsy signature to detect molecular residual disease (MRD) in stage II–III colorectal cancer (CRC) patients. Identifying patients with MRD after surgery is crucial for selecting appropriate candidates for adjuvant chemotherapy (ACT), allowing for more personalized treatment approaches and potentially improving patient outcomes.

Detailed Description

The current standard for treating stage II–III colorectal cancer involves surgical resection, often followed by adjuvant chemotherapy (ACT) for high-risk patients. However, identifying patients who would benefit most from ACT remains challenging. Molecular residual disease (MRD) in these patients is a critical factor in determining the likelihood of recurrence. This study aims to develop an exosome-based liquid biopsy assay using circulating exosomal microRNAs (exo-miRNAs) to predict the presence of MRD in postoperative patients. By analyzing exo-miRNAs from blood samples collected after surgery, the goal is to identify high-risk patients who may benefit from ACT while sparing low-risk patients from unnecessary treatment. A risk-stratification model, termed the exosome-based molecular residual disease prediction for adjuvant chemotherapy induction (EMRATI) score, will be developed to improve ACT decision-making and enhance clinical outcomes for stage II–III CRC patients.

Official Title

An Exosome-Based Liquid Biopsy Assay to Detect Molecular Residual Disease for the Identification of High-Risk Patients with Stage II–III Colorectal Cancer

Conditions

Colorectal cancer

Colorectal cancer recurrent

Other Study ID Numbers

- 23228/CRMRD

Study Start (Actual)

2023-04-01

Primary Completion (Estimated)

2024-12-30

Study Completion (Estimated)

2024-12-30

Enrollment (Estimated)

200

Study Type

Observational (patient registry)

Study Contact

Name: Takayuki Noma, MD

Phone Number: 6268418625

Email: tnoma@coh.org

This study has one location.

United States

California locations

Duarte, California, United States, 91010

Recruiting

City of Hope Medical Center

Contact:

Ajay Goel, PhD

626-218-3452 ajgoel@coh.org

Contact:
Takayuki Noma, MD
6268418625 tnoma@coh.org
Contact:
Takayuki Noma, MD
Eligibility Criteria
Description
Inclusion criteria:

1. Patients with pathologically confirmed stage II or III colorectal cancer
2. Patients who have undergone curative-intent surgery
3. Patients with no evidence of distant metastasis (stage IV)
4. Patients aged 18 years or older
5. Patients who provided written informed consent

Exclusion criteria:

1. Patients with stage IV cancer or those receiving neoadjuvant therapy
2. Patients with non-curative resection or requiring urgent surgery
3. Patients with a follow-up period of fewer than 3 years
4. Patients with severe comorbidities or who are unable to participate in follow-up assessments

Study Population
The study will enroll patients with stage II–III colorectal cancer who have undergone curative surgery and require assessment for molecular residual disease to determine whether adjuvant chemotherapy is necessary.
Ages Eligible for Study
18 Years and older (adult, older adult)
Sexes Eligible for Study
All
Accepts Healthy Volunteers
No
Sampling Method
Probability sample
Design Details
Observational model: case-control
Time perspective: cross-sectional
Target follow-up duration: 5 years
Biospecimen retention: samples without DNA
Biospecimen description: Postoperative serum samples will be used to isolate exosomal miRNAs for MRD analysis.

Groups and Interventions

Groups/cohorts
Training cohort (recurrence group) Stage II–III CRC patients who experienced postoperative recurrence (evaluated by miRNA panel)
Training cohort (non-recurrence group) Stage II–III CRC patients who did not experience postoperative recurrence (evaluated by miRNA panel)
Testing cohort (recurrence group) Validation of miRNA panel and EMRATI score in independent stage II–III CRC patients who experienced postoperative recurrence
Testing cohort (non-recurrence group) Validation of miRNA panel and EMRATI score in independent stage II–III CRC patients who did not experience postoperative recurrence

Primary Outcome Measures

Outcome measure	Measure description	Time frame
Tumor evaluation (recurrence)	Assessment of tumor recurrence through clinical and imaging evaluations	Follow-up at regular intervals during the first 3 years post-surgery

Secondary Outcome Measures

Outcome measure	Measure description	Time frame
Overall survival (OS)	Evaluation of the overall survival (OS) of patients, defined as the time from surgery to death from any cause	Patients will be monitored for overall survival for up to 5 years post-surgery.

Sponsor: City of Hope Medical Center

Investigators

- Principal investigator: Ajay Goel, PhD, City of Hope Medical Center

Publications

- Zhou H, Zhu L, Song J, Wang G, Li P, Li W, Luo P, Sun X, Wu J, Liu Y, Zhu S, Zhang Y. Liquid biopsy at the frontier of detection, prognosis and progression monitoring in colorectal cancer. Mol Cancer. 2022;21(1):86. https://doi.org/10.1186/s12943-022-01556-2.
- Ruiz-Banobre J, Roy R, Alustiza Fernandez M, Murcia O, Jover R, Pera M, Balaguer F, Lopez-Lopez R, Goel A. Clinical significance of a microRNA signature for the identification and predicting prognosis in colorectal cancers with mucinous differentiation. Carcinogenesis. 2020;41(11):1498–506. https://doi.org/10.1093/carcin/bgaa097.

- Matsuyama T, Toiyama Y, Ishikawa T, Okugawa Y, Yasuno M, Maurel J, Kinugasa Y, Uetake H, Goel A. A metastasis-associated microRNA-based liquid biopsy signature for risk-stratification in colorectal cancer: a multicenter cohort study. Clin Transl Med. 2022;12(12):e998. https://doi.org/10.1002/ctm2.998. No abstract available.
- Miyazaki K, Wada Y, Okuno K, Murano T, Morine Y, Ikemoto T, Saito Y, Ikematsu H, Kinugasa Y, Shimada M, Goel A. An exosome-based liquid biopsy signature for pre-operative identification of lymph node metastasis in patients with pathological high-risk T1 colorectal cancer. Mol Cancer. 2023;22(1):2. https://doi.org/10.1186/s12943-022-01685-8.
- Mo S, Ye L, Wang D, Han L, Zhou S, Wang H, Dai W, Wang Y, Luo W, Wang R, Xu Y, Cai S, Liu R, Wang Z, Cai G. Early Detection of Molecular Residual Disease and Risk Stratification for Stage I to III Colorectal Cancer via Circulating Tumor DNA Methylation. JAMA Oncol. 2023;9(6):770–8. https://doi.org/10.1001/jamaoncol.2023.0425.
- Yoshino T, Argiles G, Oki E, Martinelli E, Taniguchi H, Arnold D, Mishima S, Li Y, Smruti BK, Ahn JB, Faud I, Chee CE, Yeh KH, Lin PC, Chua C, Hasbullah HH, Lee MA, Sharma A, Sun Y, Curigliano G, Bando H, Lordick F, Yamanaka T, Tabernero J, Baba E, Cervantes A, Ohtsu A, Peters S, Ishioka C, Pentheroudakis G. Pan-Asian adapted ESMO Clinical Practice Guidelines for the diagnosis treatment and follow-up of patients with localised colon cancer. Ann Oncol. 2021;32(12):1496–510. https://doi.org/10.1016/j.annonc.2021.08.1752. Epub 2021 Aug 16.
- Montcusi B, Madrid-Gambin F, Marin S, Mayol X, Pascual M, Cascante M, Pozo OJ, Pera M. Circulating Metabolic Markers Identify Patients at Risk for Tumor Recurrence: A Prospective Cohort Study in Colorectal Cancer Surgery. Ann Surg. 2024;280(5):842–9. https://doi.org/10.1097/SLA.0000000000006463. Epub 2024 Aug 1.
- Kotani D, Oki E, Nakamura Y, Yukami H, Mishima S, Bando H, Shirasu H, Yamazaki K, Watanabe J, Kotaka M, Hirata K, Akazawa N, Kataoka K, Sharma S, Aushev VN, Aleshin A, Misumi T, Taniguchi H, Takemasa I, Kato T, Mori M, Yoshino T. Molecular residual disease and efficacy of adjuvant chemotherapy in patients with colorectal cancer. Nat Med. 2023;29(1):127–34. https://doi.org/10.1038/s41591-022-02115-4. Epub 2023 Jan 16.
- Tie J, Cohen JD, Lahouel K, Lo SN, Wang Y, Kosmider S, Wong R, Shapiro J, Lee M, Harris S, Khattak A, Burge M, Harris M, Lynam J, Nott L, Day F, Hayes T, McLachlan SA, Lee B, Ptak J, Silliman N, Dobbyn L, Popoli M, Hruban R, Lennon AM, Papadopoulos N, Kinzler KW, Vogelstein B, Tomasetti C, Gibbs P; DYNAMIC Investigators. Circulating Tumor DNA Analysis Guiding Adjuvant Therapy in Stage II Colon Cancer. N Engl J Med. 2022;386(24):2261–72. https://doi.org/10.1056/NEJMoa2200075. Epub 2022 Jun 4.
- Kandimalla R, Gao F, Matsuyama T, Ishikawa T, Uetake H, Takahashi N, Yamada Y, Becerra C, Kopetz S, Wang X, Goel A. Genome-wide Discovery and Identification of a Novel miRNA Signature for Recurrence Prediction in Stage II

and III Colorectal Cancer. Clin Cancer Res. 2018;24(16):3867–77. https://doi.org/10.1158/1078-0432.CCR-17-3236. Epub 2018 Mar 7.

Recruiting

Exosome-Based Liquid Biopsies for Upper Gastrointestinal Cancers Diagnosis

ClinicalTrials.gov ID NCT06278064

Sponsor: Beijing Friendship Hospital

Information provided by Min Li, Beijing Friendship Hospital (responsible party)

Last update posted: 2024-02-26

Study Overview

Brief Summary

This study constitutes a case-control investigation employing a retrospective approach. Plasma samples from individuals with esophageal cancer, benign esophageal diseases, gastric cancer, benign gastric diseases, and a healthy control group were systematically collected. Advanced data-independent acquisition (DIA) proteomics and single-vesicle membrane protein detection techniques were employed to quantify protein content within exosomes. Specific protein biomarkers indicative of early-stage upper gastrointestinal tumors were identified. External validation of these protein markers was conducted using parallel reaction monitoring (PRM) technology on an independent validation cohort. The objective is to establish protein marker predictions for early diagnosis of upper gastrointestinal tumors and prognostication of therapeutic efficacy.

Detailed Description

This study employs a multicenter, retrospective cohort design, collecting and analyzing plasma and tissue exosome protein data from patients with upper gastrointestinal tumors (stage I–II), upper gastrointestinal benign diseases, and a healthy control group who have visited Beijing Friendship Hospital and other relevant subcenter hospitals over the past 5 years. Concurrently, relevant clinical and pathological information is recorded.

Samples from the training cohort undergo traditional quantitative exosome proteomic analysis (data-independent acquisition, DIA) and single-vesicle membrane protein analysis (PBA). A comprehensive upper gastrointestinal tumor-specific exosome protein database is constructed, incorporating extensive information. Subsequently, bioinformatics methods are employed to conduct in-depth analysis of the extensive protein data, screening for proteins with high specificity for upper gastrointestinal tumors, capable of direct detection on the exosome membrane surface. By establishing and evaluating diagnostic models, we aim to quantify the diagnostic potential of these markers, providing a scientific basis for future early screening methods for upper gastrointestinal tumors.

Finally, external validation of these protein markers in an independent validation cohort ensures their reliability and stability across different patient populations. The academic significance of this research lies in its thorough exploration of exosome proteomics in early cancer diagnosis, offering potential innovative breakthroughs for academic progress and clinical practice in this field.

Official Title

Plasma Extracellular Vesicle Quantitative Proteomic Analysis for Early Diagnosis of Upper Gastrointestinal Cancers

Conditions

Gastric cancer

Esophagus cancer

Intervention/Treatment

- Other: gastric cancer
- Other: esophagus cancer

Other Study ID Numbers

- BFHHZML20240006

Study Start (Actual)

2024-02-01

Primary Completion (Estimated)

2024-12-31

Study Completion (Estimated)

2025-06-30

Enrollment (Estimated)

562

Study Type

Observational

Study Contact

Name: Li Min, Ph.D.

Phone Number: +86 13552652141

Email: minli@ccmu.edu.cn

Study Contact Backup

Name: Chenjie Xu, PhD

This study has three locations.

China

Beijing, China

Recruiting

Beijing Friendship Hospital, Capital Medical University

Contact:

Li Min, PhD

Principal investigator: Li Min, PhD

Beijing, China

Recruiting

Cancer Hospital Chinese Academy of Medical Sciences

Contact:
Yibin Xie, PhD
Hebei locations
Shijiazhuang, Hebei, China
Recruiting
The Fourth Hospital of Hebei Medical University
Contact:
Lianmei Zhao, PhD
Eligibility Criteria
Description
Inclusion criteria:

- Confirmed diagnosis of upper gastrointestinal cancers or benign upper gastrointestinal diseases through gastroscopy and pathological examination
- Collection of plasma samples prior to surgical treatment
- Availability of complete clinical data

Exclusion criteria:

- Previous reception of anti-tumor treatments (including radiotherapy, chemotherapy, etc.) before blood collection
- Coexistence of other systemic tumors
- Absence of plasma sample collection before surgical treatment
- Incomplete clinical data
- Pregnancy status

Study Population
The study population included a range of subjects with upper gastrointestinal cancers and diseases, including patients with malignant and benign upper gastrointestinal diseases and healthy controls, who were admitted to the main study center and other collaborating sub-center hospitals.
Ages Eligible for Study
Child, adult, older adult
Sexes Eligible for Study
All
Accepts Healthy Volunteers
Yes
Sampling Method
Non-probability sample
Design Details
Observational model: case-control
Time perspective: retrospective
Biospecimen retention: samples without DNA
Biospecimen description: Only proteins will be detected and analyzed in this study.

Groups and Interventions

Groups/cohorts	Intervention/treatment
Gastric cancer group Patients diagnosed with gastric cancer, including early gastric cancer and advanced gastric cancer	Other: gastric cancer Patients diagnosed with gastric cancer, including early stage gastric and advanced gastric cancer
Esophagus cancer group Patients diagnosed with esophagus cancer, including early esophagus cancer and advanced esophagus cancer	Other: esophagus cancer Patients diagnosed with esophagus cancer, including early esophagus gastric and advanced esophagus cancer
Noncancer group Patients diagnosed with benign upper gastrointestinal diseases or healthy controls	

Primary Outcome Measures

Outcome measure	Measure description	Time frame
Plasma proteins in patients with gastric cancer	The outcome will be tested by data-independent acquisition (DIA) proteomics technology	Before receiving treatment for gastric cancer
Plasma proteins in patients with esophagus cancer	The outcome will be tested by data-independent acquisition (DIA) proteomics technology	Before receiving treatment for esophagus cancer

Sponsor: Beijing Friendship Hospital

Investigators

- Principal investigator: Li Min, PhD, Beijing Friendship Hospital

Not Yet Recruiting

A Prospective, Multicenter Cohort Study of Urinary Exosome lncRNAs for Preoperative Diagnosis of Lymphatic Metastasis in Patients with Bladder Cancer

ClinicalTrials.gov ID NCT05270174

Sponsor: Sun Yat-sen Memorial Hospital of Sun Yat-sen University

Information provided by Sun Yat-sen Memorial Hospital of Sun Yat-sen University (responsible party)

Last update posted: 2023-02-21

Study Overview

Brief Summary

Bladder cancer is one of the most frequent malignant tumors of the urinary system in China, seriously threatening the life safety of patients. The main treatment methods for bladder cancer include surgical resection, radiotherapy and chemotherapy, immunotherapy, and targeted therapy, among which surgical resection is still the only reliable radical treatment at present. Lymphatic metastasis is the main mode of metastasis of bladder cancer, and preoperative diagnosis is of great significance to determine whether radical surgical treatment can be performed for some patients with advanced bladder cancer. Recent studies reveal that exosomes, as key signaling molecules in the tumor microenvironment, have been confirmed to be associated with various tumor progressions. Our previous study showed that lncRNA-ELNAT1 highly expressed in urine exosomes of bladder cancer patients can promote lymphatic metastasis of bladder cancer by inducing lymphatic angiogenesis and is associated with poor prognosis of patients. However, whether exosome ELNAT1 can be used as an independent preoperative predictor of lymph node metastasis of bladder cancer needs to be explored in further clinical trials, and this study will further clarify the association between the two. In this study, urine exosomes were collected from positive and negative control patients with lymph node metastasis of bladder cancer, and the ROC curve was statistically analyzed and fitted to determine whether exosome ELANT1 could be used as an independent predictor of lymph node metastasis of bladder cancer.

Detailed Description

1. According to the selection criteria, bladder cancer patients with informed consent in the study were first included.
2. The patients with indications of radical cystectomy were selected.
3. Urine samples were collected before radical cystectomy, and exocrine bodies were extracted to analyze the expression level of ELNAT1.
4. According to the postoperative lymph node pathological results, the above patients were further divided into two groups: lymphatic metastasis positive group and negative group.
5. We perform statistical analysis of urinary exosomal ELNAT1 to validate the performance of diagnosing lymphatic metastasis of bladder cancer

Official Title

A Prospective, Multicenter Cohort Study of Urinary Exosome lncRNAs for Preoperative Diagnosis of Lymphatic Metastasis in Patients with Bladder Cancer

Conditions

Explore whether lncRNA-ElNAT1 in urine exosomes can be used as a new target for preoperative diagnosis of lymph node metastasis

Intervention/Treatment

- Other: no intervention

Other Study ID Numbers

- SYSEC-KY-KS-2021-278

Study Start (Estimated)
2023-06-01
Primary Completion (Estimated)
2025-01-01

Study Completion (Estimated)
2025-08-01
Enrollment (Estimated)
74
Study Type
Observational
Study Contact
Name: Changhao Chen
Phone Number: +86-13631412669
Email: chenchh53@mail.sysu.edu.cn
This study has one location.
China
Guangzhou, China
Sun Yat-sen Memorial Hospital
Contact:
Changhao M Chen
+8613631412669 chenchh53@mail.sysu.edu.cn
Eligibility Criteria
Description
Inclusion criteria:

1. Patients older than 18 years old
2. Clinically diagnosed urothelial carcinoma bladder cancer
3. Patients agreed to provide the urine sample
4. Patients who voluntarily agreed to informed consent

Exclusion criteria:

1. Patients with distant metastasis
2. Patients with uncontrolled viral infection (HIV, HBV, HCV)
3. Patients who are pregnant or have the possibility of pregnancy and are lactating
4. Hypersensitivity or history of allergic to the drug being used
5. Patients with cerebrovascular disease, complications, and infections that are not medically controlled
6. Patients with a history of other malignant diseases within the past 5 years (excluding cured non-melanoma skin cancer or in situ cervical cancer)
7. Those who are taking drugs that can cause drug interactions with chemotherapy
8. Patients who withdraw consent

Study Population
Patients diagnosed with bladder cancer
Ages Eligible for Study
18 Years and older (adult, older adult)
Sexes Eligible for Study
All
Accepts Healthy Volunteers

No
Sampling Method
Probability sample
Design Details
Observational model: cohort
Time perspective: prospective

Groups and Interventions

Groups/cohorts	Intervention/treatment
lncRNA-ELNAT1 high expression group	Other: no intervention No intervention
lncRNA-ELNAT1 low expression group	Other: no intervention No intervention

Primary Outcome Measures

Outcome measure	Measure description	Time frame
Lymph node metastases in bladder cancer	Analyses of number and location of lymph node metastases based on pathological diagnosis	1 year

Secondary Outcome Measures

Outcome measure	Measure description	Time frame
Recurrence rate	The rate of recurrence will be detected after radical cystectomy by postoperative follow-up visit	3 years

Sponsor: Sun Yat-sen Memorial Hospital of Sun Yat-sen University

Recruiting

Exosome Testing as a Screening Modality for Human Papillomavirus-Positive Oropharyngeal Squamous Cell Carcinoma

ClinicalTrials.gov ID NCT02147418
Sponsor: New Mexico Cancer Research Alliance
Information provided by New Mexico Cancer Research Alliance (responsible party)
Last update posted: 2024-01-11
Study Overview
Brief Summary

Cancer of the oropharynx (middle, side and back walls of the throat; back of the tongue; soft palate, and tonsils), or oropharyngeal squamous cell carcinoma (OPSCC), has been on the rise in the United States. Human papillomavirus (HPV) has been recognized in many of these cancers, and testing for HPV has contributed to the higher reported rates of OPSCC. In this study, our goal is to develop a new test that can detect certain HPV proteins in the blood or saliva to help improve detection of OPSCC.

Detailed Description

While secondary screening strategies have successfully reduced the rate of HPV-positive cervical cancers, an effective screening modality for HPV-OPSCC does not exist. A central problem in the early diagnosis of HPV-OPSCC is the relative inaccessibility of the tonsillar crypts, where oncogenic infections are thought to originate. Unlike the relatively smooth surface of the cervix which permits mechanical sampling with Pap tests and which can be evaluated visually for evidence of dysplasia, much of the tonsillar epithelium is found below the surface in a complex network. As a consequence, any screening modality cannot depend upon direct access to malignant lesions. What is needed is a minimally invasive, diffusible or circulating marker of HPV-OPSCC, and a means to collect and detect it.

Official Title

An Observational, Single-Institution Pilot/Feasibility Study of Exosome Testing as a Screening Modality for Human Papillomavirus-Positive Oropharyngeal Squamous Cell Carcinoma

Conditions

Oropharyngeal cancer

Other Study ID Numbers

- INST 1310

Study Start (Actual)

2015-02-25

Primary Completion (Estimated)

2025-12

Study Completion (Estimated)

2027-12

Enrollment (Estimated)

30

Study Type

Observational

Study Contact

Name: Andrew Cowan, MD

Email: AnCowan@salud.unm.edu

Study Contact Backup

Name: Valerie Parks, RN

Phone Number: 505-925-0390

Email: vparks@salud.unm.edu

This study has one location.

United States
New Mexico locations
Albuquerque, New Mexico, United States, 87131-0001
Recruiting
University of New Mexico Cancer Center
Contact:
Andrew Cowan, MD
AnCowan@salud.unm.edu
Contact:
Valerie Parks, RN
505-925-0390 vparks@salud.unm.edu
Principal investigator: Andrew Cowan, MD
Eligibility Criteria
Description
Inclusion criteria (cancer patients):

- Male or female
- Age greater than or equal to 18
- Previously untreated, pathologically confirmed OPSCC (HPV+ or HPV−)
- Ability to understand study information and provide written consent for participation

Inclusion criteria (noncancer patients):

- Male or female
- Age greater than or equal to 18
- Ability to understand study information and provide written consent for participation

Exclusion criteria:

- Age less than 18 years
- Prisoners
- Pregnant women
- Patients with mental disability

Study Population

The patient population will consist of adults presenting to the Division of Otolaryngology—Head and Neck Surgery at the University of New Mexico with previously untreated OPSCC. Both HPV-positive and HPV-negative malignancies will be collected as the study and control groups, respectively. In addition, saliva samples will be collected from patients presenting with benign conditions as a further negative control.

Ages Eligible for Study
18 Years and older (adult, older adult)
Sexes Eligible for Study
All
Accepts Healthy Volunteers

Yes
Sampling Method
Non-probability sample
Design Details
Observational model: case-control
Time perspective: prospective
Biospecimen retention: samples without DNA

Biospecimen description: All oropharyngeal rinse (gargle) specimens will be processed within 24 hours of collection. Any remaining material after testing will be stored for a period not to exceed 1 year in a secure location.

Groups and Interventions

Groups/cohorts
Group 1: HPV-positive cancer Oropharyngeal cancer patients testing positive for human papillomavirus (HPV)
Group 2: HPV-positive cancer Oropharyngeal cancer patients who test positive for human papillomavirus (HPV)
Group 3: healthy controls Patients with benign conditions

Primary Outcome Measures

Outcome measure	Measure description	Time frame
Cultured cell exosome protein signature outcome measure	The presence of unique proteins obtained from primary cell cultures derived from HPV-OPSCC confirmed patients will be compared to normal tonsillar epithelial cells and established cell lines. The distribution of these protein signatures will be compared in HPV-OPSCC and normal epithelial cells.	1 month

Other Outcome Measures

Outcome measure	Measure description	Time frame
Exosome signatures oropharyngeal rinse measure	Compare exosome protein signatures generated from cells obtained through oropharyngeal rinses of patients with HPV-positive OPSCC and normal controls to identify an exosome protein marker that is absent (or present at a different, statistically significant level) in the oropharyngeal rinses of normal controls.	1 month

Sponsor: New Mexico Cancer Research Alliance

Investigators

- Principal investigator: Andrew Cowan, MD, University of New Mexico Cancer Center

Recruiting

Early Onset Colorectal Cancer Detection (ENCODE)

ClinicalTrials.gov ID NCT06342401

Sponsor: City of Hope Medical Center

Information provided by City of Hope Medical Center (responsible party)

Last update posted: 2024-10-31

Study Overview

Brief Summary

Colorectal cancer (CRC) once predominantly affected older individuals but in recent years has witnessed a progressive increase in incidence among young adults. Once rare, early-onset colorectal cancer (EOCRC, that is, a CRC diagnosed before the age of 50) now constitutes 10–15% of all newly diagnosed CRC cases and it stands as the first cause of cancer-related death in young men and the second for young women.

This study aims to detect EOCRC with a non-invasive test, using a blood-based molecular assay based on microRNA (ribonucleic acid)

Detailed Description

The rising incidence of early-onset colorectal cancer (EOCRC) is a pressing clinical issue unique to our times, and it is expected to grow with an anticipated further 90% increase in incidence by the decade's end. Challenges persist even after reducing the CRC screening age to 45: under-45s lack routine screening and compliance in the 45–50 age group remains low, partly due to invasiveness and discomfort of standard screening methods. Urgent action is warranted to develop affordable, sensitive, and feasible screening for timely detection and improved participation. A non-invasive, patient-friendly screening test, like a blood-based assay, could address these epidemiological concerns and also attract underserved populations.

This study involves the development and validation of a liquid biopsy, assessing circulating cell-free and exosomal microRNAs (cf-miRNA and exo-miRNA, respectively) for indirect sampling of tumor tissue in the bloodstream. The researchers intend to harness machine learning and bioinformatics to create an integrated panel (with both cf-miRNAs and exo-miRNAs) to enhance the inherently high sensitivity of cf-miRNAs with the distinctive specificity of exo-miRNAs. This combined approach will not only improve the performance of a diagnostic model but will also tap into the diverse tumor biology aspects of EOCRC.

The study's core goal is to develop cost-efficient, non-invasive, clinic-friendly biomarkers with high sensitivity and specificity, aiding EOCRC detection.

The researchers intend to do so in three phases:

1. To perform comprehensive small RNA-Seq from matched cf-miRNA, exo-miRNA, cancer-derived miRNA, and mucosa-derived miRNA
2. To develop and train two miRNA detection panels (cf-miRNA and exo-miRNA, respectively) based on advanced machine-learning models and, then, combine these two using several machine-learning models to obtain a final detection biomarker
3. To validate the findings in an independent cohort of EOCRC and controls

In summary, this proposal promises to improve patient care and compliance, and, ultimately, reduce mortality from EOCRC.

Official Title

Development and Validation for an Exosome-Based and Machine Learning Powered Liquid Biopsy for the Detection of Early-Onset Colorectal Cancer

Conditions

Colorectal cancer

Colorectal neoplasms

Colorectal adenocarcinoma

Colorectal cancer stage I

Intervention/Treatment

- Diagnostic test: ENCODE

Other Study ID Numbers

- 23228/ENCODE

Study Start (Actual)

2023-04-15

Primary Completion (Estimated)

2025-04-15

Study Completion (Estimated)

2025-10-15

Enrollment (Estimated)

400

Study Type

Observational

Study Contact

Name: Ajay Goel, PhD

Phone Number: 626-218-3452

Email: AJGOEL@COH.ORG

This study has thirteen locations.

United States

California locations

Duarte, California, United States, 91010

Recruiting

City of Hope Medical Center

Contact:

Ajay Goel, PhD

626-218-3452 AJGOEL@COH.ORG

Principal investigator: Alessandro Mannucci, MD

Italy

Milan, Italy

Recruiting

IRCCS San Raffaele

Contact:

Giulia Martina Cavestro, MD, PhD
cavestro.giuliamartina@hsr.it
Principal investigator: Alessandro Mannucci, MD
Japan
Kawasaki, Japan
Recruiting
Kawasaki University
Mie, Japan
Recruiting
Mie University
Tokyo, Japan
Recruiting
National Cancer Center Hospital
Tokyo, Japan
Recruiting
Tokyo Medical and Dental University
Yamagata, Japan
Recruiting
Yamagata University
Spain
Barcelona, Spain
Recruiting
Barcelona University
Contact:
Francesc Balaguer, MD, PhD
fprunes@clinic.cat
Barcelona, Spain
Recruiting
Colorectal Surgery, Vall d'Hebron University Hospital, Universitat Autonoma de Barcelona UAB
Contact:
Marc Martí-Gallostra
mmgallostra@vhebron.net
Barcelona, Spain
Recruiting
Surgery Department, Hospital del Mar, Barcelona, Spain
Contact:
Marta Jiménez-Toscano
mjimeneztoscano@psmar.cat
La Laguna, Spain
Recruiting
University of La Laguna
Madrid, Spain
Recruiting
Salamanca Biomedical Research Institute

Contact:
Jose Perea, MD
josepereag@hotmail.com
Sub-investigator: Jose Perea, MD
Salamanca, Spain
Recruiting
University of Salamanca-SACYL-CSIC, Salamanca, Spain
Contact:
Rosario Vidal-Tocino
a119121@usal.es
Eligibility Criteria
Description
Inclusion criteria:

- Stage I, II, III, and IV colorectal cancer (TNM classification, 8th edition) diagnosed before the age of 50 (EOCRC cases)
- Received standard diagnostic and staging procedures as per local guidelines, and at least one sample was drawn before receiving any curative-intent treatment
- Colonoscopy-proven cancer-free status at the time of study inclusion (non-disease controls)

Exclusion criteria:

- Hereditary colorectal cancer syndromes (identified through genetic testing)
- Inflammatory bowel diseases
- Lack of written informed consent

Study Population

Individuals younger than 50 years of age who were diagnosed with colorectal cancer before the age of 50 (cases) or were free from colorectal cancer at the time of study inclusion (controls)

Ages Eligible for Study
18 to 50 years (adult)
Sexes Eligible for Study
All
Accepts Healthy Volunteers
Yes
Sampling Method
Non-probability sample
Observational model: case-control
Time perspective: retrospective
Biospecimen retention: samples without DNA
Biospecimen description: plasma

Groups and Interventions

Groups/cohorts	Intervention/treatment
Early onset colorectal cancer (training cohort) Colorectal cancer diagnosed before the age of 50	Diagnostic test: ENCODE A panel of microRNA, both cell-free and exosomes, whose expression level is tested from plasma samples from patients with early onset colorectal cancer and non-disease controls. Other names: ENCODE (Early oNset COlorectal cancer DEtection)
Non-disease controls (training cohort) Individuals free from colorectal cancer, younger than 50 years of age	Diagnostic test: ENCODE A panel of microRNA, both cell-free and exosomes, whose expression level is tested from plasma samples from patients with early onset colorectal cancer and non-disease controls. Other names: ENCODE (Early oNset COlorectal cancer DEtection)
Early onset colorectal cancer (validation cohort) Colorectal cancer diagnosed before the age of 50	Diagnostic test: ENCODE A panel of microRNA, both cell-free and exosomes, whose expression level is tested from plasma samples from patients with early onset colorectal cancer and non-disease controls Other names: ENCODE (Early oNset COlorectal cancer DEtection)
Non disease controls (validation cohort) Individuals free from colorectal cancer, younger than 50 years of age	Diagnostic test: ENCODE A panel of microRNA, both cell-free and exosomes, whose expression level is tested from plasma samples from patients with early onset colorectal cancer and non-disease controls Other names: ENCODE (Early oNset COlorectal cancer DEtection)

Primary Outcome Measures

Outcome measure	Measure description	Time frame
Sensitivity	True positive rate: the probability of a positive test result, conditioned on the individual truly being positive	Through study completion, an average of 1 year

Secondary Outcome Measures

Outcome measure	Measure description	Time frame
Specificity	True negative rate: the probability of a negative test result, conditioned on the individual truly being negative	Through study completion, an average of 1 year
Proportion of correct predictions (true positives and true negatives) among the total cases (i.e., accuracy)	A measure of trueness: proportion of correct predictions (both true positives and true negatives) among the total number of cases examined	Through study completion, an average of 1 year

Sponsor: City of Hope Medical Center

Investigators

- Principal investigator: Ajay Goel, PhD, City of Hope Medical Center

Publications

- Bray F, Ferlay J, Soerjomataram I, Siegel RL, Torre LA, Jemal A. Global cancer statistics 2018: GLOBOCAN estimates of incidence and mortality worldwide for 36 cancers in 185 countries. CA Cancer J Clin. 2018;68(6):394–424. https://doi.org/10.3322/caac.21492. Epub 2018 Sep 12. Erratum In: CA Cancer J Clin. 2020;70(4):313. https://doi.org/10.3322/caac.21609.
- Sung H, Ferlay J, Siegel RL, Laversanne M, Soerjomataram I, Jemal A, Bray F. Global Cancer Statistics 2020: GLOBOCAN Estimates of Incidence and Mortality Worldwide for 36 Cancers in 185 Countries. CA Cancer J Clin. 2021;71(3):209–49. https://doi.org/10.3322/caac.21660. Epub 2021 Feb 4.
- Patel SG, Karlitz JJ, Yen T, Lieu CH, Boland CR. The rising tide of early-onset colorectal cancer: a comprehensive review of epidemiology, clinical features, biology, risk factors, prevention, and early detection. Lancet Gastroenterol Hepatol. 2022;7(3):262–74. https://doi.org/10.1016/S2468-1253(21)00426-X. Epub 2022 Jan 26.
- Akimoto N, Ugai T, Zhong R, Hamada T, Fujiyoshi K, Giannakis M, Wu K, Cao Y, Ng K, Ogino S. Rising incidence of early-onset colorectal cancer – a call to action. Nat Rev Clin Oncol. 2021;18(4):230–43. https://doi.org/10.1038/s41571-020-00445-1. Epub 2020 Nov 20.
- Keum N, Giovannucci E. Global burden of colorectal cancer: emerging trends, risk factors and prevention strategies. Nat Rev Gastroenterol Hepatol. 2019;16(12):713–32. https://doi.org/10.1038/s41575-019-0189-8. Epub 2019 Aug 27.
- Cavestro GM, Mannucci A, Balaguer F, Hampel H, Kupfer SS, Repici A, Sartore-Bianchi A, Seppala TT, Valentini V, Boland CR, Brand RE, Buffart TE, Burke CA, Caccialanza R, Cannizzaro R, Cascinu S, Cercek A, Crosbie EJ, Danese S, Dekker E, Daca-Alvarez M, Deni F, Dominguez-Valentin M, Eng C, Goel A, Guillem JG, Houwen BBSL, Kahi C, Kalady MF, Kastrinos F, Kuhn F, Laghi L, Latchford A, Liska D, Lynch P, Malesci A, Mauri G, Meldolesi E, Moller P, Monahan KJ, Moslein G, Murphy CC, Nass K, Ng K, Oliani C, Papaleo E, Patel SG, Puzzono M, Remo A, Ricciardiello L, Ripamonti CI, Siena S, Singh SK, Stadler ZK, Stanich PP, Syngal S, Turi S, Urso ED, Valle L, Vanni VS, Vilar E, Vitellaro M, You YN, Yurgelun MB, Zuppardo RA, Stoffel EM; Associazione Italiana Familiarita Ereditarieta Tumori; Collaborative Group of the Americas on Inherited Gastrointestinal Cancer; European Hereditary Tumour Group, and the International Society for Gastrointestinal Hereditary Tumours. Delphi Initiative for Early-Onset Colorectal Cancer (DIRECt) International Management Guidelines. Clin Gastroenterol Hepatol. 2023;21(3):581–603.e33. https://doi.org/10.1016/j.cgh.2022.12.006. Epub 2022 Dec 20.
- Ullah F, Pillai AB, Omar N, Dima D, Harichand S. Early-Onset Colorectal Cancer: Current Insights. Cancers (Basel). 2023;15(12):3202. https://doi.org/10.3390/cancers15123202.

- Syed H, Sommovilla J, Burke CA, McGee S, Macaron C, Heald B, Lyu R, Schmit SL, Nair K, Kamath S, Krishnamurthi S, Khorana AA, Liska D. Referral, Uptake, and Outcome of Genetic Counseling and Testing in Patients With Early-Onset Colorectal Cancer. J Natl Compr Canc Netw. 2023;21(11):1156–63.e5. https://doi.org/10.6004/jnccn.2023.7057.
- Boardman LA, Vilar E, You YN, Samadder J. AGA Clinical Practice Update on Young Adult-Onset Colorectal Cancer Diagnosis and Management: Expert Review. Clin Gastroenterol Hepatol. 2020;18(11):2415–24. https://doi.org/10.1016/j.cgh.2020.05.058. Epub 2020 Jun 7.
- Rogers CR, Brooks E, Curtin K, De Vera MA, Qeadan F, Rogers TN, Petersen E, Gallagher P, Pesmen C, Johnson W, Henley C, Hickman W, Newcomb E, Korous KM, Handley MA. Protocol for #iBeatCRC: a community-based intervention to increase early-onset colorectal cancer awareness using a sequential explanatory mixed-methods approach. BMJ Open. 2021;11(12):e048959. https://doi.org/10.1136/bmjopen-2021-048959.

Recruiting

Correlation Between Various Urinary Exosomal Protein Biomarkers and Pathological Manifestation in Thyroid Follicular Neoplasm: Early and Pre-operative Diagnosis of Follicular Thyroid Cancer

ClinicalTrials.gov ID NCT05463107

Sponsor: National Taiwan University Hospital

Information provided by National Taiwan University Hospital (responsible party)

Last update posted: 2024-03-19

Study Overview

Brief Summary

Thyroid cancer is the most common endocrine malignancy in the world. Generally, thyroid cancer could be divided into well-differentiated and poorly differentiated. Well-differentiated thyroid cancers usually have two different patterns, including papillary thyroid cancer and follicular thyroid cancer. Thyroid sonography is convenient to obtain repeatedly for the images of nodular goiter. However, cytology and pathology are still the golden rules to make the final diagnosis. Under the basis of sono-guided fine-needle aspiration cytology, diagnosis of papillary thyroid cancer is typically using fine-needle aspiration cytology based on the presentation of typical cytologic features. On the other hand, thyroid follicular lesion cannot be interpretated via cytology because the evidence of capsular invasion or vascular permeation of capsule will not be available in fine-needle aspiration cytology. Surgical intervention with pathological specimens is the only pathway to make the final diagnosis. Interestingly, both patterns of well-differentiated thyroid cancer shared the same follow-up tumor marker, i.e., serum thyroglobulin. Up to date, preoperative diagnosis of follicular thyroid cancer is still one of the unresolved issues in endocrine oncology.

Detailed Description

Thyroid cancer is one of the most popular malignancies in the past several decades all over the world. For poorly-differentiated thyroid cancer, therapeutic strategy of costly target therapy together with immune therapy will be the pivotal one because of its poor prognosis. The average 5-year relative survival rate of anaplastic thyroid cancer is only 3% to 31 % on the stage from distant metastasis to localized disease.

However, it will be very different for well-differentiated thyroid cancer, and the average 5-year relative survival rate of both thyroid papillary or follicular thyroid cancer is more than 98 %. Therefore, the most important treatment strategy for endocrinologists will consider the development of biomarkers for early diagnosis and postoperative follow-up, rather than measuring serum thyroglobulin alone, which is the only biomarker in the current medical guidelines, and there is no choice. Our research team tried to find the newer biomarker together with serum thyroglobulin for postoperative longitudinal follow-up of well-differentiated thyroid cancer in the past 5 years. The investigators used urinary exosomal proteins as target and did find several peptides to be helpful, including our published urinary exosomal thyroglobulin (UExTg). In Taiwan, goiter and thyroid cancer are prevalent diseases. Although papillary thyroid cancer could be diagnosed via reliable sono-guided fine-needle aspiration cytology, follicular thyroid cancer is still an unresolved issue in daily medical practice, especially in cytology. the investigators need to find a practicably earlier biomarker, which should be convenient, non-invasive and repeatable in sample collection. In our previous research and published data, urine will be a reliable source of data.

Exosomes are nano-vesicles, containing DNA, RNA, and proteins, and usually secreted by cells into extracellular spaces. Generally, the vesicles of exosomes are only 40 to 150 nm in diameter. Exosomes may carry and transfer the messages between different tissues. Now, the existing evidences revealed that exosomes may represent certain messages from malignant cells, including diagnosed biomarkers or prognostic predictors. Previously, published data of exosomal studies in thyroid cancer focused on serum microRNA, long coding RNA, and circular RNA, but only few published data on peptides, which were named as liquid biopsy. However, cell-secreted exosomes of malignancy could be collected not only from plasma and body fluid but also from urine, which is the non-invasive pathway but valuable wastes of human body. Our research group had developed experienced technique to collect urinary exosomes via our pilot study in the past several years.

Since the investigators proved the role of urinary exosomal thyroglobulin, UExTg, in postoperative follow-up in well-differentiated thyroid cancer in the past 3 years, from 2018 to 2020, the investigators also found several peptides to be the candidates of prognostic predictors in our preliminary studies, including calprotectin A8/A9, annexin-2, and angiopoietin-1.

Official Title

Correlation Between Various Urinary Exosomal Protein Biomarkers and Pathological Manifestation in Thyroid Follicular Neoplasm: Early and Pre-operative Diagnosis of Follicular Thyroid Cancer
Conditions
Thyroid cancer
Follicular thyroid cancer
Other Study ID Numbers

- 202110076RINB

Study Start (Actual)
2022-08-01
Primary Completion (Estimated)
2025-07-31
Study Completion (Estimated)
2028-07-31
Enrollment (Estimated)
50
Study Type
Observational
Study Contact
Name: Chih-Yuan Wang, Doctor
Phone Number: +886-2-23123456 ext 265371
Email: cyw1965@gmail.com
Study Contact Backup
Name: Pei-Jie Huang, Bachelor
Phone Number: +886-2-23123456 ext 265051
Email: pylaff1920@gmail.com
This study has one location.
Taiwan
Taipei, Taiwan
Recruiting
National Taiwan University Hospital
Contact:
Chih-Yuan Wang
+886 2 23123456 ext 265371 cyw1965@gmail.com
Eligibility Criteria
Description
Inclusion criteria:

- Diagnosed patients with nodular goiter or multinodular goiter, thyroid papillary, and follicular and anaplastic thyroid cancer, preoperation

Exclusion criteria:

- Unclearly diagnosed patients with thyroid papillary, follicular, and anaplastic thyroid cancer

Study Population

Clinical study was designed as having a prospective pattern and enrolled patients with nodular goiter or multinodular goiter, who had received fine-needle aspiration cytology and/or thyroidectomy. Cytology and complete surgical pathology survey will be recorded for cytological and surgical samples. This study will enroll 50 consecutive patients with nodular goiter or multinodular goiter in second and third years.

Ages Eligible for Study

20 to 80 years (adult, older adult)

Sexes Eligible for Study

All

Accepts Healthy Volunteers

No

Sampling Method

Probability sample

Design Details

Observational model: cohort

Time perspective: prospective

Primary Outcome Measures

Outcome measure	Measure description	Time frame
Change of serum thyroglobulin level	Thyroid function test	Within 36 months
Change of serum-free T4 level	Thyroid function test	Within 36 months
Change of serum TSH level	Thyroid function test	Within 36 months
Change of anti-thyroglobulin level	Thyroid function test	Within 36 months
Urinary exosomal thyroglobulin detection	Urinary exosomal biomarker	Within 36 months
Urinary exosomal galectin-3 detection	Urinary exosomal biomarker	Within 36 months
Urinary exosomal calprotectin A9 detection	Urinary exosomal biomarker	Within 36 months
Urinary exosomal transketolase detection	Urinary exosomal biomarker	Within 36 months
Urinary exosomal keratin 19 detection	Urinary exosomal biomarker	Within 36 months
Urinary exosomal angiopoietin-1 detection	Urinary exosomal biomarker	Within 36 months
Urinary exosomal tissue inhibitor of metalloproteinase detection	Urinary exosomal biomarker	Within 36 months
Urinary exosomal keratin 8 detection	Urinary exosomal biomarker	Within 36 months
Urinary exosomal calprotectin A8 detection	Urinary exosomal biomarker	Within 36 months
Urinary exosomal annexin II detection	Urinary exosomal biomarker	Within 36 months
Urinary exosomal afamin detection	Urinary exosomal biomarker	Within 36 months

Secondary Outcome Measures

Outcome measure	Measure description	Time frame
Thyroid fine needle aspiration cytology	Urinary exosomal biomarker	Within 36 months
Ultrasonography of thyroid nodules	Urinary exosomal biomarker	Within 36 months

Sponsor: National Taiwan University Hospital

Investigators

- Principal investigator: Chih-Yuan Wang, Doctor, Department of Internal Medicine, National Taiwan University Hospital

Recruiting

Urinary Exosomal Biomarkers of Thyroglobulin and Galectin-3 for Prognosis and Follow-up in Patients of Thyroid Cancer

ClinicalTrials.gov ID NCT04948437

Sponsor: National Taiwan University Hospital

Information provided by National Taiwan University Hospital (responsible party)

Last update posted: 2024-06-26

Study Overview

Brief Summary

Now, the investigators carried out a prospective study enrolling patients with thyroid cancer, who had received ablative thyroidectomy and/or radioactive iodine therapy for 2 more years. The investigators' study already enrolled 73 patients with thyroid cancer, and the investigators plan to enroll 30 new patients in this consecutive research study. All patients received total thyroidectomy under clinically surgical judgement in initial therapeutic option. The investigators also further found some difference between papillary thyroid cancer and follicular thyroid cancer, and the investigators will continue annually to closely monitor the change of U-Ex Tg and urinary exosomal galectin-3 between differently cellular types of thyroid cancers.

Detailed Description

Although, most thyroid cancers are clinically endocrine tumors of low malignancy, most patients usually receive radioactive iodine-131 treatment and thyroidectomy. Such patients are followed up with thyroid ultrasound and continuous serum thyroglobulin assessment after surgery. Previous studies have shown that one third of well-differentiated thyroid cancers may be transformed into poorly differentiated or even fatal malignant tumors during disease progression, but the efficacy of surgery, chemotherapy, and external radiation therapy is not significant. In other words, effective treatment strategies and tracking models will be very important, including surgical removal of thyroid cancer, radioactive iodine-131 treatment, and tracking of biomarkers in thyroid cancer.

When thyroid cancer cells are poorly differentiated, cell dedifferentiation is a key factor for malignant transformation and invasion. Usually, in papillary thyroid carcinoma and follicular thyroid carcinoma, the cancer cells will gradually dedifferentiate, and undifferentiated thyroid carcinoma is the final result. Therefore, the investigators try to find biomarkers and therapeutic tracking targets based on the expression of exosomal proteins in urine. The basis of this clinical study depends on the previous basic experiments of culturing undifferentiated thyroid cancer cells.

Exosomes are nanosomes that are secreted into the extracellular environment. Cancer cell-derived exosomes can be found in the plasma, saliva, urine, and other body fluids of cancer patients. The investigators will analyze exosomal proteins in urine, including thyroglobulin and galectin-3, and discover early prognostic biomarkers in urine through the prospective observation study. The investigators have published preliminary research papers on 16 patients with thyroid mastoid carcinoma and follicular carcinoma in international scientific journals. During the period of surgery and further radioactive iodine-131 therapy, including before and 1 day, 3 months, and 6 months after surgery, the urinary biomarkers of thyroglobulin and galectin-3 in the urine were analyzed at different stages. A prospective study currently in progress has enrolled 73 patients with thyroid mastoid carcinoma and follicular carcinoma. After thyroidectomy, urine was collected during outpatient follow-up and analyzed for exosome biomarkers in the urine. During the first 2 years of this project, such new urinary biomarkers of thyroid papillary carcinoma and thyroid follicular carcinoma had shown certain different patterns. The investigators' research team expects to enroll 30 new thyroid cancer patients in this consecutive plan. Under continuous follow-up research, in addition to identifying the clinical application of new biomarker as prognostic predictors for future thyroid cancer patients after surgery, the investigators also plan to observe current patients with thyroid follicular cancer. Up to date, follicular thyroid cancer cannot be diagnosed preoperatively via images or aspiration cytology, because pathology after surgery is the only diagnostic golden rule. According to the observations conducted in the current experiment, the urine exosomal thyroglobulin has the opportunity to be a way to diagnose thyroid follicular carcinoma before surgery.

Official Title

Urinary Exosomal Biomarkers of Thyroglobulin and Galectin-3 for Prognosis and Follow-up in Patients of Well-differentiated Thyroid Cancer

Conditions

Thyroid cancer

Papillary thyroid cancer

Follicular thyroid cancer

Other Study ID Numbers

- 202012036RIND

  Study Start (Actual)
  2021-08-19
  Primary Completion (Estimated)
  2024-10-31
  Study Completion (Estimated)
  2026-10-31
  Enrollment (Estimated)
  103
  Study Type
  Observational
  Study Contact
  Name: Chih-Yuan Wang, Doctor
  Phone Number: +886-2-23123456 ext 65371
  Email: cyw1965@gmail.com
  Study Contact Backup
  Name: Pei-Jie Huang, Bachelor
  Phone Number: +886-2-23123456 ext 65051
  Email: pylaff1920@gmail.com
  This study has one location.
  Taiwan
  Taipei, Taiwan
  Recruiting
  Chih-Yuan Wang, MD
  Contact:
  Chih-Yuan Wang, Doctor
  +886-2-23123456 ext 65371
  Eligibility Criteria
  Description
  Inclusion criteria:

- Diagnosed patients with thyroid papillary, follicular, and anaplastic thyroid cancer, post-operation follow-up

  Exclusion criteria:

- Unclearly diagnosed patients with thyroid papillary, follicular and anaplastic thyroid cancer

  Study Population

The investigators carried out a prospective study enrolling patients with thyroid cancer, who had received ablative thyroidectomy and/or radioactive iodine therapy for 2 more years. The study already enrolled seventy-three patients with thyroid cancer, and the investigators plan to enroll 30 new patients in this consecutive research study. All patients received total thyroidectomy under clinically surgical judgement in initial therapeutic option. The investigators also further found some difference between papillary thyroid cancer and follicular thyroid cancer, and we will continue annually to closely monitor the change of U-Ex Tg and urinary exosomal galectin-3 between differently cellular types of thyroid cancers.

Ages Eligible for Study
20 to 80 years (adult, older adult)
Sexes Eligible for Study
All
Accepts Healthy Volunteers
No
Sampling Method
Probability sample
Design Details
Observational model: cohort
Time perspective: prospective

Primary Outcome Measures

Outcome measure	Measure description	Time frame
Change of serum thyroglobulin level	Thyroid function test	Within 36 months
Change of serum-free T4 level	Thyroid function test	Within 36 months
Change of serum TSH level	Thyroid function test	Within 36 months
Change of anti-thyroglobulin level	Thyroid function test	Within 36 months
Urinary exosomal thyroglobulin detection	Urinary exosomal biomarker	Within 36 months
Urinary exosomal galectin-3 detection	Urinary exosomal biomarker	Within 36 months
Urinary exosomal calprotectin A9 detection	Urinary exosomal biomarker	Within 36 months
Urinary exosomal transketolase detection	Urinary exosomal biomarker	Within 36 months
Urinary exosomal keratin 19 detection	Urinary exosomal biomarker	Within 36 months
Urinary exosomal angiopoietin-1 detection	Urinary exosomal biomarker	Within 36 months
Urinary exosomal tissue inhibitor of metalloproteinase detection	Urinary exosomal biomarker	Within 36 months
Urinary exosomal keratin 8 detection	Urinary exosomal biomarker	Within 36 months
Urinary exosomal calprotectin A8 detection	Urinary exosomal biomarker	Within 36 months
Urinary exosomal annexin II detection	Urinary exosomal biomarker	Within 36 months
Urinary exosomal afamin detection	Urinary exosomal biomarker	Within 36 months

Sponsor: National Taiwan University Hospital

Investigators

- Principal investigator: Chih-Yuan Wang, Doctor, Department of Internal Medicine, National Taiwan University Hospital

Recruiting

Early Detection of Advanced Adenomas and Colorectal Cancer (AACRC)

ClinicalTrials.gov ID NCT06342440

Sponsor: City of Hope Medical Center

Information provided by City of Hope Medical Center (responsible party)

Last update posted: 2024-06-07

Study Overview

Brief Summary

This study aims to develop a highly sensitive, specific, and cost-effective blood assay for early detection of colorectal adenomas and cancer, using advanced machine learning and state-of-the-art biological analyses.

Detailed Description

Colorectal cancer (CRC) is a significant global health concern, ranking third in diagnosis and second in mortality. Despite being potentially preventable, it remains a leading cause of cancer-related deaths. Traditional screening methods like fecal immunochemical testing (FIT) have shown benefits in reducing late-stage diagnoses but have not effectively prevented CRC incidence. This is because tests like FIT can effectively detect the cancers, but not the precursor lesions, called adenomas. On the other hand, endoscopy-first approaches offer higher sensitivity for such adenomas and, therefore, lower the risk of developing CRC but face challenges such as invasiveness, cost, and patient compliance.

Non-invasive tests are more appealing to patients than invasive tests and can increase participation rates. Biomarker studies have shown promise, but existing tests lack sensitivity for early-stage CRC and advanced adenomas (AAs). This is likely because they assume the same analyte can detect both CRC and AAs, which may not be accurate due to differences in analyte release and the biological changes that occur during the adenoma-carcinoma sequence.

This study proposes developing an innovative liquid biopsy test tailored for AAs and CRC to address this. An ideal screening test should be minimally invasive, highly sensitive, and cost-effective. This test would optimize patient compliance and resource allocation by detecting both conditions from a single blood draw. More specifically, circulating microRNA (miRNA) analysis shows promise: tests based on cell-free microRNA (cf-miRNA) have demonstrated high sensitivity, while those based on exosome-derived microRNA (exo-miRNA) offer high specificity. Therefore, combining both analytes in a single test could maximize sensitivity and specificity.

This study will develop a non-invasive blood test for AA and CRC in four phases:

1. Genome-wide profiling of cf-miRNA and exo-miRNA and selecting the best candidates for biomarker panels
2. Utilizing machine learning to identify promising candidates and train algorithms for detecting AAs and CRC separately, based on results from quantitative polymerase chain reaction (qPCR) analysis

3. Combining these algorithms to create detection signatures for both conditions
4. Independently validating these signatures using diverse cohorts to ensure broad applicability and compare the effectiveness of the blood assay to standard care through retrospective and prospective studies

This study aims to develop a highly sensitive, specific, and cost-effective liquid biopsy for early detection of AAs and CRC. Success could transform clinical practice by preventing CRC through early detection of premalignant lesions. Innovations include incorporating premalignant lesions into screening and combining cf-miRNA and exo-miRNA biomarkers for accuracy. This approach could reduce CRC mortality and incidence and pave the way for new clinical trials.

Official Title

A Liquid Biopsy Assay for the Non-Invasive Early Detection of Advanced Adenomas and Colorectal Cancer

Conditions

Colorectal cancer

Colorectal neoplasms

Colorectal polyp

Colorectal adenocarcinoma

Intervention/Treatment

- Diagnostic test: DENEB

Other Study ID Numbers

- 23228/AACRC

Study Start (Actual)

2020-03-15

Primary Completion (Estimated)

2025-12-15

Study Completion (Estimated)

2025-12-15

Enrollment (Estimated)

2000

Study Type

Observational

Study Contact

Name: Ajay Goel, PhD

Phone Number: 6262183452

Email: AJGOEL@COH.ORG

This study has six locations.

United States

California locations

Monrovia, California, United States, 91016

Recruiting

City of Hope Medical Center

Contact:
Ajay Goel, PhD
626-218-3452 AJGOEL@COH.ORG
Principal investigator: Ajay Goel, PhD
San Diego, California, United States, 92093
Recruiting
University of California San Diego
Contact:
C Richard Boland, MD, PhD
Sub-investigator: C Richard Boland, MD, PhD
China
Dalian, China
Recruiting
The First Affiliated Hospital of Dalian Medical University
Contact:
Jing Zhang
Sub-investigator: Jing Zhang
Italy
Milan, Italy
Recruiting
IRCCS San Raffaele
Contact:
Giulia Martina Cavestro, MD, PhD
cavestro.giuliamartina@hsr.it
Sub-investigator: Giulia Martina Cavestro
Japan
Mie, Japan
Recruiting
Mie University
Contact:
Yuji Toiyama
Sub-investigator: Yuji Toiyama
Spain
Barcelona, Spain
Recruiting
Barcelona University
Contact:
Francesc Balaguer, MD, PhD
fprunes@clinic.cat
Sub-investigator: Francesco Balaguer
Eligibility Criteria
Description
Inclusion criteria:

- All individuals included in the study need to have had a colonoscopy at the time of blood sampling
- Received standard diagnostic and staging (as necessary) procedures as per local guidelines, and at least one sample was drawn before receiving any curative-intent treatment
- Received standard pathological and endoscopic diagnosis and assessment for cohort assignment

Exclusion criteria:

- Hereditary colorectal cancer syndromes (identified through genetic testing)
- Inflammatory bowel diseases
- Lack of written informed consent

Study Population
Three independent cohorts of individuals who belong to one of the following four

- Negative colonoscopy findings
- Low-risk adenomas (at most)
- Advanced adenomas (at most)
- Colorectal cancer

Ages Eligible for Study
18 Years and older (adult, older adult)
Sexes Eligible for Study
All
Accepts Healthy Volunteers
Yes
Sampling Method
Non-probability sample
Design Details
Observational model: case-control
Time perspective: retrospective
Biospecimen retention: samples without DNA
Biospecimen description: serum

Groups and Interventions

Groups/cohorts	Intervention/treatment
Non-disease controls (discovery cohort) Individuals who underwent colonoscopy and were found not to have any adenomas or cancer	
Low-risk adenoma (discovery cohort) Individuals who underwent colonoscopy and were found to only have low-risk adenomas, defined as all of the following: 1 to 4 adenomas at most All adenomas have low-grade dysplasia at most. All adenomas are <10 mm in diameter.	
Advanced adenoma (discovery cohort) Individuals who underwent colonoscopy and were found to have high-risk adenomas, defined as one or more of the following: 5 or more adenomas One or more adenomas have high-grade dysplasia. One or more adenomas are >10 mm in diameter.	
Colorectal cancer (discovery cohort) Individuals who underwent colonoscopy and were found to have colorectal cancer.	
Non-disease controls (training cohort) Individuals who underwent colonoscopy and were found not to have any adenomas or cancer	Diagnostic test: DENEB A panel of circulating microRNA, whose expression level is tested in cell-free and exosome-derived samples. Other names: DENEB (DEtection of colorectal NEoplasias in blood)
Low-risk adenoma (training cohort) Individuals who underwent colonoscopy and were found to only have low-risk adenomas, defined as follows: 1 to 4 adenomas at most All adenomas have low-grade dysplasia at most. All adenomas are <10 mm in diameter.	Diagnostic test: DENEB A panel of circulating microRNA, whose expression level is tested in cell-free and exosome-derived samples. Other names: DENEB (DEtection of colorectal NEoplasias in blood)
Advanced adenoma (training cohort) Individuals who underwent colonoscopy and were found to have high-risk adenomas, defined as one or more of the following: 5 or more adenomas One or more adenomas have high-grade dysplasia One or more adenomas are >10 mm in diameter.	Diagnostic test: DENEB A panel of circulating microRNA, whose expression level is tested in cell-free and exosome-derived samples. Other names: DENEB (DEtection of colorectal NEoplasias in blood)

(continued)

Groups/cohorts	Intervention/treatment
Colorectal cancer (training cohort) Individuals who underwent colonoscopy and were found to have colorectal cancer	Diagnostic test: DENEB A panel of circulating microRNA, whose expression level is tested in cell-free and exosome-derived samples Other names: DENEB (DEtection of colorectal NEoplasias in blood)
Non-disease controls (validation cohort) Individuals who underwent colonoscopy and were found not to have any adenomas or cancer	Diagnostic test: DENEB A panel of circulating microRNA, whose expression level is tested in cell-free and exosome-derived samples Other names: DENEB (DEtection of colorectal NEoplasias in blood)
Low-risk adenoma (validation cohort) Individuals who underwent colonoscopy and were found to only have low-risk adenomas, defined as follows: 1 to 4 adenomas at most All adenomas have low-grade dysplasia at most. All adenomas are <10 mm in diameter.	Diagnostic test: DENEB A panel of circulating microRNA, whose expression level is tested in cell-free and exosome-derived samples Other names: DENEB (DEtection of colorectal NEoplasias in blood)
Advanced adenoma (validation cohort) Individuals who underwent colonoscopy and were found to have high-risk adenomas, defined as one or more of the following: 5 or more adenomas One or more adenomas have high-grade dysplasia. One or more adenomas are >10 mm in diameter.	Diagnostic Test: DENEB A panel of circulating microRNA, whose expression level is tested in cell-free and exosome-derived samples. Other names: DENEB (DEtection of colorectal NEoplasias in blood)
Colorectal cancer (validation cohort) Individuals who underwent colonoscopy and were found to have colorectal cancer	Diagnostic test: DENEB A panel of circulating microRNA, whose expression level is tested in cell-free and exosome-derived samples Other names: DENEB (DEtection of colorectal NEoplasias in blood)

Primary Outcome Measures

Outcome measure	Measure description	Time frame
Sensitivity	True positive rate: the probability of a positive test result, conditioned on the individual truly being positive	Through study completion, an average of 1 year

Secondary Outcome Measures

Outcome measure	Measure description	Time frame
Specificity	True negative rate: the probability of a negative test result, conditioned on the individual truly being negative	Through study completion, an average of 1 year
Proportion of correct predictions (true positives and true negatives) among the total number of cases (i.e., accuracy)	A measure of trueness: proportion of correct predictions (both true positives and true negatives) among the total number of cases examined	Through study completion, an average of 1 year

Sponsor: City of Hope Medical Center

Investigators

- Principal investigator: Ajay Goel, PhD, City of Hope Medical Center

Publications

- Ahlquist DA, Sargent DJ, Loprinzi CL, Levin TR, Rex DK, Ahnen DJ, Knigge K, Lance MP, Burgart LJ, Hamilton SR, Allison JE, Lawson MJ, Devens ME, Harrington JJ, Hillman SL. Stool DNA and occult blood testing for screen detection of colorectal neoplasia. Ann Intern Med. 2008;149(7):441–50, W81. https://doi.org/10.7326/0003-4819-149-7-200810070-00004.
- Aziz Z, Wagner S, Agyekum A, Pumpalova YS, Prest M, Lim F, Rustgi S, Kastrinos F, Grady WM, Hur C. Cost-Effectiveness of Liquid Biopsy for Colorectal Cancer Screening in Patients Who Are Unscreened. JAMA Netw Open. 2023;6(11):e2343392. https://doi.org/10.1001/jamanetworkopen.2023.43392.
- Barnell EK, Kang Y, Wurtzler EM, Griffith M, Chaudhuri AA, Griffith OL; Geneoscopy Scientists. Noninvasive Detection of High-Risk Adenomas Using Stool-Derived Eukaryotic RNA Sequences as Biomarkers. Gastroenterology. 2019;157(3):884–7.e3. https://doi.org/10.1053/j.gastro.2019.05.058. Epub 2019 May 30. No abstract available.
- Barnell EK, Wurtzler EM, La Rocca J, Fitzgerald T, Petrone J, Hao Y, Kang Y, Holmes FL, Lieberman DA. Multitarget Stool RNA Test for Colorectal Cancer Screening. JAMA. 2023;330(18):1760–8. https://doi.org/10.1001/jama.2023.22231. Erratum In: JAMA. 2024 Mar 12;331(10):888. https://doi.org/10.1001/jama.2024.1637.
- Bettegowda C, Sausen M, Leary RJ, Kinde I, Wang Y, Agrawal N, Bartlett BR, Wang H, Luber B, Alani RM, Antonarakis ES, Azad NS, Bardelli A, Brem H, Cameron JL, Lee CC, Fecher LA, Gallia GL, Gibbs P, Le D, Giuntoli RL, Goggins M, Hogarty MD, Holdhoff M, Hong SM, Jiao Y, Juhl HH, Kim JJ, Siravegna G, Laheru DA, Lauricella C, Lim M, Lipson EJ, Marie SK, Netto GJ, Oliner KS, Olivi A, Olsson L, Riggins GJ, Sartore-Bianchi A, Schmidt K, Shih IM, Oba-Shinjo SM, Siena S, Theodorescu D, Tie J, Harkins TT, Veronese S, Wang TL, Weingart JD, Wolfgang CL, Wood LD, Xing D, Hruban RH, Wu J, Allen PJ, Schmidt CM, Choti MA, Velculescu VE, Kinzler KW, Vogelstein B,

Papadopoulos N, Diaz LA Jr. Detection of circulating tumor DNA in early- and late-stage human malignancies. Sci Transl Med. 2014;6(224):224ra24. https://doi.org/10.1126/scitranslmed.3007094.

- Bosch LJW, de Wit M, Pham TV, Coupe VMH, Hiemstra AC, Piersma SR, Oudgenoeg G, Scheffer GL, Mongera S, Sive Droste JT, Oort FA, van Turenhout ST, Larbi IB, Louwagie J, van Criekinge W, van der Hulst RWM, Mulder CJJ, Carvalho B, Fijneman RJA, Jimenez CR, Meijer GA. Novel Stool-Based Protein Biomarkers for Improved Colorectal Cancer Screening: A Case-Control Study. Ann Intern Med. 2017;167(12):855–66. https://doi.org/10.7326/M17-1068. Epub 2017 Nov 21.
- Brenner H, Heisser T, Cardoso R, Hoffmeister M. Reduction in colorectal cancer incidence by screening endoscopy. Nat Rev Gastroenterol Hepatol. 2024;21(2):125–33. https://doi.org/10.1038/s41575-023-00847-3. Epub 2023 Oct 4.
- Carethers JM. Stool-Based Screening Tests for Colorectal Cancer. JAMA. 2023;329(10):839–40. https://doi.org/10.1001/jama.2023.0547.
- Carethers JM. Improving Noninvasive Colorectal Cancer Screening. N Engl J Med. 2024;390(11):1045–46. https://doi.org/10.1056/NEJMe2400366. No abstract available.
- Chung DC, Gray DM 2nd, Singh H, Issaka RB, Raymond VM, Eagle C, Hu S, Chudova DI, Talasaz A, Greenson JK, Sinicrope FA, Gupta S, Grady WM. A Cell-free DNA Blood-Based Test for Colorectal Cancer Screening. N Engl J Med. 2024;390(11):973–83. https://doi.org/10.1056/NEJMoa2304714.
- Church TR, Wandell M, Lofton-Day C, Mongin SJ, Burger M, Payne SR, Castanos-Velez E, Blumenstein BA, Rosch T, Osborn N, Snover D, Day RW, Ransohoff DF; PRESEPT Clinical Study Steering Committee, Investigators and Study Team. Prospective evaluation of methylated SEPT9 in plasma for detection of asymptomatic colorectal cancer. Gut. 2014;63(2):317–25. https://doi.org/10.1136/gutjnl-2012-304149. Epub 2013 Feb 13.
- de Klaver W, Wisse PHA, van Wifferen F, Bosch LJW, Jimenez CR, van der Hulst RWM, Fijneman RJA, Kuipers EJ, Greuter MJE, Carvalho B, Spaander MCW, Dekker E, Coupe VMH, de Wit M, Meijer GA. Clinical Validation of a Multitarget Fecal Immunochemical Test for Colorectal Cancer Screening : A Diagnostic Test Accuracy Study. Ann Intern Med. 2021;174(9):1224–31. https://doi.org/10.7326/M20-8270. Epub 2021 Jul 20.
- de Klerk CM, Wieten E, Lansdorp-Vogelaar I, Bossuyt PM, Spaander MC, Dekker E. Performance of two faecal immunochemical tests for the detection of advanced neoplasia at different positivity thresholds: a cross-sectional study of the Dutch national colorectal cancer screening programme. Lancet Gastroenterol Hepatol. 2019;4(2):111–8. https://doi.org/10.1016/S2468-1253(18)30319-4. Epub 2018 Nov 27.
- Fu B, Yan P, Zhang S, Lu Y, Pan L, Tang W, Chen S, Chen S, Zhang A, Liu W. Cell-Free Circulating Methylated SEPT9 for Noninvasive Diagnosis and Monitoring of Colorectal Cancer. Dis Markers. 2018;2018:6437104. https://doi.org/10.1155/2018/6437104. eCollection 2018.

- Gagrat ZD, Krockenberger M, Bhattacharya A, Gagrat BZ, Leduc CM, Matter MB, Fourrier KD, Mahoney DW, Edwards V DK, Lidgard GP, Limburg PJ, Johnson SC, Domanico MJ, Kisiel JB. Next-generation Multi-target Stool DNA Panel Accurately Detects Colorectal Cancer and Advanced Precancerous Lesions. Cancer Prev Res (Phila). 2024;17(3):119–26. https://doi.org/10.1158/1940-6207.CAPR-23-0285.
- Grobbee EJ, Wisse PHA, Schreuders EH, van Roon A, van Dam L, Zauber AG, Lansdorp-Vogelaar I, Bramer W, Berhane S, Deeks JJ, Steyerberg EW, van Leerdam ME, Spaander MC, Kuipers EJ. Guaiac-based faecal occult blood tests versus faecal immunochemical tests for colorectal cancer screening in average-risk individuals. Cochrane Database Syst Rev. 2022;6(6):CD009276. https://doi.org/10.1002/14651858.CD009276.pub2.
- Gupta S, Lieberman D, Anderson JC, Burke CA, Dominitz JA, Kaltenbach T, Robertson DJ, Shaukat A, Syngal S, Rex DK. Recommendations for Follow-Up After Colonoscopy and Polypectomy: A Consensus Update by the US Multi-Society Task Force on Colorectal Cancer. Gastrointest Endosc. 2020;91(3):463–85.e5. https://doi.org/10.1016/j.gie.2020.01.014. Epub 2020 Feb 7. No abstract available.
- Imperiale TF, Gruber RN, Stump TE, Emmett TW, Monahan PO. Performance Characteristics of Fecal Immunochemical Tests for Colorectal Cancer and Advanced Adenomatous Polyps: A Systematic Review and Meta-analysis. Ann Intern Med. 2019;170(5):319–29. https://doi.org/10.7326/M18-2390. Epub 2019 Feb 26.
- Imperiale TF, Kisiel JB, Itzkowitz SH, Scheu B, Duimstra EK, Statz S, Berger BM, Limburg PJ. Specificity of the Multi-Target Stool DNA Test for Colorectal Cancer Screening in Average-Risk 45-49 Year-Olds: A Cross-Sectional Study. Cancer Prev Res (Phila). 2021;14(4):489–96. https://doi.org/10.1158/1940-6207.CAPR-20-0294. Epub 2021 Jan 12.
- Imperiale TF, Porter K, Zella J, Gagrat ZD, Olson MC, Statz S, Garces J, Lavin PT, Aguilar H, Brinberg D, Berkelhammer C, Kisiel JB, Limburg PJ; BLUE-C Study Investigators. Next-Generation Multitarget Stool DNA Test for Colorectal Cancer Screening. N Engl J Med. 2024;390(11):984–93. https://doi.org/10.1056/NEJMoa2310336.
- Kim ER, Kwon HN, Nam H, Kim JJ, Park S, Kim YH. Urine-NMR metabolomics for screening of advanced colorectal adenoma and early stage colorectal cancer. Sci Rep. 2019;9(1):4786. https://doi.org/10.1038/s41598-019-41216-y.
- Lo YMD. Cell-free DNA for Colorectal Cancer Screening. N Engl J Med. 2024;390(11):1047–50. https://doi.org/10.1056/NEJMe2311101. No abstract available.
- Luan Y, Zhong G, Li S, Wu W, Liu X, Zhu D, Feng Y, Zhang Y, Duan C, Mao M. A panel of seven protein tumour markers for effective and affordable multi-cancer early detection by artificial intelligence: a large-scale and multicentre case-control study. EClinicalMedicine. 2023;61:102041. https://doi.org/10.1016/j.eclinm.2023.102041. eCollection 2023 Jul.

- Pardini B, Ferrero G, Tarallo S, Gallo G, Francavilla A, Licheri N, Trompetto M, Clerico G, Senore C, Peyre S, Vymetalkova V, Vodickova L, Liska V, Vycital O, Levy M, Macinga P, Hucl T, Budinska E, Vodicka P, Cordero F, Naccarati A. A Fecal MicroRNA Signature by Small RNA Sequencing Accurately Distinguishes Colorectal Cancers: Results From a Multicenter Study. Gastroenterology. 2023;165(3):582–99.e8. https://doi.org/10.1053/j.gastro.2023.05.037. Epub 2023 May 30.
- Wang H, Tso V, Wong C, Sadowski D, Fedorak RN. Development and validation of a highly sensitive urine-based test to identify patients with colonic adenomatous polyps. Clin Transl Gastroenterol. 2014;5(3):e54. https://doi.org/10.1038/ctg.2014.2.
- Wisse PHA, de Klaver W, van Wifferen F, van Maaren-Meijer FG, van Ingen HE, Meiqari L, Huitink I, Bierkens M, Lemmens M, Greuter MJE, van Leerdam ME, Spaander MCW, Dekker E, Coupe VMH, Carvalho B, de Wit M, Meijer GA. The multitarget faecal immunochemical test for improving stool-based colorectal cancer screening programmes: a Dutch population-based, paired-design, intervention study. Lancet Oncol. 2024;25(3):326–37. https://doi.org/10.1016/S1470-2045(23)00651-4. Epub 2024 Feb 9.
- Zhao F, Bai P, Xu J, Li Z, Muhammad S, Li D, Zhang Z, Gao Y, Liu Q. Efficacy of cell-free DNA methylation-based blood test for colorectal cancer screening in high-risk population: a prospective cohort study. Mol Cancer. 2023;22(1):157. https://doi.org/10.1186/s12943-023-01866-z.
- Zhang Z, Liu X, Yang X, Jiang Y, Li A, Cong J, Li Y, Xie Q, Xu C, Liu D. Identification of faecal extracellular vesicles as novel biomarkers for the non-invasive diagnosis and prognosis of colorectal cancer. J Extracell Vesicles. 2023;12(1):e12300. https://doi.org/10.1002/jev2.12300.
- Wender R, Brooks D, Sharpe K, Doroshenk M. The National Colorectal Cancer Roundtable: Past Performance, Current and Future Goals. Gastrointest Endosc Clin N Am. 2020;30(3):499–509. https://doi.org/10.1016/j.giec.2020.02.013. Epub 2020 Apr 16.

Recruiting

ExoLuminate Study for Early Detection of Pancreatic Cancer

ClinicalTrials.gov ID NCT05625529

Sponsor: Biological Dynamics

Information provided by Harmeet Dhani, Biological Dynamics (responsible party)

Last update posted: 2023-11-28

Study Overview

Brief Summary

ExoLuminate is a nationally enrolling registry study designed for earlier detection of cancer in patients at elevated risk or clinically-suspicious for pancreatic ductal adenocarcinoma (PDAC).

Those with elevated risk for PDAC can include individuals with intraductal papillary mucinous neoplasms, family history of pancreatic cancer, germline mutations in genes known to be associated with cancer, and a personal or family history of pancreatitis.

The goal of the study is to compare the performance of ExoVerita™ assay in early detection of PDAC to current standard-of-care methods of surveillance.

Detailed Description

Biological Dynamics, Inc. has developed a non-invasive blood test ("liquid biopsy") that can identify early-stage disease with high sensitivity and specificity. The proprietary ExoVerita™ assay uses alternating current electric (ACE) field to isolate extracellular vesicles (EVs) for differentiated multiomics applications and includes an optimized machine learning algorithm to identify a panel of EV-bound protein biomarkers in patient's plasma in order to detect PDAC at earlier stages.

ExoLuminate is a prospective, multicenter, observational registry study designed to evaluate the non-inferiority of the performance of the ExoVerita™ assay in detecting pancreatic ductal adenocarcinoma (PDAC) in high-risk or clinically suspicious populations in comparison to standard-of-care methods.

The study is planned to recruit a minimum of 1000 U.S. adults over 3 years (with a 2-year follow-up for data collection).

Eligible subjects will be evaluated using the ExoVerita™ assay through blood donation(s) at specified time intervals. Overall, this study poses minimal risk to subject.

Official Title

Exoluminate Study: Observational Registry Study to Assess Exo-PDAC Assay Performance for Detection of Pancreatic Adenocarcinoma (PDAC) in High-Risk or Clinically Suspicious Patients

Conditions

Pancreatic cancer

Exosomes

Extracellular vesicles

Pancreatic neoplasms

Other Study ID Numbers

- BioDyn-011

Study Start (Actual)

2022-12-19

Primary Completion (Estimated)

2026-01-01

Study Completion (Estimated)

2027-01-01

Enrollment (Estimated)

1000

Study Type
Observational (patient registry)
Study Contact
Name: Harmeet Dhani, MD, MSc
Phone Number: 858-202-6150
Email: exoluminate@biologicaldynamics.com
This study has eight locations.
United States
California locations
La Jolla, California, United States, 92093
Recruiting
University of California, San Diego
Contact:
Rebekah White, MD
San Diego, California, United States, 92121
Recruiting
Biological Dynamics
Contact:
Harmeet Dhani, MD
Contact:
858-202-6150
Santa Monica, California, United States, 90404
Recruiting
Saint John's Cancer Institute at Providence Saint John's Health Center
Contact:
Hoon David, PhD
Contact:
310-449-5267
Van Nuys, California, United States, 91405
Recruiting
Dr. Lomis Comprehensive Surgical Center
Contact:
Thomas Lomis, MD
District of Columbia locations
Washington, District of Columbia, United States, 20010
Recruiting
MedStar Health Research Institute
Contact:
Priyanka Kanth, MD
Florida locations
Gainesville, Florida, United States, 32610
Recruiting
University of Florida
Contact:
Steven Hughes, MD

Port Orange, Florida, United States, 32127
Recruiting
Bhanu Visvalingam
Contact:
Bhanu Visvalingam, MD
Contact:
386-304-7070
Massachusetts locations
Boston, Massachusetts, United States, 02136
Recruiting
Dana Farber Cancer Institute
Contact:
Sapna Syngal, MD
Contact:
857-215-1892
Eligibility Criteria
Description
Inclusion criteria:

- ≥18 years old
- Meeting criteria for one of the study cohorts
- Capable of giving informed consent
- Able to provide a blood sample

Exclusion criteria:

- < 18 years old
- Pregnancy
- Active cancer (other than pancreatic cancer) and/or undergoing treatment for an active cancer diagnosis (except for skin malignancies)
- Prior organ transplant or bone marrow transplant
- History of fainting or other adverse effects when blood is drawn
- Any condition that, in the opinion of the investigator, should preclude enrollment

Study Population
Individuals at high risk of pancreatic cancer or with stage I–II pancreatic cancer (or clinical suspicion). See cohorts under Groups and Interventions for details.
Ages Eligible for Study
18 Years and older (adult, older adult)
Sexes Eligible for Study
All
Accepts Healthy Volunteers
No
Sampling Method
Non-probability sample
Design Details
Observational model: cohort

Time perspective: prospective
Target follow-up duration: 3 years
Biospecimen retention: samples without DNA
Biospecimen description: double-spun plasma, EDTA tubes

Groups and Interventions

Groups/cohorts
Cohort 1 Individuals without history of PDAC meeting any of the following criteria: A. 2+ relatives with PDAC on same side of family; 2 are first-degree related to each other and at least 1 is first-degree related to subject; age ≥ 50 years or ≤ 10 years younger than earliest PDAC in family at diagnosis. B. 2+ first-degree relatives with PDAC; age ≥ 50 years or ≤ 10 years younger than earliest PDAC in family at diagnosis. C. BRCA1, BRCA2, PALB2, ATM, MLH1, MSH2, MSH6, PMS2, EPCAM pathogenic or likely pathogenic variant, AND 1 first- or second-degree relative with PDAC; age ≥ 50 years or ≤ 10 years younger than earliest PDAC in family at diagnosis D. Familial atypical moles and malignant melanoma (FAMMM) with pathogenic or likely pathogenic CDKN2A variant; age ≥ 40 years. E. Peutz-Jegher syndrome with STK11 pathogenic or likely pathogenic variant; age ≥35 years. F. Hereditary pancreatitis with PRSS1 pathogenic or likely pathogenic variant and history of pancreatitis; age ≥ 40 years.
Cohort 2 Individuals without history of PDAC meeting any of the following criteria: A. ATM, BRCA1, BRCA2, or PALB2 pathogenic or likely pathogenic variant regardless of family history; age ≥50 years. B. Two or more (2+) relatives with PDAC on the same side of family, any degree of relation, not meeting other criteria above; age ≥50 years or ≤10 years younger than earliest PDAC in family at time of diagnosis C. One (1) first-degree relative with PDAC at age ≤45 years; ≤10 years younger than PDAC diagnosis in family member at time of diagnosis
Cohort 3 A. Individuals meeting criteria for Cohorts 1 or 2 EXCEPT age (i.e., too young to qualify for Cohorts 1 or 2); age ≥ 18 years
Cohort 4 A. Individuals without history of PDAC presenting for evaluation who do not meet any criteria for the other cohorts after collection of full family history and/or germline testing, e.g., they have only 1 relative with PDAC; age ≥ 18 years
Cohort 5—Personal history of PDAC Individuals with a personal history of PDAC meeting any of the following criteria (age ≥ 18 years for all subgroups): A. Family history includes at least one first-degree relative with PDAC, or 2 relatives with PDAC who are first degree related to each other B. Personal or family history of a pathogenic or likely pathogenic germline variant in ATM, BRCA1, BRCA2, CDKN2A, EPCAM, MLH1, MSH2, MSH6, PALB2, PMS2, PRSS1, and STK11 C. Diagnosed with PDAC at ≤ age 45

(continued)

Groups/cohorts
Cohort 6—Pancreatic cysts Individuals with pancreatic cysts (age ≥ 18 years for all subgroups): A. Individuals with a pancreatic cystic neoplasm (IPMN) and/or mucinous cystic neoplasm (MCN) and/or PanIN not meeting any criteria for Cohorts 1–3 or 6 (no personal history of PDAC, no known family history of PDAC, no known pathogenic germline variants linked to PDAC risk present in cohorts 1C, 2A, 1D, 1E, and 1F). B. Individuals with a pancreatic cystic neoplasm (IPMN) and/or MCN and/or PanIN without PDAC and with at least one of the pathogenic or likely pathogenic gene mutations present in cohorts 1C, 2A, 1D, 1E, and 1F and/or a first-degree relative with PDAC
Cohort 7—Acute or chronic pancreatitis Individuals with a personal history of pancreatitis meeting any of the following criteria (age ≥ 18 years for all subgroups): A. Chronic pancreatitis B. At least 2 episodes of acute pancreatitis
Cohort 8—PDAC stages I–II or clinical suspicion Individuals with one of the following conditions and treatment naïve (age ≥ 18 years for all subgroups): A. Biopsy-proven, clinical stage I–II PDAC and candidate for surgical resection B. Clinical findings suspicious for early stage PDAC prior to biopsy

Primary Outcome Measures

Outcome measure	Measure description	Time frame
Clinical performance of ExoVerita™ assay	Specificity	36 months or until diagnostic resolution

Secondary Outcome Measures

Outcome measure	Measure description	Time frame
Clinical performance of ExoVerita™ assay	Sensitivity	36 months or until diagnostic resolution
Stage Shift	Evaluation of stage distribution (SEER) at diagnosis	36 months or until diagnostic resolution

Sponsor: Biological Dynamics

Collaborators

- Medical College of Wisconsin
- Dana-Farber Cancer Institute

Investigators

- Principal investigator: Harmeet Dhani, MD, M.Sc. Biological Dynamics

Publications

- Hinestrosa JP, Kurzrock R, Lewis JM, Schork NJ, Schroeder G, Kamat AM, Lowy AM, Eskander RN, Perrera O, Searson D, Rastegar K, Hughes JR, Ortiz V,

Clark I, Balcer HI, Arakelyan L, Turner R, Billings PR, Adler MJ, Lippman SM, Krishnan R. Early-stage multi-cancer detection using an extracellular vesicle protein-based blood test. Commun Med (Lond). 2022;2:29. https://doi.org/10.1038/s43856-022-00088-6. eCollection 2022.

- Hinestrosa JP, Sears RC, Dhani H, Lewis JM, Schroeder G, Balcer HI, Keith D, Sheppard BC, Kurzrock R, Billings PR. Development of a blood-based extracellular vesicle classifier for detection of early-stage pancreatic ductal adenocarcinoma. Commun Med (Lond). 2023;3(1):146. https://doi.org/10.1038/s43856-023-00351-4.

Recruiting

Interrogation of Exosome-mediated Intercellular Signaling in Patients with Pancreatic Cancer

ClinicalTrials.gov ID NCT02393703

Sponsor: Memorial Sloan Kettering Cancer Center

Information provided by Memorial Sloan Kettering Cancer Center (responsible party)

Last update posted: 2024-11-15

Study Overview

Brief Summary

The purpose of this study is to isolate and analyze exosomes, which are tiny carriers of important proteins and nucleic acids that serve as messenger systems in the blood and tissue. Blood and tissue from patients with pancreatic cancer will be compared with blood and tissue from patients with noncancerous pancreatic disease. Including patients without cancer will allow the investigators to establish "normal" values, which currently do not exist. The investigators will then look to see whether exosome activity has a connection to disease recurrence and outcomes in patients. The results of this study will be the basis for future studies exploring this area.

Official Title

Interrogation of Exosome-mediated Intercellular Signaling in Patients with Pancreatic Cancer

Conditions

Pancreatic cancer

Benign pancreatic disease

Other Study ID Numbers

- 15-015

Study Start (Actual)

2015-03

Primary Completion (Estimated)

2025-03
Study Completion (Estimated)
2025-03
Enrollment (Estimated)
111
Study Type
Observational
Study Contact
Name: William Jarnagin, MD
Phone Number: 212-639-7601
Study Contact Backup
Name: Peter Kingham, MD
Phone Number: 212-639-5260
This study has one location.
United States
New York locations
New York, New York, United States, 10065
Recruiting
Memorial Sloan Kettering Cancer Center
Contact:
William R Jarnagin, MD
212-639-7601
Contact:
Peter Kingham, MD
212-639-5260
Principal investigator: William R Jarnagin, MD
Eligibility Criteria
Description
Inclusion criteria:

- All patients ≥ 18 years of age undergoing pancreaticoduodenectomy, partial or complete pancreatectomy, and duodenal ampullectomy for presumed ductal adenocarcinoma, intraductal papillary mucinous neoplasm (IPMN), or pancreatic neuroendocrine tumors, without an invasive component or other benign pancreatic disease will be eligible.

Exclusion criteria:

- The presence of metastatic disease or disease that precludes resection.
- Receipt of neoadjuvant chemotherapy or radiation for the index cancer within 6 months of being enrolled in the study.
- INR >2.
- Known clotting factor deficiency or hypercoagulable state.
- Any patient with the need or anticipated need for full anti-coagulation during hospitalization for the resection.

- Receipt of antiplatelet agents (other than aspirin) in the preceding week prior to resection.
- IPMN or pancreatic neuroendocrine tumors by radiographic imaging with high suspicion for invasive component. Additionally, if at the discretion of the operating surgeon, blood collection would lead to undue morbidity, the patient will be excluded and replaced.

Study Population
MSKCC clinic
Ages Eligible for Study
18 Years and older (adult, older adult)
Sexes Eligible for Study
All
Accepts Healthy Volunteers
Yes
Sampling Method
Non-probability sample
Design Details
Observational model: cohort
Time perspective: prospective
Biospecimen retention: samples with DNA
Biospecimen description: blood, pancreatic fluid, and pancreas tissue

Primary Outcome Measures

Outcome measure	Measure description	Time frame
Successful isolation of exosomes	Isolation of at least 100,000 microvesicles is needed for exosomes purification for downstream applications such as proteomics and RNA sequencing.	1 year

Secondary Outcome Measures

Outcome measure	Measure description	Time frame
Evaluation of the liver microenvironment	For alterations in cellular infiltrate and ECM using IF and IHC	1 year

Sponsor: Memorial Sloan Kettering Cancer Center

Collaborators

- Weill Medical College of Cornell University
- National Institutes of Health (NIH)
- University of Pittsburgh

Investigators

- Principal investigator: William Jarnagin, MD, Memorial Sloan Kettering Cancer Center

Enrolling By Invitation

Plasma Exosome RNA to Diagnose Prostate Cancer (exo-PRECISE)

ClinicalTrials.gov ID NCT06604130
Sponsor: Xijing Hospital
Information provided by Xijing Hospital (responsible party)
Last update posted: 2024-09-19
Study Overview
Brief Summary
The aim of the present study is to investigate an RNA combination to diagnose prostate cancer.
Official Title
Plasma Exosome RNA Combination for Diagnosing Prostate Cancer: A Prospective, Multicenter Diagnostic Trial
Conditions
Prostate cancer
Intervention/Treatment

- Diagnostic test: prostate cancer screening decision

Other Study ID Numbers

- KY20242271-C-1
- NSFC(China) Study Start (Actual)

2021-03-12
Primary Completion (Estimated)
2025-07-01
Study Completion (Estimated)
2025-07-31
Enrollment (Estimated)
1200
Study Type
Interventional
Phase
Not applicable
This study has one location.
China
Shaanxi locations
Xian, Shaanxi, China, 710032

Xijing Hospital
Eligibility Criteria
Description
Inclusion criteria:

1. Blood prostate-specific antigen PSA $>$ 4ng/dl.
2. Patients suspected of having prostate cancer through clinical symptoms, digital rectal examination, ultrasound examination, magnetic resonance imaging, and PSMA PET/CT examination.
3. The patient is willing to undergo prostate biopsy.

Exclusion criteria:

1. Previous diagnosis of prostate cancer through prostate biopsy.
2. History of other malignant tumors in the past 2 years.
3. According to the research physician's judgment, serious complications may occur and affect the normal conduct of the experiment.

Ages Eligible for Study
18 Years and older (adult, older adult)
Sexes Eligible for Study
Male
Accepts Healthy Volunteers
Yes
Study Plan
Design Details
Primary purpose: diagnostic
Allocation: N/A
Interventional model: sequential assignment
Masking: none (open label)

Arms and Interventions

Participant group/arm	Intervention/treatment
Experimental: the experimental arm receiving diagnosis from serum RNA combination	Diagnostic test: prostate cancer screening decision The subjects would receive serum PSA test.

Primary Outcome Measures

Outcome measure	Measure description	Time frame
The diagnostic efficacy of plasma exo-RNA panel alone in diagnosing PCa	The primary outcome is to investigate a plasma-exosome RNA panel in diagnosing prostate cancer and evaluate its diagnostic efficacy, sensitivity, specificity, positive predictive value (PPV), negative predictive value (NPV), and accuracy in diagnosing PCa. Descriptive statistics were calculated and presented as the frequency (percentage) for categorical variables, the mean (standard deviation) for continuous variables with a normal distribution, and the median (quartile) for continuous variables with a skewed distribution. Two-sample *t* tests were used to assess continuous variables with a normal distribution, and the Wilcoxon signed-rank test was used to assess continuous variables with a skewed distribution. The Mann-Whitney *U* test was used to compare means from two samples. The correlation between two samples was analyzed by Spearman's ρ test. The receiver operating characteristic (ROC) curve was used to determine the cutoff value of exo-RNA panel for diagnosing patients with PCa.	The time of prostate biopsy and after 6 months follow-up

Secondary Outcome Measures

Outcome measure	Measure description	Time frame
Diagnostic efficacy of plasma exo-RNA panel in diagnosing csPCa, insignPCa and its comparison with other imaging methods or blood tests	The secondary outcome is to evaluating the performance of exo-RNA panel in identifying grade group 2 (GG2) or higher clinically significant prostate cancer (csPCa) tumors, clinically insignificant PCa (insignPCa; GG1), and compare the diagnostic performance of the plasma-exosome RNA panel with other imaging methods or blood tests in identifying prostate cancer patients; Whether the exo-RNA panel could predict the PCa patients with higher Gleason score (GS). The comparison between diagnostic performance of exo-RNA panel and other imaging or blood tests is performed in ROC curves. The ICC analysis was performed by reliability analysis. All statistical analyses were conducted using IBM SPSS statistics software, version 23.0 (IBM, Inc., Chicago, IL, USA) and GraphPad Prism software, version 8.0 (GraphPad Software, Inc., La Jolla, CA, USA. All hypothesis tests were two-sided, and $P < 0.05$ was considered to indicate statistical significance.	The time of prostate biopsy and after 6 months follow-up

Sponsor: Xijing Hospital

Not Yet Recruiting

Exosomes Detection for the Prediction of the Efficacy and Adverse Reactions of Anlotinib in Patients with Advanced NSCLC

ClinicalTrials.gov ID NCT05218759

Sponsor: Shanghai Chest Hospital

Information provided by Aiqin Gu, Shanghai Chest Hospital (responsible party)

Last update posted: 2022-02-01

Study Overview

Brief Summary

Exosomes detection for the prediction of the efficacy and adverse reactions of anlotinib in patients with advanced NSCLC

Detailed Description

Explore blood exosomal miRNA as a biomarker for predicting the efficacy or risk of serious adverse reactions in patients with advanced lung adenocarcinoma (or lung squamous cell carcinoma) after anlotinib treatment.

Official Title

Exosomes Detection for the Prediction of the Efficacy and Adverse Reactions of Anlotinib in Patients with Advanced NSCLC

Conditions

Non-small cell lung cancer

Intervention/Treatment

- Drug: anlotinib

Other Study ID Numbers

- KS(Y)21217

Study Start (Estimated)

2022-02-21

Primary Completion (Estimated)

2025-05-31

Study Completion (Estimated)

2025-10-31

Enrollment (Estimated)

30

Study Type

Interventional

Phase

Not applicable

Study Contact

Name: Aiqin Gu, MD

Phone Number: +86-18017321300

Email: Guaiqin11@126.com

No location data

Eligibility Criteria
Description
Inclusion criteria:

1. Patients who have signed informed consent.
2. Male or female, age between 18 and 75 years old.
3. Patients with advanced lung adenocarcinoma who failed standard treatment.
4. Complete prognostic assessment information.
5. Efficacy evaluation: PR/SD/PD.
6. Anlotinib single drug administration.
7. ECOG PS score: 0–1.
8. Patient's expected survival time is greater than 12 weeks.
9. The functions of main organs meets the following criteria: (1) absolute neutrophil count (ANC) ≥1.5 × 10^9/L, (2) white blood cell count (WBC) ≥3.0 × 10^9/L, (3) platelet (PLT) ≥100 × 10^9/L, (4) hemoglobin (Hb) ≥90g/L, (5) creatinine clearance ≥50ml/min or serum creatinine (Cr) ≤1.5× upper limit of normal (ULN), (6)serum total bilirubin (TBIL) ≤1.5× ULN, (7) alanine aminotransferase (ALT) and aspartate aminotransferase (AST) ≤2.5× ULN, (8) left ventricular ejection fraction (LVEF) ≥ the lower limit of the normal (50%), (9) serum Cr ≤1.5 ULN or creatinine clearance (CCr) ≥ 60ml/min, (10) ALT and AST ≤ 5ULN, and (11) activated partial coagulation activity enzyme time (APTT), international normalized ratio (INR), and prothrombin time (PT) ≤1.5× ULN.
10. Women of childbearing age should make sure their pregnancy test is negative within 2 weeks before the study and keep using contraceptive methods during the study and within 24 weeks after the last administration of anlotinib. For men, they must agree to use contraceptive methods during the study period and also 24 weeks after the last administration of anlotinib.

Exclusion criteria:

1. Patients whose plasma is not qualified for the test (hemolysis, precipitation, etc.)
2. Patients who have used anlotinib before
3. Pathological diagnosis results do not meet the requirements for entry
4. Patients who have never used TKIs
5. Patients with hemoptysis, more than 50mL per day
6. Patients with other kinds of malignancies within 5 years
7. Patients who have taken systemic therapy (immunotherapy, cytotoxic therapy, or other targeted therapies) within 6 weeks before grouping
8. Patients who have symptoms of diseases that affect the patient's medication
9. Patients who have suffered non-relieving toxicity from previous treatment
10. Patients who have habitus of hemorrhage, the history of ulcer or fracture, and nonhealing wounds
11. Patients who have suffered arterial/venous thrombosis within 24 weeks
12. Patients who have been diagnosed with mental disorder

13. Patients who have suffered other diseases that may affect the patient's life safety and the results of this experiment

Ages Eligible for Study
18 to 75 years (adult, older adult)
Sexes Eligible for Study
All
Accepts Healthy Volunteers
No
Study Plan
Design Details
Primary purpose: diagnostic
Allocation: randomized
Interventional model: parallel assignment
Masking: none (open label)

Arms and Interventions

Participant group/arm	Intervention/treatment
Experimental: arm A Progressive disease (PD) after anlotinib administration	Drug: anlotinib Anlotinib administration at a dose of 10 mg daily Other names: H20180004
Experimental: arm B Stable disease (SD) after anlotinib administration	Drug: anlotinib Anlotinib administration at a dose of 10 mg daily Other Names: H20180004

Primary Outcome Measures

Outcome measure	Measure description	Time frame
PD	Progressive disease (PD) after anlotinib administration	At the time of 2 months (2 cycles after treatment)
SD	Stable disease (SD) after anlotinib administration	At the time of 2 months (2 cycles after treatment)

Secondary Outcome Measures

Outcome measure	Measure description	Time frame
Severe adverse reaction group	Severe adverse reaction group after anlotinib administration	At the time of 2 months (2 cycles after treatment)
Adverse reaction non-serious group	Adverse reaction non-serious group after anlotinib administration	At the time of 2 months (2 cycles after treatment)

Sponsor: Shanghai Chest Hospital

Collaborators

- 3D Medicines

  Investigators

- Principal investigator: Aiqin Gu, Chief Physician, Shanghai Chest Hospital, Shanghai, China, 200030

  Recruiting

A Prospective Feasibility Study Evaluating Extracellular Vesicles Obtained by Liquid Biopsy for Neoadjuvant Treatment Response Assessment in Rectal Cancer (RECC-EV)

ClinicalTrials.gov ID NCT04852653

Sponsor: University Hospital, Bordeaux

Information provided by University Hospital, Bordeaux (responsible party)

Last update posted: 2024-03-20

Study Overview

Brief Summary

Routine clinical and radiological assessment of response of patients with rectum cancer to neoadjuvant chemoradiotherapy does not allow accurate identification of complete pathological response, and leads to frequent false positive and negative results. Molecular markers reflecting the initial and post-nCRT status of the tumor would be ideal to select patients eligible for organ preservation. This project will test the detection of tumor extracellular vesicles (EVs) in liquid biopsy as a reliable marker for the identification of poor versus good responders to nCRT.

Detailed Description

Neoadjuvant treatment (NT) followed by total mesorectum excision (TME) constitutes the gold standard for locally advanced carcinoma of the low and middle rectum. When good clinical response to NT is obtained, strategies with organ preservation, including close surveillance without immediate surgery or transanal local excision, can spare patients with the highly morbid and functional cost of TME. Current assessment of good responders relies on the downstaging and/or downsizing of the tumor as evaluated by MRI imaging and clinical exam. This strategy is prone to errors in more than 1/3 cases. Better assessment of tumor response to NT would better select patients eligible for organ preservation strategies. This study will use the detection of tumor extracellular vesicles (EVs) in liquid biopsy to identify good response of rectum cancer to neoadjuvant treatment. Tumor EVs will be detected in the blood of the patients at different times of their regular management (before, during, and after NT). Protein content or tumor DNA in EVs will be detected after tumor DNA sequencing in the primary biopsies. Response will be assessed according to tumor EV presence or absence in the blood. As EV quantification is possible, kinetics of their detection will help response assessment and patient follow-up.

Official Title

A Prospective Feasibility Study Evaluating Extracellular Vesicles Obtained by Liquid Biopsy for Neoadjuvant Treatment Response Assessment in Rectal Cancer

Conditions

Rectal cancer

Liquid biopsy

Intervention/Treatment

- Procedure: supplementary blood samples collection during the normal follow-up of the patients

Other Study ID Numbers

- CHUBX 2020/21

Study Start (Actual)

2021-09-21

Primary Completion (Estimated)

2025-03

Study Completion (Estimated)

2025-03

Enrollment (Estimated)

40

Study Type

Observational

Study Contact

Name: Samuel Amintas

Phone Number: +33 (0)5 57 62 32 89

Email: samuel.amintas@chu-bordeaux.fr

Study Contact Backup

Name: Véronique Vendrely

Phone Number: +33 (0)5 57 62 33 13

Email: veronique.vendredly@chu-bordeaux.fr

This study has one location.

France

Bordeaux, France

Recruiting

CHU Bordeaux

Contact:

Samuel Amintas

samuel.amintas@chu-bordeaux.fr

Eligibility Criteria

Description

Inclusion criteria:

- Adenocarcinoma of rectum histologically proven
- Location ≤10 cm from the anal margin

  - Stage T3, T4, or T2 if low rectal cancer
  - With indication of radiochemotherapy alone or chemotherapy followed by chemoradiotherapy prior to total mesorectal surgery or transanal surgery

- No metastasis
- Operable patient
- Patient ≥ 18 years old
- Patient likely to receive radiation therapy and chemotherapy
- No history of pelvic radiotherapy for any reason
- No history of chemotherapy unless it was more than 10 years ago
- Effective contraception for patients of childbearing age: male and non-menopausal women must agree to use two medically validated methods of contraception (one for the patient and the other for the partner) during treatment and less up to 6 months for men and 4 months for women after last treatment
- Patient information and obtaining free, informed, and written consent, signed by the patient and his investigator
- Affiliate subject or beneficiary of a social security scheme of a member country of the European Community (article L1121-11 of the Code of Public Health)

Exclusion criteria:

- Tumor of the upper rectum (>10 cm from the anal margin)
- Metastatic disease
- T1 stage tumor
- History of pelvic radiotherapy and chemotherapy
- Contraindication to chemotherapy and/or radiotherapy
- Insufficient tumoral sample on initial rectal biopsy for performing molecular analysis of tumor by NGS.
- Other concomitant cancer or history of cancer other than treated in situ cervix cancer or basal cell or squamous cell carcinoma
- Pregnant woman, likely to be pregnant, or breastfeeding

  - Symptomatic cardiac and/or coronary insufficiency
  - Severe renal impairment (creatinine clearance less than 30ml/min)
  - Full or partial deficiency in dihydropyrimidine dehydrogenase (DPD) (uracilemia ≥16 ng/ml)
  - Peripheral neuropathy > grade 1
  - Treatment with St. John's Wort
  - Treatment with yellow fever vaccine
  - Treatment with prophylactic phenytoin
  - Treatment with sorivudine or its chemically analogues related, such as brivudine
  - Active infection or other serious underlying disease likely to prevent the patient from receiving treatment
  - Persons deprived of their liberty, or under measure of judicial protection (curatorship or guardianship) or incapable of giving their consent

– Impossibility of submitting to the medical follow-up of the test for geographical, social or psychological reasons

Study Population
Patients with adenocarcinoma of rectum histologically proven
Ages Eligible for Study
18 Years and older (adult, older adult)
Sexes Eligible for Study
All
Accepts Healthy Volunteers
No
Sampling Method
Non-probability sample
Design Details
Observational model: cohort
Time perspective: prospective

Groups and Interventions

Groups/cohorts	Intervention/treatment
Patients with adenocarcinoma of rectum histologically proven	Procedure: supplementary blood samples collection during the normal follow-up of the patients Supplementary blood samples collection during the normal follow-up of the patients

Primary Outcome Measures

Outcome measure	Measure description	Time frame
Positivity of the liquid biopsy	Presence of onco-exosomes and/or exoDNA according to the response to the neoadjuvant treatment by chemotherapy alone or followed by radiochemotherapy of rectal cancer	6 months

Secondary Outcome Measures

Outcome measure	Measure description	Time frame
Prediction of the response of rectal cancer to neoadjuvant treatment	To evaluate whether the kinetics of detection of oncoexosomes and exoDNA is a predictor of the response of rectal cancer to neoadjuvant treatment	6 months
Genetic profile of the primary tumor predictive of the response to nCRT	To evaluate whether the initial mutational profile of the tumor is a predictor of the response of rectal cancer to chemotherapy and radiochemotherapy neoadjuvant treatment	6 months

Sponsor: University Hospital, Bordeaux

Chapter 3
Cardiac Exosome Trials

Recruiting

ExosoMe as Integrative Tool for pRognostic Stratification of Adverse Cardiac remodeLing in stEmi Patients: the MIRACLE Study (MIRACLE)

ClinicalTrials.gov ID NCT06070974

Sponsor: Centro Cardiologico Monzino

Information provided by Centro Cardiologico Monzino (responsible party)

Last update posted: 2023-10-06

Study Overview

Brief Summary

This is a multicenter observational prospective study aimed to assess whether plasma exosomes can help identify, at an early stage, patients at high risk of adverse remodeling after STEMI (ST-elevation myocardial infarction), thus accelerating proper patient management in order to reduce the risk of future cardiovascular events. In order to study the correlation between exosome profile and severity of myocardial infarction, consecutive STEMI patients will be enrolled 3 days after percutaneous coronary intervention (PCI).

Detailed Description

Adverse cardiac remodeling is a process of structural and functional changes associated with worse clinical outcomes and increased mortality, which occurs in response to sustained pathophysiological stimuli, such as ST-elevation myocardial infarction (STEMI). Despite the progresses achieved with reperfusion therapy in STEMI, a significant portion of patients still develops adverse remodeling. Cardiovascular magnetic resonance (CMR) is the gold standard for clinical

J. N. Weiss, *Global Exosome Trials*, https://doi.org/10.1007/978-3-031-96420-6_3

diagnosis of adverse remodeling, as it provides reliable and reproducible information on ventricular size, function, and tissue damage. However, CMR is not always applicable, due to resources and availability reasons and to patients' contraindications. Therefore, additional markers for the early detection of patients at risk for adverse remodeling after STEMI are needed. Exosomes are small extracellular vesicles released by cells and detectable in all body fluids, including plasma. Their release and cargo are influenced by cellular microenvironment, thus mirroring cell/organ status. Previous study demonstrated that concentration and cargo of plasma exosomes released during STEMI well reflect the pathophysiology of the disease, suggesting their potential as biomarkers. Whether exosome profile analysis could predict adverse remodeling after STEMI remains to be investigated.

The relevant hypothesis to be tested is whether plasma exosomes may help to identify, in an early phase, patients at high risk of adverse remodeling after STEMI, accelerating proper patient management in order to reduce risk of further cardiovascular events and improve outcomes. Overall, this new knowledge will pave the way toward a new strategy to predict adverse remodeling in STEMI patients and to develop patient-tailored therapy.

Official Title

ExosoMe as Integrative Tool for pRognostic Stratification of Adverse Cardiac remodeLing in stEmi Patients: the MIRACLE Study

Conditions

STEMI

Intervention/Treatment

- Diagnostic test: CMR and blood collection

Other Study ID Numbers

- CCM 1931

Study Start (Actual)
2023-05-03
Primary Completion (Estimated)
2026-04-30
Study Completion (Estimated)
2026-04-30
Enrollment (Estimated)
100
Study Type
Observational
Study Contact
Name: Andrea Baggiano, MD
Phone Number: 0258002139
Email: andrea.baggiano@cardiologicomonzino.it
Study Contact Backup
Name: Marta Zarà, PhD
Phone Number: 0258002755

Email: marta.zara@cardiologicomonzino.it
This study has two locations.
Italy
Milano, Italy, 20149
Recruiting
Istituto Auxologico Italiano
Contact:
Silvia Castelletti, MD
s.castelletti@auxologico.it
Milan Locations.
Milano, Milan, Italy, 20138
Recruiting
IRCCS Centro Cardiologico Monzino
Contact:
Andrea Baggiano, MD
0258002139 andrea.baggiano@cardiologicomonzino.it
Contact:
Marta Zarà, PhD
0258002755 marta.zara@cardiologicomonzino.it
Eligibility Criteria
Description
Inclusion criteria:

- Chest pain suggestive of myocardial ischemia lasting >30 min
- Electrocardiogram (ECG) showing ST-segment elevation > 0.1 mV in more or equal to 2 limb leads or > 0.2 mV in more or equal to 2 contiguous precordial leads, or presumed new left bundle-branch block
- Successful treatment with pPCI within 12 h from the onset of symptoms

Exclusion criteria:

- Previous myocardial infarction (MI)
- Time to pPCI >12 h
- Atrial fibrillation
- Renal failure with glomerular filtration <30 ml/min
- Claustrophobia
- Other contraindications to CMR

Study Population

Consecutive patients with acute STEMI will be screened for study eligibility by site personnel to identify those who meet all selection criteria

Ages Eligible for Study
18 Years and older (adult, older adult)
Sexes Eligible for Study
All
Sampling Method
Non-probability sample

Design Details
Observational model: cohort
Time perspective: prospective
Biospecimen retention: samples without DNA
Biospecimen description: blood collection for exosome isolation and analysis

Groups and Interventions

Groups/cohorts	Intervention/treatment
Single-arm study STEMI patients, who meet all the inclusion and none of the exclusion criteria, will be enrolled 3 days after PCI to study the correlation between exosome profile and severity of myocardial infarction.	Diagnostic test: CMR and blood collection All patients enrolled will undergo 2 CMR examination (within 3–5 days post PCI and after 6 months), and blood collection on the third day after PCI (T0). Patients recruited at Centro Cardiologico Monzino will be subjected to a blood withdrawal also at different time points: 1, 3, and 6 months after STEMI (T1, T2, and T3, respectively).

Primary Outcome Measures

Outcome measure	Measure description	Time frame
Verify whether the profile of circulating plasma exosomes reflects CMR-assessed STEMI severity at hospital discharge	Assess the ability of exosome profile, detected in the blood sample 3 days after PCI (T0), to reflect STEMI severity as assessed by CMR and evaluate the correlation of T0 exosome profile with clinicopathological features	Within 3–5 days post PCI
Evaluate whether exosome profile in the acute phase of hospitalization after STEMI predicts adverse remodeling at 6 months	Assess the ability of T0 exosomes to predict adverse cardiac remodeling, both alone or in combination with CMR analysis and discover new exosome candidates able to predict adverse cardiac remodeling	6 months
Assess whether changes in exosomes profile a different time points following STEMI (1, 3, and 6 months) reflects clinical outcome	Evaluate the change of exosomes profile during time and test the correlation of exosomes change during time or at specific time points with clinical complication and outcome	6 months

Sponsor: Centro Cardiologico Monzino

Collaborators

- Istituto Auxologico Italiano

Investigators

- Principal investigator: Andrea Baggiano, MD, IRCCS Centro Cardiologico Monzino

Publications

- Pontone G, Carita P, Rabbat MG, Guglielmo M, Baggiano A, Muscogiuri G, Guaricci AI. Role of cardiac magnetic resonance imaging in myocardial infarction. Curr Cardiol Rep. 2017;19(10):101. https://doi.org/10.1007/s11886-017-0907-1.

- Masci PG, Pavon AG, Pontone G, Symons R, Lorenzoni V, Francone M, Zalewski J, Barison A, Guglielmo M, Aquaro GD, Galea N, Muscogiuri G, Muller O, Carbone I, Baggiano A, Iglesias JF, Nessler J, Andreini D, Camici PG, Claus P, de Luca L, Agati L, Janssens S, Schwitter J, Bogaert J. Early or deferred cardiovascular magnetic resonance after ST-segment-elevation myocardial infarction for effective risk stratification. Eur Heart J Cardiovasc Imaging. 2020;21(6):632–639. https://doi.org/10.1093/ehjci/jez179.
- Kalluri R, LeBleu VS. The biology, function, and biomedical applications of exosomes. Science. 2020;367(6478):eaau6977. https://doi.org/10.1126/science.aau6977.
- Zara M, Campodonico J, Cosentino N, Biondi ML, Amadio P, Milanesi G, Assanelli E, Cerri S, Biggiogera M, Sandrini L, Tedesco CC, Veglia F, Trabattoni D, Blandini F, Tremoli E, Marenzi G, Barbieri SS. Plasma exosome profile in ST-Elevation myocardial infarction patients with and without out-of-hospital cardiac arrest. Int J Mol Sci. 2021;22(15):8065. https://doi.org/10.3390/ijms22158065.

Recruiting

Study of Role of Blood Microvesicles and Exosomes in Patients with Graft Occlusion After Aortocoronary Bypass Surgery (MVBYPASS)

ClinicalTrials.gov ID NCT05411445

Sponsor: Maria Cecilia Hospital

Information provided by Maria Cecilia Hospital (responsible party)

Last update posted: 2024-08-28

Study Overview

Brief Summary

Coronary artery bypass graft (CABG) surgery is still the standard treatment of coronary revascularization for patients with severe coronary artery disease (CAD). Graft patency, together with completeness of revascularization, is a major determinant of long-term outcome following CABG. The surgical procedure elicits a persistent systemic inflammatory response associated with the activation of the hemostatic system leading to perturbation of endothelial and vascular function and activation of platelets and leukocytes. All of these events are the main players responsible for the early and late graft failure in a significant percentage of patients.

Detailed Description

Circulating microvesicles (MVs) have received increasing attention during the last years as novel players in cardiovascular disease. MVs are small membrane vesicles involved in cell-to-cell communication acting as biological messengers. MVs of different origin are present in the circulation of healthy subjects, and their number increases in several pathological conditions contributing to the development, progression, and clinical outcome of diseases. They have been proposed as biomarkers of thrombosis, vascular injury, and inflammation in atherothrombosis and myocardial infarction, where elevated levels have been correlated with disease severity. Among the circulating MVs, those expressing phosphatidylserine are defined as procoagulant MVs. A subgroup of procoagulant MVs also express tissue factor (TF), the key activator of the blood coagulation cascade. These procoagulant MVs have a role in the prediction of cardiovascular events and are able to identify patients at high recurrence risk. Thus far, many studies have generated compelling data on the sensitivity of circulating MVs as biomarkers of cardiovascular disease progression and events. The usefulness of MVs in patients undergoing CABG, however, has only been tested in one study that highlighted their importance in surgical hemostasis. No information is so far available on the association between the amount or pattern of circulating MVs and CABG outcome. Thus, we carried out this study to investigate potential functional role of MVs and exosomes in graft occlusion based on their protein profile as well as their procoagulant potential.

Official Title

Study of Role of Blood Microvescicles and Exosomes in Patients with Graft Occlusion After Aortocoronary Bypass Surgery

Conditions

Coronary Artery Bypass Surgery

Other Study ID Numbers

- MCH 2022-01

Study Start (Actual)

2022-06-01

Primary Completion (Estimated)

2025-06-01

Study Completion (Estimated)

2025-09-01

Enrollment (Estimated)

300

Study Type

Observational

Study Contact

Name: Alberto Albertini, MD

Phone Number: +39 0545 217693

Email: aalbertini@gvmnet.it

Study Contact Backup

Name: Elena Tenti

Email: etenti@gvmnet.it

This study has one location.

Italy

Ravenna Locations

Cotignola, Ravenna, Italy, 48033

Recruiting

MCH
Contact:
Alberto Albertini, MD
aalbertini@gvmnet.it
Eligibility Criteria
Description
Inclusion criteria:

- Between the ages of 40 and 80
- Ejection fraction >30%
- Coronary artery bypass surgery
- Informed consent
- Willingness to carry out the follow-up visits and the assessments required by the protocol

Exclusion criteria:

- Emergency intervention
- Changes in liver or kidney function
- Changes in coagulation factors
- Associated interventions (valve replacement, carotid endarterectomy)

Study Population
Patients undergoing elective CABG (coronary artery bypass graft)
Ages Eligible for Study
40 to 80 years (adult, older adult)
Sexes Eligible for Study
All
Accepts Healthy Volunteers
No
Sampling Method
Non-probability sample
Design Details
Observational model: case-only
Time perspective: prospective
What is the Study Measuring?

Primary Outcome Measures

Outcome measure	Measure description	Time frame
Confirmation and validation of the potential role of blood MV and exosomes as predictors of bypass occlusions		From 15 to 21 months

Sponsor: Maria Cecilia Hospital

Recruiting

Exploring of Serum Biomarkers of Delirium After Cardiovascular Surgery

ClinicalTrials.gov ID NCT06007755

Sponsor: Huazhong University of Science and Technology

Information provided by Hua Zheng, Huazhong University of Science and Technology (responsible party)

Last update posted: 2023-10-03

Study Overview

Brief Summary

The incidence of postoperative delirium in patients after cardiovascular surgery is very high, which seriously affects the short-term and long-term prognosis of patients, but its mechanism is not clear. Recent studies have found that lactic acid participates in the process of sepsis by inducing histone lactation in macrophages. Histone H3 lysine 18 lactylation (H3K18la) is significantly associated with the severity of disease and inflammatory response. Inflammation plays an important role in postoperative delirium. We therefore hypothesized that macrophage H3K18la also plays a role in postoperative delirium. At the same time, the latest literature shows that the early markers of Alzheimer's disease (AD), such as Aβ, exosomes, and phosphorylated tau, etc., can also be detected in the serum of AD patients. Given the obvious correlation between Alzheimer's disease and postoperative delirium, we hypothesized that serum biomarkers of AD could also be used as serum biomarkers for postoperative delirium.

The objectives of this study were to investigate the correlation between H3K18 in serum monocytes and postoperative delirium and its severity in patients undergoing cardiovascular surgery. Meanwhile, we also detect the serum levels of biomarkers of AD, such as Aβ, tau, and exosomes etc., in patients undergoing major cardiac surgery. We aim to find the serum biomarkers of delirium after major cardiac surgery, so as to provide a more convenient diagnostic basis for the prevention of postoperative delirium.

Official Title

Exploring of Serum Biomarkers of Delirium After Cardiovascular Surgery

Conditions

Delirium

Other Study ID Numbers

- TJMZK202301

Study Start (Actual)

2023-09-01

Primary Completion (Estimated)

2024-10-01

Study Completion (Estimated)

2025-12-31

Enrollment (Estimated)

113
Study Type
Observational
Study Contact
Name: Hua Zheng, Dr.
Phone Number: 0086-27-83663173
Email: hzheng@hust.edu.cn
This study has one location.
China
Hubei Locations
Wuhan, Hubei, China, 430030
Recruiting
Department of Anesthesiology, Tongji Hospital, Tongji Medical College, Huazhong University of Science and Technology
Contact:
Hua Zheng, Dr
+86 18672750530 hzheng@hust.edu.cn
Eligibility Criteria
Description
Inclusion criteria:

- Patients who receive cardiovascular surgery
- Patients who participated voluntarily and signed informed consent

Exclusion Criteria:

- Past medical history of neurological and psychiatric diseases; severe visual or hearing impairment

Study Population
Patients aged over 18 years undergoing cardiovascular surgery
Ages Eligible for Study
18 Years and older (adult, older adult)
Sexes Eligible for Study
All
Accepts Healthy Volunteers
No
Sampling Method
Probability sample
Design Details
Observational model: cohort
Time perspective: prospective

Groups and Interventions

Groups/cohorts
Delirium is determined by 3D-CAM score
No delirium is determined by 3D-CAM score

Primary Outcome Measures

Outcome measure	Measure description	Time Frame
Incidence of postoperative delirium	The incidence of postoperative delirium was determined according to the 3-Minute Diagnostic Interview for Confusion Assessment Method (3D-CAM) diagnostic algorithm. The algorithm consists of four clinical criteria: (1) acute onset and fluctuating course, (2) inattention, and either (3) disorganized thinking or (4) altered level of consciousness. To define a patient as having delirium, both the first and the second criteria have to be present, as well as either the third or the fourth criteria.	After surgery through to postoperative day 7

Secondary Outcome Measures

Outcome measure	Measure description	Time frame
The level of H3K18 in serum monocytes of postoperative delirium and un-delirium patients	Lactylation levels of all proteins and H3K18 from peripheral blood mononuclear (PBMC) were determined by western blotting and serum levels of inflammatory cytokines by flow cytometry.	Perioperative data
The level of Aβ in serum of postoperative delirium and un-delirium patients	The level of Aβ in serum was determined by colorimetric and surface-enhanced Raman scattering (SERS) dual-mode magnetic immunosensor.	Perioperative data
The level of tau in serum of postoperative delirium and un-delirium patients	The level of tau in serum was determined by colorimetric and surface-enhanced Raman scattering (SERS) dual-mode magnetic immunosensor.	Perioperative data
The level of exosomes in serum of postoperative delirium and un-delirium patients	The level of exosomes in serum was determined by colorimetric and surface-enhanced Raman scattering (SERS) dual-mode magnetic immunosensor.	Perioperative data

Sponsor: Huazhong University of Science and Technology

Chapter 4
Renal Exosome Trials

Recruiting

Effect of Mesenchymal Stem Cells-Derived Exosomes in Decompensated Liver Cirrhosis

ClinicalTrials.gov ID NCT05871463

Sponsor: Research Institute for Gastroenterology and Liver Diseases (RIGLD)

Information provided by Research Institute for Gastroenterology and Liver Diseases (RIGLD) (responsible party)

Last update posted: 2023-05-23

Study Overview

Brief Summary

Decompensated liver cirrhosis (LC), a life-threatening complication of chronic liver disease, is one of the major indications for liver transplantation. Recently, mesenchymal stem cell (MSC) transfusion has been shown to lead to the regression of liver fibrosis in mice and humans. However, little is known about MSC-exosome therapy. We will evaluate the therapeutic potential of mesenchymal stem cell exosomes as an alternative to cell therapy in cirrhotic patients. This study examined the safety and efficacy of umbilical cord-derived MSC-exosomes in patients with decompensated LC.

Detailed Description

Liver fibrosis is the major cause of morbidity and mortality in patients with liver disorders. Liver fibrosis can be reverted with the removal of the underlying etiology. However, if chronic inflammation and injury persist, liver fibrosis is likely to progress to liver cirrhosis (LC). LC is generally characterized by the formation and accumulation of an extracellular matrix, which lead to the progressive distortion of the hepatic architecture. LC usually progresses irreversibly into a decompensated

J. N. Weiss, *Global Exosome Trials*, https://doi.org/10.1007/978-3-031-96420-6_4

stage, which is characterized by a series of clinical manifestations, including ascites, variceal hemorrhage, and hepatic encephalopathy, while ascites is the most common clinical symptom in such patients. Although ascites might be treated with diuretics, periodic paracentesis, or a transjugular intrahepatic portosystemic shunt, liver transplantation is the only option that can improve the survival of these patients. However, the severe shortage of donor livers, high costs, and potential serious complications have restricted the availability of liver transplantation worldwide. Therefore, alternative strategies are under intense investigation. Mesenchymal stem cells (MSC) have self-renewal abilities and multidirectional differentiation potentials. They also interact with various types of immune cells, leading to immunomodulation. MSCs have been used therapeutically in clinical trials for graft-versus-host disease and appear to be effective in immune-mediated tissue injury, transplantation, and autoimmunity. In particular, MSCs have also been used to treat liver diseases in animal models and patients. Studies from animal models have shown that bone marrow-derived MSC (BM-MSC) infusion ameliorates liver fibrosis and reverses fulminant hepatic failure. In clinical trials, autologous MSC infusion has been demonstrated to be safe and feasible and can improve the liver function of some LC patients. In addition, BM-MSC from patients with chronic HBV infection suffer from proliferative deficiency and might not be the best choice. In contrast, human umbilical cord-derived MSC (UC-MSC) are free from these limitations related to autologous BM-MSC. In addition, UC-MSC can be obtained from the discarded UC and, therefore, can be produced on a large scale. It has been reported that human UC-MSC infusion can improve liver fibrosis in rats. It has been shown that UC-MSC have potential to be used in clinical scenarios for the treatment of human liver diseases. In the present study, the investigators examine the safety and efficacy of UC-MSC–derived exosomes in decompensated LC patients. Fifteen enrolled patients will receive standard medication plus MSC-derived exosomes at a final dose of 40 mg in 3 weeks.

Official Title

Clinical Trial Phase IIa, on Amelioration of Decompensated Liver Cirrhosis with Mesenchymal Stem Cells-derived Exosomes

Conditions

Decompensated liver cirrhosis

Intervention/Treatment

- Biological: MSC-derived exosomes

Other Study ID Numbers

- 1208

Study Start (Estimated)

2023-05-26

Primary Completion (Estimated)

2023-08-11

Study Completion (Estimated)

2023-12-11

Enrollment (Estimated)
15
Study Type
Interventional
Phase
Phase 2
Study Contact
Name: Kaveh Baghaei, Ph.D.
Phone Number: +98 21 2243 2516
Email: kavehbaghai@gmail.com
This study has one location.
Islamic Republic of Iran
Tehran, Iran, Islamic Republic of, 1985714711
Recruiting
Research Institute of Gastroenterology & Liver Diseases
Contact:
Kaveh Baghaei, Ph.D.+98 21 2243 2516 kavehbaghai@gmail.com
Principal investigator: Behzad Hatami, MD
Eligibility Criteria
Description
Inclusion criteria

- Able to understand and willing to voluntarily sign an informed consent form (ICF) authorization
- Males or females between 18 and 75 years old with a clinically confirmed diagnosis of liver cirrhosis with any etiology, except viral cirrhosis
- Child score class B or C

Exclusion criteria

- Known cardiovascular disease
- (a) History of hepatocellular carcinoma (HCC). (b) History of malignancy within the past 5 years or ongoing malignancy other than basal cell carcinoma, or resected noninvasive cutaneous squamous carcinoma at the time of screening visit. (c) Active, serious infections that require parenteral antibiotic or antifungal therapy within 30 days prior to screening visit
- Females who are pregnant or breastfeeding
- Current or anticipated treatment with radiation therapy, cytotoxic chemotherapeutic agents, and immunomodulating agents (such as systemic corticosteroids, interleukins, and interferons)
- Use of any experimental medications within the last 6 months of screening visit
- Any other clinically significant disorders or prior therapy that, in the opinion of the investigator, would make the subject unsuitable for the study or unable to comply with the dosing and protocol requirements
- Weight loss of >5% within 6 months prior to screening, based on subject's reporting

- Currently or participated in a weight loss program within the last 6 months
- Any history of bariatric surgery
- Diabetes mellitus Type I
- Daily alcohol intake >20 ml (2 units)/day for women and 30 ml (3 units)/day for men (on average), as per Alcohol Use Disorders Identification Test (AUDIT) questionnaire at Screening and plan to consume the same alcohol amount referenced above during the trial
- Use of any immunosuppressive medication, anti-inflammatory monoclonal antibody treatment, or chronic systemic corticosteroids >10 mg prednisone equivalent concurrently or within 1 year prior to screening
- Uncontrolled or clinically unstable thyroid disease, in the judgment of the principal investigator
- Uncontrolled arterial hypertension
- Any severe, acute, or chronic medical or psychiatric condition that may increase the risk associated with study participation or study drug administration, may interfere with the informed consent process and/or with compliance with the requirements of the study, or may interfere with the interpretation of study results and, in the investigator's opinion, would make the subject inappropriate for entry into this study

Ages Eligible for Study
18 to 75 years (adult, older adult)
Sexes Eligible for Study
All
Accepts Healthy Volunteers
No
Design Details
Primary purpose: treatment
Allocation: Not applicable
Interventional model: single group assignment
Masking: none (open label)

Arms and Interventions

Participant group/arm	Intervention/treatment
Experimental: exosome Standard medication + MSC-derived exosomes at a final dose of 40 mg in three weeks	Biological: MSC-derived exosomes Patients will receive standard medication plus MSC-derived exosomes at a final dose of 40 mg in 3 weeks. Standard medication includes the following: (a) treatment of the underlying cause of cirrhosis such as drug treatment of hepatitis B and C; (b) symptomatic treatment of port complications such as ascites, prevention of variceal bleeding, and treatment and prevention of hepatic encephalopathy.

Primary Outcome Measures

Outcome measure	Measure description	Time frame
Liver function by MELD score	Calculation of MELD score based on patient's laboratory values for serum creatinine, bilirubin, international normalized ratio for prothrombin time, and sodium	Baseline
Liver function by MELD score	Calculation of MELD score based on patient's laboratory values for serum creatinine, bilirubin, international normalized ratio for prothrombin time, and sodium	After 2 months of the trial
Liver function by MELD score	Calculation of MELD score based on patient's laboratory values for serum creatinine, bilirubin, international normalized ratio for prothrombin time, and sodium	After 4 months of the trial
Liver function by CHILD score	Calculation of CHILD score based on patient's laboratory values for serum bilirubin, albumin, international normalized ratio for prothrombin time, ascites, and encephalopathy	Baseline
Liver function by CHILD score	Calculation of CHILD score based on patient's laboratory values for serum bilirubin, albumin, international normalized ratio for prothrombin time, ascites, and encephalopathy	After 2 months of the trial
Liver function by CHILD score	Calculation of CHILD score based on patient's laboratory values for serum bilirubin, albumin, international normalized ratio for prothrombin time, ascites, and encephalopathy	After 4 months of the trial

Secondary Outcome Measures

Outcome measure	Measure description	Time frame
Change in liver enzyme AST	Blood test	Baseline, after 2 and 4 months of the trial
Change in liver enzyme ALT	Blood test	Baseline, after 2 and 4 months of the trial
International normalized ratio (INR) for prothrombin time	Blood test	Baseline, after 2 and 4 months of the trial
Bilirubin	Blood test	Baseline, after 2 and 4 months of the trial

Sponsor: Research Institute for Gastroenterology and Liver Diseases (RIGLD)

Investigators

- Principal investigator: Behzad Hatami, MD, Research Institute for Gastroenterology and Liver Diseases, Shahid Beheshti Medical University, Tehran, Iran

Chapter 5
Diabetes Exosome Trials

Recruiting

Phase 2a Multi-Center Prospective, Randomized Trial to Evaluate the Safety & Efficacy of Topical PEP-TISSEEL for Diabetic Foot Ulcers (DFU)

ClinicalTrials.gov ID NCT06319287

Sponsor: Rion Inc.

Information provided by Rion Inc. (responsible party)

Last update posted: 2024-11-15

Study Overview

Brief Summary

A phase 2a multicenter, prospective, randomized, controlled study to evaluate the safety and efficacy of topically applied PEP-TISSEEL in subjects with diabetic foot ulcers (DFU)

Detailed Description

The objective of this multicenter, prospective, randomized controlled study is to evaluate the safety and efficacy of PEP-TISSEEL+ standard of care (SOC) compared to SOC only treatment in 40 subjects (20 subjects PEP-TISSEEL + SOC and 20 subjects SOC only), specifically for the treatment of their non-healing DFU.

Treatment for the PEP-TISSEEL+SOC arm is as follows:

- PEP-TISSEEL
- Mepitel dressing followed by Tegaderm®
- 3M Cavilon® (may be used on the borders prior to placing the Tegaderm®)
- Padded three-layer secondary outer layer dressing (Profore (Smith and Nephew (Memphis, TN)); and

J. N. Weiss, *Global Exosome Trials*, https://doi.org/10.1007/978-3-031-96420-6_5

- Offloaded with an offloading Controlled Ankle Movement (CAM) Boot (FootDefender (Miami, FL) or total contact Cast (TCC))

Treatment for the standard of care (SOC) only arm is as follows:

- Fibracol
- Mepitel dressing followed by Tegaderm® (or equivalent)
- 3M Cavilon® (may be used on the borders prior to placing the Tegaderm® or equivalent)
- Padded three-layer secondary outer layer dressing (Profore (Smith and Nephew (Memphis, TN)) or equivalent); and
- Offloaded with an offloading CAM Boot (FootDefender (Miami, FL) or TCC)

Enrolled subjects will be randomized in a 1:1 ratio with 20 subjects receiving 2 vials PEP delivered in 10 mL TISSEEL plus SOC and the other 20 subjects receiving SOC only.

Before randomization, subjects must complete a two (2) week run-in period (screening) in which they will be evaluated for inclusion and exclusion criteria and will receive standard of care treatment with required off-loading CAM Boot (FootDefender, Miami FL) or TCC. The investigator will choose and document the appropriate type of off-loading modality based on their clinical judgement and the subject's diabetic foot ulcer off-loading requirements.

Official Title

A Phase 2a Multi-Center, Prospective, Randomized Controlled Study to Evaluate the Safety and Efficacy of Topically Applied PEP-TISSEEL in Subjects with Diabetic Foot Ulcers (DFU)

Conditions

Diabetic foot ulcer

Intervention/Treatment

- Biological: PEP (purified exosome product)/TISSEEL

Other Study ID Numbers

- PRO-00125

Study Start (Actual)

2024-02-27

Primary Completion (Estimated)

2025-04-05

Study Completion (Estimated)

2025-07-12

Enrollment (Estimated)

40

Study Type

Interventional

Phase

Phase 2

Study Contact
Name: Shariq Khan, M.S.
Phone Number: 847-702-4063
Email: khan@riontx.com
Study Contact Backup
Name: Maureen Merrifield, Ph.D.
Phone Number: 281-914-6228
Email: merrifield@riontx.com
This study has one location.
United States
Ohio locations
Blue Ash, Ohio, United States, 45242
Recruiting
Professional Education & Research Institute (PERI)
Contact:
Charles Zelen, M.D.
540-344-3668 cmzelen@mriedu.com
Contact:
Morgan Zelen
203-671-5915 mzelen@periedu.com
Eligibility Criteria
Description
Inclusion criteria:

1. Males and females ≥18 years of age
2. Properly obtained written informed consent
3. Documented history of type I or type II diabetes mellitus, requiring oral and/or insulin replacement therapy
4. The index ulcer is classified as Wagner grade 1 ulcer and remains Wagner 1 Grade between screening and randomization/baseline visit (visit 1 through visit 3)
5. These ulcers are superficial, full-thickness ulcers limited to the dermis, not extending to the subcutaneous tissue
6. Area of index ulcer must be between 1 and 15 cm^2 post debridement at screening and baseline
7. The index ulcer must be located anatomically on the foot with ≥50% of the wound area below the medial or lateral malleolus
8. Presence of a persistent nonhealing DFU for at least 4 weeks from randomization and not more than 1 year that has failed to respond to SOC at any point during this timeframe
9. Adequate vascular perfusion as evidenced by one of the following:
   (a) Dorsal transcutaneous oxygen measurement (TCOM/TcPO2) measurement of ≥40 mmHg within 90 days of screening (visit 1 or 2)
   (b) Ankle Branchial Index (ABI) between 0.7 and 1.3 within 90 days of screening (Visit 1 or 2) using the extremity on which the index ulcer is located

(c) Arterial Doppler ultrasound evaluating for biphasic or triphasic dorsalis pedis and/or posterior tibial vessels at the level of the ankle or a TBI (Toe Brachial Index) of >0.6 is acceptable within 90 days of screening (visit 1 or 2)

10. The index ulcer has been offloaded with protocol defined offloading device during screening (run-in) period through randomization/baseline visit.
11. Must meet one of the following criteria:

    (a) Female subjects of non-childbearing potential defined as: (i) postmenopausal for at least 1 year (subject verbal confirmation acceptable), or surgically sterilized (i.e., hysterectomy or bilateral oophorectomy more than 3 months prior to screening (visit 1 or 2)), or (ii) bilateral tubal ligation more than 6 months prior to Screening (Visit 1 or 2), or (iii) Must have a negative serum β-hCG pregnancy test at visit 1 and not be breastfeeding prior to being administered with the study drug
    (b) Male subjects of non-childbearing potential are defined as those vasectomized subjects whose vasectomy was performed 6 months prior to screening (visit 1 or 2) or those diagnosed as sterile by a physician
    (c) Females and males of childbearing potential who practice an acceptable method of contraception defined as the use of any form of hormonal contraceptive, a barrier method with spermicide, condoms, intrauterine device, or abstinence from sexual intercourse starting at least 60 days prior to screening and continuing at least 30 days following the last treatment

        Females will undergo a negative serum β-hCG pregnancy test at visit 1 and an additional urine test at baseline/randomization (visit 3 or day 0) and must not be breastfeeding prior to being administered with the study drug
12. Ability to comply with the study protocol as per investigator discretion

Exclusion criteria:

1. Actively undergoing chemotherapy treatment (localized radiation treatment is allowed if it is not on the DFU wound site and in remission based on scans, bloodwork or some other kind of test, such as a breast biopsy or a bone marrow biopsy)
2. Ulceration with exposed tendon, capsule, or bone
3. Suspicion of bone or joint infection by clinical or other criteria as per STONEES criteria below:

    (a) STONEES criteria for infection: (i) size increase, (ii) temperature elevation, (iii) os (probe to bone), (iv) new areas of breakdown, (v) exudative, (vi) erythema/edema, (vii) smell

4. Unable or unwilling to utilize the protocol defined offloading device
5. Subjects who have undergone endovascular or open revascularization of the index limb within the last 30 days from screening.
6. Index ulcer has decreased in area by ≥30% between screening (visit 1) and baseline visits

7. Any subject that is currently on/or requires oral, systemic or topical antibiotics, or is anticipated to require their use during the course of the study
8. Any subject that has vascular compromise requiring surgical intervention or has undergone vascular reconstruction or angioplasty less than 1 month prior to randomization. Any planned surgical procedures during the study participation
9. Serum creatinine level > 3.0 mg/dL
10. Hemoglobin A1c (HbA1c) >12%
11. Aspartate aminotransferase (AST, GOT) and/or alanine aminotransferase (ALT, GPT) >3× the upper limit of normal
12. Acute active Charcot foot
13. The location of the index ulcer is within 2 cm of any other ulcer
14. Any subject that would be unable to safely monitor the infection status of the index ulcer at home and return for scheduled visits
15. History of immunosuppression or taking immunosuppressive agents including systemic corticosteroids, except stable daily doses of 5 mg/day or less for chronic conditions for up to 5 days
16. Any subject with a life expectancy ≤6 months
17. Pregnancy, including a positive pregnancy test at baseline, or lactation/breast-feeding at anytime
18. Use of investigational drugs or biologics within 28 days prior to screening (visit 1 or 2)
19. History of a concurrent condition that, in the investigator's opinion, would jeopardize the safety of the subject or compliance with the protocol
20. Known or suspected active abuse of alcohol, or non-prescription drugs
21. Participation in another interventional clinical study or study in the past 30 days of screening (visit 1 or 2) or concurrent participation in another interventional clinical study
22. Subjects who have untreated Hep C
23. Subjects who are HIV positive
24. Subjects on anticoagulation that are not maintained within the International Normalized Ratio (INR) of >3.0

Ages Eligible for Study
18 Years and older (adult, Older adult)
Sexes Eligible for Study
All
Accepts Healthy Volunteers
No
Design Details
Primary purpose: treatment
Allocation: randomized
Interventional model: parallel assignment

Interventional model description: multicenter, open label, randomized controlled clinical trial Evaluating the effect of PEP/TISSEEL in the treatment of diabetic foot ulcers

Masking: none (open label)
Masking description: open label

Arms and Interventions

Participant group/arm	Intervention/treatment
Active comparator: PEP-TISSEEL+SOC Treatment for the PEP-TISSEEL+SOC arm is as follows: PEP-TISSEEL Mepitel dressing followed by Tegaderm® (Mepilex can be used if subjects are allergic to Tegaderm) 3M Cavilon® (may be used on the borders prior to placing the Tegaderm or Mepilex) Padded three-layer secondary outer layer dressing (Profore (Smith and Nephew (Memphis, TN)); and Offloaded with an offloading controlled ankle movement (CAM) boot (Foot Defender (Miami, FL) or total contact cast (TCC)) Use of an alternate offloading device (e.g., Charcot Restraint Orthotic Walker (CROW) boot, custom shoe, etc.) may be approved on a case-by-case basis	Biological: PEP (purified exosome product)/TISSEEL PEP drug product is a lyophilized powder contained within a 10R glass vial. PEP drug product is a lyophilized powder derived from apheresed platelets in plasma. The powder cake weighs approximately 75 mg per vial. This protocol will evaluate 2 vials of PEP drug product delivered in 10 mL TISSEEL fibrin sealant (15 mg/mL PEP-TISSEEL) for 12 weeks. TISSEEL is a fibrin sealant indicated as an adjunct to standard surgical techniques (such as suture and ligature) to prevent leakage from colonic anastomoses following the reversal of temporary colostomies Other names: Extracellular vesicles
Sham comparator: standard of care Fibracol Mepitel dressing followed by Tegaderm (Mepilex can be used if subjects are allergic to Tegaderm) 3M Cavilon (may be used on the borders prior to placing the Tegaderm or Mepilex) Padded three-layer secondary outer layer dressing (Profore (Smith and Nephew (Memphis, TN)) or equivalent); and Offloaded with an offloading CAM Boot (Foot Defender (Miami, FL) or TCC) Use of an alternate offloading device (e.g., Charcot Restraint Orthotic Walker (CROW) boot, custom shoe, etc.) may be approved on a case-by-case basis	Biological: PEP (purified exosome product)/TISSEEL PEP drug product is a lyophilized powder contained within a 10R glass vial. PEP drug product is a lyophilized powder derived from apheresed platelets in plasma. The powder cake weighs approximately 75 mg per vial. This protocol will evaluate 2 vials of PEP drug product delivered in 10 mL TISSEEL fibrin sealant (15 mg/mL PEP-TISSEEL) for 12 weeks. TISSEEL is a fibrin sealant indicated as an adjunct to standard surgical techniques (such as suture and ligature) to prevent leakage from colonic anastomoses following the reversal of temporary colostomies Other names: Extracellular vesicles

Primary Outcome Measures

Outcome measure	Measure description	Time frame
Wound closure	Complete wound closure (wound healing) by 12 weeks (efficacy; landmark analysis)	12 weeks
Safety	Count dose limiting toxicity events (incidence of treatment-emergent adverse event)	6 months

Secondary Outcome Measures

Outcome measure	Measure description	Time frame
Percent area reduction of wound at 12 Weeks	Percentage area reduction (PAR) at 12 weeks	12 weeks

Other Outcome Measures

Outcome measure	Measure description	Time frame
Visual analog scale (VAS) for pain over 12 weeks	VAS pain (mean difference between baseline and 12 weeks) from 0 (no pain) to 10 (worst possible pain)	12 weeks
Semmes-Weinstein Score	Semmes-Weinstein score (mean difference between baseline and 12 weeks)	12 weeks
Wound-Q Scale	Wound-Q (domains: wound characteristics and health-related quality of life; mean difference between baseline and 12 weeks)	12 weeks

Sponsor: Rion Inc.

Collaborators

- Professional Education and Research Institute

Recruiting

Effect of Dietary Protein on the Regulation of Exosome microRNA Expression in Patients with Insulin Resistance

ClinicalTrials.gov ID NCT05318898

Sponsor: Instituto Nacional de Ciencias Medicas y Nutricion Salvador Zubiran

Information provided by Martha Guevara Cruz, Instituto Nacional de Ciencias Medicas y Nutricion Salvador Zubiran (responsible party)

Last update posted: 2023-10-23

Study Overview

Brief Summary

miRNAs are small non-coding RNAs of approximately 22 nucleotides in length, which have the function of regulating gene expression at the post-transcriptional level through base complementation of protein-coding transcripts, and this interaction leads to translational repression by destabilizing the messenger RNA. Evidence demonstrates an association between differences in miRNA expression and the development of various pathologies, including obesity, type 2 diabetes, cardiovascular disease, neurodegenerative disorders, and cancer. Other factors that could also modulate miRNA expression include nutritional status, diet, and even exercise. The aim of this study is to identify exosome microRNAs that modify their expression in plasma from patients with insulin resistance fed different dietary protein sources. A randomized controlled clinical trial will be performed where the selected participants will be assigned by lottery to a dietary intervention of usual diet with protein of plant or animal origin for 4 weeks. The study will consist of 3 visits where anthropometric parameters, body composition, systolic and diastolic blood pressure, dietary compliance through 24-hour recall and food logs, biochemical tests (insulin, glucose, triglycerides, total cholesterol, HDL, LDL), the relative expression of plasma exosome miRNAs, and markers of oxidative stress will be evaluated. Participants will receive a weekly food pantry during the first two visits in order to improve compliance to the dietary intervention.

Detailed Description

The study will evaluate the effect of two dietary interventions on the regulation of plasma exosome microRNA expression in patients with insulin resistance.

Study Program

The study will consist of three visits.

Planned (selection of participants)

1. Participants will be invited through advertisements.
2. Participants will be corroborated to ensure that they meet the criteria for selection.
3. If they are candidates for the protocol, participants will be provided with the letter of consent to read carefully and any doubts that may arise will be resolved. Participants will be informed about the characteristics of the study as well as the expected risks and benefits. If they agree, the participant will be asked to sign the consent form.
4. Anthropometric measurements such as weight, height, blood pressure, and body composition will be determined by means of bioelectrical impedance.
5. A 24-hour reminder of food consumption will be made.
6. A whole blood sample will be taken for glucose and insulin determination, in order to determine the HOMA-Insulin Resistance index.

Once the insulin resistance patients are identified (HOMA- Insulin Resistance $\geq$2.5), the study will begin and participants will be randomized into two intervention groups.

Visit 1 (baseline)

1. A medical and nutritional assessment will be performed.

2. The physical activity questionnaire (IPAQ long version) will be administered and participants will be advised not to change their physical activity.
3. Anthropometric and blood pressure measurements will be taken.
4. Oral glucose tolerance test will be performed for 2 hours after a 12-hour fast to determine the area under the insulin and glucose curve and determination of insulinemic and glycemic indices.
5. A blood sample will be obtained to determine plasma exosome microRNA expression and C-reactive protein as a confounding variable for concurrent infection.
6. The patient will be assigned to an intervention group (vegetable protein vs. animal protein) by block randomization.
7. The participants will continue their usual diet, and the consumption of animal protein or the consumption of vegetable protein will be recommended, according to the assigned group. They will be given and explained a list of foods that provide proteins of animal and vegetable origin, which they could integrate into their usual diet; these lists will indicate which foods to consume and which not to consume, according to the intervention group to which they were assigned.
8. They will be given a logbook to write down their daily food consumption, and they will be taught how to fill it out.
9. An online questionnaire will be explained how to fill out every third day to detect the consumption of recommended and non-recommended foods from the list provided, according to the assigned group.
10. They will be given a pantry with foods rich in protein only (animal protein vs. vegetable protein) according to the assigned group (explained in the section on pantries).

Visit 2 (intermediate)

1. Consumption logs will be collected.
2. The weekly pantry will be delivered.
3. Clarification of doubts.

Visit 3 (final)

1. A medical and nutritional assessment will be performed.
2. The physical activity questionnaire (IPAQ long version) will be completed.
3. Anthropometric and blood pressure measurements will be performed.
4. Oral glucose tolerance test will be performed for 2 hours after a 12-hour fast to determine the area under the insulin and glucose curve and determination of insulinemic and glycemic indices.
5. A blood sample will be obtained to determine plasma exosome microRNA expression and C-reactive protein as a confounding variable for concurrent infection.
6. Body temperature will be determined, and if female, the date of last menstrual period will be questioned as a confounding variable.
7. The food log will be collected.
8. Clarification of doubts and thanks will be given for their participation.

Official Title
Effect of Dietary Protein on the Regulation of Exosome microRNA Expression in Patients
Conditions
Insulin resistance
Intervention/Treatment

- Other: vegetal protein
- Other: animal protein

Other Study ID Numbers

- 3986-22-22-1

Study Start (Actual)
2023-09-15
Primary Completion (Estimated)
2024-07-01
Study Completion (Estimated)
2024-12-01
Enrollment (Estimated)
40
Study Type
Interventional
Phase
Not applicable
Study Contact
Name: Martha Guevara-Cruz, Doctor
Phone Number: 525554870900 ext 2802
Email: marthaguevara8@yahoo.com.mx
Study Contact Backup
Name: Laura M Velazquez-Villegas, Doctor
Phone Number: 525554870900 ext 2802
Email: laura.velazquezv@incmnsz.mx
This study has two locations.
Mexico
Mexico City, Mexico, 14060
Recruiting
Martha Guevara Cruz
Contact:
Martha Guevara Cruz, Dr
5554870900 marthaguevara8@yahoo.com.mx
Mexico City, Mexico, 14080
Recruiting
Instituto Nacional de Ciencias Médicas y Nutrición Salvador Zubirán
Contact:
Martha Guevara-Cruz, Dr

55 5487 0900 ext 2802 marthaguevara8@yahoo.com.mx
Sub-investigator: Karla Guadalupe Hernández-Gómez, M.S.
Eligibility Criteria
Description
Inclusion criteria:

- Adults (men and women) between the ages of 18 and 60.
- Patients with obesity (BMI ≥ 30 and ≤ 50 kg/m^2) and with insulin resistance (HOMA—Insulin Resistance Index ≥2.5).
- Signature of letter of consent.

Exclusion criteria:

- Patients with any type of diabetes.
- Patients with kidney disease diagnosed by a medical or with creatinine >1.3 mg/dL for men and > 1.1 mg/dL for women and/or blood urea nitrogen >20 mg/dL.
- Patients with acquired diseases that produce obesity and diabetes secondarily.
- Patients who have suffered a cardiovascular event.
- Patients with weight loss >3 kg in the last 3 months.
- Patients with any catabolic diseases.
- Gravidity status.
- Positive smoking and alcoholism.
- Treatment with any medication.

Ages Eligible for Study
18 to 60 years (adult)
Sexes Eligible for Study
All
Accepts Healthy Volunteers
No
Study Plan
Design details
Primary purpose: treatment
Allocation: randomized
Interventional model: parallel assignment
Masking: single (outcomes assessor)

Masking description: The person performing the analysis of the study results should be unaware of the assigned intervention so that such knowledge does not influence the results. Therefore, it will be a person outside the study.

Arms and Interventions

Participant group/arm	Intervention/treatment
Experimental: regular diet with vegetable protein Nutritional recommendations will be given to ensure that the patient consumes a regular diet where the protein intake will be mostly from vegetable protein sources.	Other: vegetal protein Nutritional recommendations will be given to ensure that the patient consumes a regular diet where the protein intake will be mostly from vegetal protein sources.
Active Comparator: regular diet with animal protein Nutritional recommendations will be given to ensure that the patient consumes a regular diet where the protein intake will be mostly from animal protein sources.	Other: animal protein Nutritional recommendations will be given to ensure that the patient consumes a regular diet where the protein intake will be mostly from animal protein sources.

Primary Outcome Measures

Outcome measure	Measure description	Time frame
Change in the expression profile of microRNAs from exosomes with real-time quantitative polymerase chain reaction in fold change	Fold change in the expression profile of microRNAs from exosomes after 4 weeks of usual diet with consumption of different protein sources (vegetable vs. animal) with real-time quantitative polymerase chain reaction	4 weeks

Secondary Outcome Measures

Outcome measure	Measure description	Time frame
Change on HOMA index	Change in the HOMA index after 4 weeks of usual diet with consumption of different protein sources (vegetable vs. animal)	4 weeks
Change in body weight in kg	Change in the body weight in kg after 4 weeks of usual diet with consumption of different protein sources (vegetable vs. animal) using a standard calibrated electronic balance	4 weeks
Change in biochemical parameters in mg/dL	Change the biochemical parameters in mg/dL (glucose, total cholesterol, triglycerides, HDL cholesterol, and LDL cholesterol) after 4 weeks of usual diet with consumption of different protein sources (vegetable vs. animal) analyzed by an enzymatic colorimetric method using the Cobas C111 analyzer (Roche Diagnostic, Indianapolis, IN).	4 weeks
Change in body composition in percentage	Change in the body composition in percentage after 4 weeks of usual diet with consumption of different protein sources (vegetable vs. animal) by multifrequency bioimpedance analysis	4 weeks
Change in C-reactive protein in mg/L	Change in C-reactive protein in mg/L after 4 weeks of usual diet with consumption of different protein sources (vegetable vs. animal) analyzed by an enzymatic colorimetric method using the Cobas C111 analyzer (Roche Diagnostic, Indianapolis, IN).	4 weeks

(continued)

Outcome measure	Measure description	Time frame
Amino acid profile in mmol/L	Change in amino acid profile in mmol/L after 4 weeks of usual diet with consumption of different protein sources (vegetable vs. animal) determined by high-performance liquid chromatography	4 weeks
Change in the area under curve of glucose in mg/dL per 2 hours	Change in the area under curve of glucose in mg/dL per 2 hours after 4 weeks of usual diet with consumption of different protein sources (vegetable vs. animal)	4 weeks
Change in the area under curve of insulin in microIU/mL per 2 hours	Change in the area under curve of insulin in microIU/mL per 2 hours after 4 weeks of usual diet with consumption of different protein sources (vegetable vs. animal)	4 weeks
Change in the waist circumference in centimeters	Change in the waist circumference in centimeters after 4 weeks of usual diet with consumption of different protein sources (vegetable vs. animal) using a flexible tape measure.	4 weeks
Change in the blood pressure in mmHg	Change in the blood pressure in mmHg after 4 weeks of usual diet with consumption of different protein sources (vegetable vs. animal)	4 weeks
Change in the Malondialdehyde in micromol/L	Change in the malondialdehyde in micromol/L after 4 weeks of usual diet with consumption of different protein sources (vegetable vs. animal) measured by ELISA	4 weeks

Sponsor: Instituto Nacional de Ciencias Medicas y Nutricion Salvador Zubiran

Investigators

- Principal investigator: Martha Guevara-Cruz, Doctor, Instituto Nacional de Ciencias Médicas y Nutrición Salvador Zubiran

Publications

- Lasser C. Mapping extracellular RNA sheds lights on distinct carriers. Cell. 2019;177(2):228–30. https://doi.org/10.1016/j.cell.2019.03.027.
- Mori MA, Ludwig RG, Garcia-Martin R, Brandao BB, Kahn CR. Extracellular miRNAs: from biomarkers to mediators of physiology and disease. Cell Metab. 2019;30(4):656–73. https://doi.org/10.1016/j.cmet.2019.07.011. Epub 2019 Aug 22.
- Safdar A, Tarnopolsky MA. Exosomes as mediators of the systemic adaptations to endurance exercise. Cold Spring Harb Perspect Med. 2018;8(3):a029827. https://doi.org/10.1101/cshperspect.a029827.
- Huang Y, Yan Y, Xv W, Qian G, Li C, Zou H, Li Y. A new insight into the roles of MiRNAs in metabolic syndrome. Biomed Res Int. 2018;2018:7372636. https://doi.org/10.1155/2018/7372636. eCollection 2018.
- Castano C, Kalko S, Novials A, Parrizas M. Obesity-associated exosomal miRNAs modulate glucose and lipid metabolism in mice. Proc Natl Acad Sci U S A. 2018;115(48):12158–63. https://doi.org/10.1073/pnas.1808855115. Epub 2018 Nov 14.

- Jimenez-Lucena R, Alcala-Diaz JF, Roncero-Ramos I, Lopez-Moreno J, Camargo A, Gomez-Delgado F, Quintana-Navarro GM, Vals-Delgado C, Rodriguez-Cantalejo F, Luque RM, Delgado-Lista J, Ordovas JM, Perez-Martinez P, Rangel-Zuniga OA, Lopez-Miranda J. MiRNAs profile as biomarkers of nutritional therapy for the prevention of type 2 diabetes mellitus: from the CORDIOPREV study. Clin Nutr. 2021;40(3):1028–38. https://doi.org/10.1016/j.clnu.2020.06.035. Epub 2020 Jul 15.
- Min KH, Yang WM, Lee W. Saturated fatty acids-induced miR-424-5p aggravates insulin resistance via targeting insulin receptor in hepatocytes. Biochem Biophys Res Commun. 2018;503(3):1587–93. https://doi.org/10.1016/j.bbrc.2018.07.084. Epub 2018 Jul 20.

Active, Not Recruiting

Expression Analysis of Urinary Exosome in Type 2 Diabetic Nephropathy and Evaluation of Its Clinical Diagnostic Value

ClinicalTrials.gov ID NCT06097351

Sponsor: Yipeng Liu

Information provided by Yipeng Liu, Qianfoshan Hospital (responsible party)

Last update posted: 2023-10-26

Study Overview

Brief Summary

Expression analysis of urinary exosome miR-142-3p in type 2 diabetic nephropathy and evaluation of its clinical diagnostic value

Detailed Description

1. Preliminary screening of miRNAs: Through GEO database and reading related literature, miRNAs differentially expressed in type 2 diabetes and diabetic nephropathy were selected as potential candidate biomarkers for follow-up verification.
2. Collection and treatment of clinical samples: Urine of diabetic patients was collected from the First Affiliated Hospital of Shandong First Medical University in strict accordance with the drainage standard, and the basic information of patients was registered. Meanwhile, the collected samples were divided into type 2 diabetes group and diabetic nephropathy group according to whether the urine was accompanied by UACR≥30/g. Subsequently, the collected samples were centrifuged and retained for supernatant.
3. Isolation and identification of urinary exosomes: Ultrafast centrifugation method was used to separate the treated urine samples of exosomes, and then identified by transmission electron microscopy, nanoparticle analysis, and Western blot, respectively.

4. Real-time PCR was used to detect the changes in urinary exosomal miRNA expression levels of the two groups of patients, and statistical analysis and correlation analysis of clinical indicators of the differentially expressed m-rnas were performed.

Target gene prediction and enrichment pathway analysis of differentially expressed m-rnas were performed to screen out pathways that might be related to the occurrence and development of DKD, and then the relevant pathways were verified by immunofluorescence, immunoprecipitate, Western blot, real-time PCR, and other methods.

Official Title

Expression Analysis of Urinary Exosome miR-142-3p in Type 2 Diabetic Nephropathy and Evaluation of Its Clinical Diagnostic Value

Conditions

Diabetic nephropathy

Intervention/Treatment

- Other: grouping based on previous laboratory results, no intervention

Other Study ID Numbers

- YXLL-KY-2023(106)

Study Start (Actual)

2020-06-01

Primary Completion (Estimated)

2023-12-30

Study Completion (Estimated)

2024-01-31

Enrollment (Estimated)

44

Study Type

Observational

This study has one location.

China

Shandong locations

Jinan, Shandong, China, 250000

Qianfoshan Hospital

Eligibility Criteria

Description

Inclusion criteria:

1. Age ≥ 18 years old
2. Previously diagnosed with type 2 diabetes
3. Typical diabetic symptoms (polydipsia, polydipsia, polyuria and weight loss) plus random blood glucose ≥11.1 mmol/l
4. Fasting blood glucose ≥7.0 mmol/l, fasting is defined as at least 8 hours without intake of calories

5. Oral glucose tolerance test (OGTT) 2-hour blood glucose ≥11.1 mmol/l, using a glucose load equivalent to 75 grams of anhydrous glucose dissolved in water (venous blood was drawn in all patients
6. With or without UACR≥30 mg/g

Exclusion criteria:

(1) Refused to enroll patients; (2) type 1 diabetic nephropathy and other special types of diabetic nephropathy; (3) patients with kidney stones and urinary system infection; (4) patients with autoimmune system diseases, malignant tumors, and blood system diseases; (5) patients with severe chronic cardiopulmonary disease, chronic liver, and kidney disease; (6) patients with severe infectious diseases; (7) use of glucocorticoids, immunosuppressants or cytotoxic drugs.

Study Population

Patients with a clinically confirmed diagnosis of type 2 diabetes during hospitalization in the Department of Nephrology and Endocrinology from December 2020 to June 2022.

Ages Eligible for Study

18 to 90 years (adult, older adult)

Sexes Eligible for Study

All

Accepts Healthy Volunteers

No

Sampling Method

Non-probability sample

Design Details

Observational model: cohort

Time perspective: retrospective

Groups and Interventions

Groups/cohorts	Intervention/treatment
Type 2 diabetes group The group was based on the clinically confirmed diagnosis of type 2 diabetes	Other: grouping based on previous laboratory results, no intervention. The patients were grouped according to the results of previous inpatient tests, and no intervention measures were taken

(continued)

Groups/cohorts	Intervention/treatment
Diabetic nephropathy group The group was based on the clinically confirmed diagnosis of type 2 diabetes. Patients were re-screened strictly according to the following admission criteria: persistent albuminuria and/or decreased eGFR, while other causes of chronic kidney disease (CKD) were excluded. When diabetes mellitus is identified as the cause of kidney damage and other primary and secondary glomerular diseases and systemic diseases are excluded, at least one of the following conditions can be diagnosed as DKD: (1) urinary albumin/creatinine ratio (UACR) $\geq$ 30 mg/g or urinary albumin excretion rate (UAER) $\geq$ 30 mg/24 h. The UACR or UAER was checked again within 3 to 6 months, and 2 out of 3 times reached or exceeded the critical value; eliminate other interfering factors such as infection; (2) eGFR< 60 ml min^{-1} (1.73 m^2) $^{-1}$ for more than 3 months; (3) renal biopsy was consistent with DKD pathological changes	Other: Grouping based on previous laboratory results, no intervention. The patients were grouped according to the results of previous inpatient tests, and no intervention measures were taken.

Primary Outcome Measures

Outcome measure	Measure description	Time Frame
Preliminary screening of miRNA	Through GEO database and reading related literature, m-rnas that are differentially expressed in type 2 diabetes and diabetic nephropathy were selected as potential candidate biomarkers for follow-up verification.	2020–2024
Clinical sample collection and processing	(2) The urine of diabetic patients was collected from the First Affiliated Hospital of Shandong First Medical University in strict accordance with the drainage standard, and the basic information of patients was registered. Meanwhile, the collected samples were divided into type 2 diabetes group and diabetic nephropathy group according to whether the urine was accompanied by UACR≥30/g. Subsequently, the collected samples were centrifuged and retained for supernatant.	2020–2024
Statistical analysis and target gene prediction of misexpressed mirnas and enrichment pathway analysis	Statistical analysis and correlation analysis of clinical indicators of differentially expressed m-rnas were performed to further evaluate their clinical diagnostic value. Subsequently, the target genes of the m-rnas differentially expressed in urinary exosomes of the two groups were analyzed by miRTarBase database and R software package, and the relevant pathways were screened out through KEGG enrichment pathway analysis. Subsequently, the relevant pathways were verified by immunofluorescence, immunocoprecipitation, Western blot, real-time PCR, and other methods.	2020–2024

Sponsor: Yipeng Liu

Investigators

- Study chair: Yipeng Liu, Qianfoshan Hospital

Active, Not Recruiting

Expression Analysis of Urinary Exosome in Type 2 Diabetic Kidney Disease and Evaluation of Its Clinical Diagnostic Value

ClinicalTrials.gov ID NCT06123871

Sponsor: Yipeng Liu

Information provided by Yipeng Liu, Qianfoshan Hospital (responsible party)

Last update posted: 2023-11-13

Study Overview

Brief Summary

Expression analysis of urinary exosome miR-136-5p in type 2 diabetic nephropathy and evaluation of its clinical diagnostic value

Detailed Description

1. Preliminary screening of miRNAs: Through GEO database and reading related literature, miRNAs differentially expressed in type 2 diabetes and diabetic nephropathy were selected as potential candidate biomarkers for follow-up verification.
2. Collection and treatment of clinical samples: Urine of diabetic patients was collected from the First Affiliated Hospital of Shandong First Medical University in strict accordance with the drainage standard, and the basic information of patients was registered. Meanwhile, the collected samples were divided into type 2 diabetes group and diabetic nephropathy group according to whether the urine was accompanied by UACR≥300/g. Subsequently, the collected samples were centrifuged and retained for supernatant.
3. Isolation and identification of urinary exosomes: Ultrafast centrifugation method was used to separate the treated urine samples of exosomes, and then identified by transmission electron microscopy, nanoparticle analysis, and Western blot, respectively.
4. Real-time PCR was used to detect the changes in urinary exosomal miRNA expression levels of the two groups of patients, and statistical analysis and correlation analysis of clinical indicators of the differentially expressed m-rnas were performed.
5. Target gene prediction and enrichment pathway analysis of differentially expressed m-rnas were performed to screen out pathways that might be related to the occurrence and development of DKD, and then, the relevant pathways were verified by immunofluorescence, immunoprecipitate, Western blot, real-time PCR, and other methods.

Official Title

Expression Analysis of Urinary Exosome miR-136-5p in Type 2 Diabetic Nephropathy and Evaluation of Its Clinical Diagnostic Value

Conditions
Diabetic nephropathy
Intervention/Treatment

- Other: grouping based on previous laboratory results, no intervention

Other Study ID Numbers

- YXLL-KY-2023(127)

Study Start (Actual)
2020-06-01
Primary Completion (Estimated)
2023-12-30
Study Completion (Estimated)
2024-01-31
Enrollment (Estimated)
30
Study Type
Observational
This study has one location.
China
Shandong locations
Jinan, Shandong, China, 250000
Qianfoshan Hospital
Eligibility Criteria
Description
Inclusion criteria:

1. Age ≥ 18 years old
2. Previously diagnosed with type 2 diabetes
3. Typical diabetic symptoms (polydipsia, polydipsia, polyuria and weight loss) plus random blood glucose ≥11.1 mmol/l
4. Fasting blood glucose ≥7.0 mmol/l, fasting is defined as at least 8 hours without intake of calories
5. Oral glucose tolerance test (OGTT) 2-hour blood glucose ≥11.1 mmol/l, using a glucose load equivalent to 75 grams of anhydrous glucose dissolved in water (venous blood was drawn in all patients
6. With or without UACR≥300 mg/g

Exclusion criteria:

1. Refused to enroll patients
2. Type 1 diabetic nephropathy and other special types of diabetic nephropathy
3. Patients with kidney stones and urinary system infection
4. Patients with autoimmune system diseases, malignant tumors, and blood system diseases

5. Patients with severe chronic cardiopulmonary disease, chronic liver, and kidney disease
6. Patients with severe infectious diseases
7. Use of glucocorticoids, immunosuppressants, or cytotoxic drugs

Study Population

Patients with a clinically confirmed diagnosis of type 2 diabetes during hospitalization in the Department of nephrology and Endocrinology from December 2020 to June 2022.

Ages Eligible for Study

18 to 90 years (adult, older adult)

Sexes Eligible for Study

All

Accepts Healthy Volunteers

No

Sampling Method

Non-probability sample

Design Details

Observational model: cohort

Time perspective: retrospective

Groups and Interventions

Groups/cohorts	Intervention/treatment
Type 2 diabetes group The group was based on the clinically confirmed diagnosis of type 2 diabetes	Other: grouping based on previous laboratory results, no intervention The patients were grouped according to the results of previous inpatient tests, and no intervention measures were taken.
Diabetic nephropathy group The group was based on the clinically confirmed diagnosis of type 2 diabetes. The group was based on the clinically confirmed diagnosis of type 2 diabetes. Patients were re-screened strictly according to the following admission criteria: persistent albuminuria and/or decreased eGFR, while other causes of chronic kidney disease (CKD) were excluded. When diabetes mellitus is identified as the cause of kidney damage and other primary and secondary glomerular diseases and systemic diseases are excluded, at least one of the following conditions can be diagnosed as DKD: (1) urinary albumin/creatinine ratio(UACR) $\geq$ 30 mg/g or urinary albumin excretion rate (UAER) $\geq$ 30 mg/24 h. The UACR or UAER was checked again within 3 to 6 months, and 2 out of 3 times reached or exceeded the critical value; eliminate other interfering factors such as infection; (2) eGFR< 60 ml min^{-1} $(1.73\ m^2)^{-1}$ for more than 3 months; (3) renal biopsy was consistent with DKD pathological changes.	Other: Grouping based on previous laboratory results, no intervention The patients were grouped according to the results of previous inpatient tests, and no intervention measures were taken.

Primary Outcome Measures

Outcome measure	Measure description	Time frame
Preliminary screening of miRNA	Through GEO database and reading related literature, m-rnas that are differentially expressed in type 2 diabetes and diabetic nephropathy were selected as potential candidate biomarkers for follow-up verification.	2020–2024
Clinical sample collection and processing	The urine of diabetic patients was collected from the First Affiliated Hospital of Shandong First Medical University in strict accordance with the drainage standard, and the basic information of patients was registered. Meanwhile, the collected samples were divided into type 2 diabetes group and diabetic nephropathy group according to whether the urine was accompanied by UACR≥300/g. Subsequently, the collected samples were centrifuged and retained for supernatant.	2020–2024
Statistical analysis and target gene prediction of misexpressed m-rnas and enrichment pathway analysis	Statistical analysis and correlation analysis of clinical indicators of differentially expressed m-rnas were performed to further evaluate their clinical diagnostic value. Subsequently, the target genes of the m-rnas differentially expressed in urinary exosomes of the two groups were analyzed by miRTarBase database and R software package, and the relevant pathways were screened out through KEGG enrichment pathway analysis. Subsequently, the relevant pathways were verified by immunofluorescence, immunoprecipitation, Western blot, real-time PCR, and other methods.	2020–2024

Sponsor: Yipeng Liu

Investigators

- Study chair: Yipeng Liu, Qianfoshan Hospital

Recruiting

Small Extracellular Vesicles and Insulin Action (SEV)

ClinicalTrials.gov ID NCT05933707

Sponsor: Washington University School of Medicine

Information provided by Washington University School of Medicine (responsible party)

Last update posted 2024-07-17

Study Overview

Brief Summary

The goals of this research study are to (1) understand why some people with obesity are protected from developing conditions such as type 2 diabetes and cardiovascular disease while others are more likely to develop obesity-related conditions and (2) assess the effect of small extracellular vesicles (sEVs also called exosomes), obtained from human participants, on metabolic function in cultured cells and in mice.

Detailed Description

Insulin resistance is commonly associated with obesity and is a major contributor to the development of obesity-related metabolic diseases, including nonalcoholic fatty liver disease, metabolic syndrome, and type 2 diabetes (T2D). Most persons with obesity are "metabolically unhealthy" (MUO), often defined by having insulin resistance and the metabolic syndrome. However, a subset of people with obesity are metabolically healthy (MHO) and protected from the adverse metabolic effects of excess adiposity. The mechanisms that determine the differences in metabolic health between people with MUO and MHO are not unclear. This project will examine the effects of plasma and adipose tissue small extracellular vesicles (sEVs) on multi-organ insulin action. The investigators will isolate sEVs from subcutaneous abdominal adipose tissue biopsies and blood samples obtained from human participants with MHO, with MUO, or who are metabolically healthy and lean (MHL) and examine the effects of these sEVs on insulin resistance in muscle, liver, and fat cells in culture and on multi-organ insulin sensitivity in lean and obese mice. The investigators will also identify differences in the potential bioactive molecules, namely miRNA and bioactive lipids, that are carried by sEVs. The results from this study will help determine whether plasma or adipose tissue sEVs in people who are MHL, MHO, or MUO are involved in regulating liver, muscle, and adipose tissue insulin sensitivity. These results could identify novel pathways that regulate metabolic health in people and provide the foundation for exploring the potential of sEVs as a therapeutic target to prevent and treat the metabolic complications of obesity.

Official Title

Effect of Small Extracellular Vesicles from Adipose Tissue on Insulin Action

Conditions

Obesity

Insulin resistance

Metabolically healthy obesity

Obesity

Metabolically benign

Intervention/Treatment

- Behavioral: people with metabolically unhealthy obesity—low calorie diet

Other Study ID Numbers

- 202005117

Study Start (Actual)

2023-06-08

Primary Completion (Estimated)

2028-10

Study Completion (Estimated)

2028-12

Enrollment (Estimated)

72
Study Type
Interventional
Phase
Not applicable
Study Contact
Name: Johanna Sonnenschein
Phone Number: 3142731879
Email: nutritionresearch@wustl.edu
Study Contact Backup
Name: Beth Henk
Phone Number: 3143628250
Email: bhenk@wustl.edu
This study has one location.
United States
Missouri locations
Saint Louis, Missouri, United States, 63110
Recruiting
Washington University School of Medicine
Contact:
Johanna Sonnenschein
314-273-1879 nutritionresearch@wustl.edu
Contact:
Beth Henk
3143628250 bhenk@wustl.edu
Principal investigator: Dmitri Samovski, PhD
Eligibility Criteria
Description
Inclusion criteria:

- Metabolically healthy lean subjects must have a BMI ≥18.5 and ≤ 24.9 kg/m^2; subjects with obesity must have a BMI ≥30.0 and ≤ 50.0 kg/m^2
- Metabolically healthy lean and people with metabolically healthy obesity must have intrahepatic triglyceride (IHTG) content ≤5%; fasting plasma glucose concentration < 100 mg/dl, 2-hour oral glucose tolerance plasma glucose concentration < 140 mg/dl, hemoglobin A 1C (HbA1c) ≤5.6%, and HOMA-IR <2.5.
- People with metabolically unhealthy obesity must have intrahepatic triglyceride (IHTG) content ≥5.6%; HOMA-IR ≥2.5, and HbA1c 5.7–6.4%, or fasting plasma glucose concentration ≥ 100 mg/dl, or 2-hour oral glucose tolerance test (OGTT) plasma glucose concentration ≥ 140 mg/dl.

Exclusion criteria:

- History of diabetes, liver disease other than NAFLD, or other serious diseases
- Consume excessive amounts of alcohol (>21 units/week for men and > 14 units/week for women)

- Take medications that could affect the study outcome measures, engage in regular exercise (>120 min/week)
- Are pregnant or lactating

Ages Eligible for Study
25 to 55 years (adult)
Sexes Eligible for Study
All
Accepts Healthy Volunteers
Yes
Design Details
Primary purpose: basic science
Allocation: non-randomized
Interventional model: parallel assignment
Masking: none (open label)

Arms and Interventions

Participant group/arm	Intervention/treatment
No intervention: metabolically healthy lean—baseline testing only Metabolically healthy lean—lean individuals that have good glucose (sugar) control (defined as normal fasting glucose, glucose tolerance and hemoglobin A1c), normal insulin sensitivity (defined as homeostatic model assessment of insulin resistance (HOMA-IR) <2.5) and normal intrahepatic triglyceride (fat) levels. Dietary intervention—none	
No intervention: people with metabolically healthy obesity—baseline testing only People with metabolically healthy obesity—persons with obesity that have good glucose (sugar) control, normal insulin sensitivity, and normal intrahepatic triglyceride (fat) levels. Dietary intervention—none.	
Experimental: people with metabolically unhealthy obesity—low calorie diet People with metabolically unhealthy obesity—persons with obesity with plasma glucose and intrahepatic triglyceride (fat) levels higher than recommended in combination with insulin resistance (defined as HOMA-IR ≥2.5). Dietary intervention—low calorie diet	Behavioral: people with metabolically unhealthy obesity—low calorie diet Consumption of a low-calorie diet with caloric intake reduced by ~25% to achieve ~10% weight loss in about 4 to 5 months. Other names: Dietary weight loss

Primary Outcome Measures

Outcome measure	Measure description	Time frame
Effect of exosomes on insulin sensitivity in cultured cells	Exosomes obtained from the plasma and adipose tissue of metabolically healthy lean participants, and participants with metabolically healthy or metabolically unhealthy obesity will be tested in cultured cells and mice to determine their effect on insulin sensitivity.	Baseline only (cross-sectional comparison of metabolically healthy lean, and of people with metabolically healthy or metabolically unhealthy obesity).
Change in the effect of exosomes on insulin sensitivity	Exosomes obtained from the plasma and adipose tissue of participants with metabolically unhealthy obesity before and after 10% weight loss will be tested in cultured cells and mice to determine their effect on insulin sensitivity.	Before and after ~10% weight loss (~4–5 months) in people with metabolically abnormal obesity

Secondary Outcome Measures

Outcome measure	Measure description	Time frame
Differences in the content of microRNAs within exosomes obtained from plasma and adipose tissue	Exosomes obtained from the plasma and adipose tissue of metabolically healthy lean participants, and participants with metabolically healthy or metabolically unhealthy obesity will be analyzed to determine their microRNA composition.	Baseline only (cross-sectional comparison of metabolically healthy lean, and of people with metabolically healthy or metabolically unhealthy obesity).
Differences in the content of lipids within exosomes obtained from plasma and adipose tissue	Exosomes obtained from the plasma and adipose tissue of metabolically healthy lean participants, and participants with metabolically healthy or metabolically unhealthy obesity will be analyzed to determine their lipid composition.	Baseline only (cross-sectional comparison of metabolically healthy lean, and of people with metabolically healthy or metabolically unhealthy obesity).
Changes in the content of microRNAs within exosomes obtained from plasma and adipose tissue	Exosomes obtained from the plasma and adipose tissue of metabolically unhealthy obesity before and after weight loss will be analyzed to determine changes in their microRNA content after weight loss.	Before and after ~10% weight loss (~4–5 months) in people with metabolically abnormal obesity
Changes in the content of lipids within exosomes obtained from plasma and adipose tissue	Exosomes obtained from the plasma and adipose tissue of metabolically unhealthy obesity before and after weight loss will be analyzed to determine changes in their lipid content after weight loss.	Before and after ~10% weight loss (~4–5 months) in people with metabolically abnormal obesity
Insulin sensitivity	Whole-body insulin sensitivity will be assessed by using the hyperinsulinemic-euglycemic clamp procedure	Baseline only (cross-sectional comparison of metabolically healthy lean, and people with metabolically healthy or metabolically unhealthy obesity).

(continued)

Outcome measure	Measure description	Time frame
Change in insulin sensitivity	Whole-body insulin sensitivity will be assessed by using the hyperinsulinemic-euglycemic clamp procedure	Before and after ~10% weight loss (~4–5 months) in people with metabolically abnormal obesity
Fat mass and fat-free mass	Fat mass and fat-free mass will be assessed using dual-energy X-ray absorptiometry (DXA)	Baseline only (cross-sectional comparison of metabolically healthy lean, and people with metabolically healthy or metabolically unhealthy obesity).
Change in fat mass and fat-free mass	Fat mass and fat-free mass will be assessed using dual-energy X-ray absorptiometry (DXA)	Before and after 10% weight loss (~4–5 months) in people with metabolically abnormal obesity
Abdominal adipose tissue volumes	Abdominal subcutaneous and intra-abdominal adipose tissue volumes will be assessed by magnetic resonance imagining (MRI)	Baseline only (cross-sectional comparison of metabolically healthy lean, and people with metabolically healthy or metabolically unhealthy obesity).
Change in abdominal adipose tissue volumes	Abdominal subcutaneous and intra-abdominal adipose tissue volumes will be assessed by magnetic resonance imagining (MRI)	Before and after ~10% weight loss (~4–5 months) in people with metabolically abnormal obesity
Intrahepatic triglyceride content	Intrahepatic triglyceride content will be assessed by magnetic resonance techniques	Baseline only (cross-sectional comparison of metabolically healthy lean, and people with metabolically healthy or metabolically unhealthy obesity).
Change in intrahepatic triglyceride content	Intrahepatic triglyceride content will be assessed by magnetic resonance techniques	Before and after ~10% weight loss (~4–5 months) in people with metabolically abnormal obesity

Sponsor: Washington University School of Medicine

Investigators

- Principal investigator: Dmitri Samovski, PhD, Washington University School of Medicine

Chapter 6
Miscellaneous Exosome Trials

Amyotrophic Lateral Sclerosis

Recruiting

Exploring Nasal Drop Therapy with Small Extracellular Vesicles for ALS (de-ALS)

ClinicalTrials.gov ID NCT06598202

Sponsor Xuanwu Hospital, Beijing

Information provided by Junwei Hao, MD, Xuanwu Hospital, Beijing (Responsible Party)

Last Update Posted 2024-10-31

Study Overview

Brief Summary

This is a multicenter, randomized, double-blinded, placebo-controlled, dose-escalation trial. The goal of this clinical trial is to evaluate the safety and preliminary efficacy of nasal drop exosomes derived from human umbilical cord blood mesenchymal stem cells (hUC-MSC-sEV-001) in amyotrophic lateral sclerosis (ALS).

Detailed Description

This is a multicenter, randomized, double-blinded, placebo-controlled, dose-escalation trial. The study will consist of two parts: Part 1 will be a dose-escalation study, and Part 2 will be an expanded safety study based on the findings from Part 1.

A traditional 3+3 dose-escalation design will be implemented in Part 1. Cohort 1 will receive low dose, Cohort 2 will receive middle dose, and Cohort 3 will receive high dose. (Cohort 1 to Cohort 3 will receive a dose of 1 mL per nostril, administered once daily, twice a week, for a total of two weeks.) If no dose-limiting toxicities (DLTs) are observed for 2 weeks after the administration of the first nasal drop, a new cohort will be enrolled at the next planned dose level. If DLTs are observed in one participant in the cohort, an additional three participants will be treated at the

J. N. Weiss, *Global Exosome Trials*, https://doi.org/10.1007/978-3-031-96420-6_6

same dose level. Dose escalation will be stopped if DLTs are observed in more than 33% of the participants.

In Part 2, 20 subjects will be randomized in a 1:1 ratio [exosome (n = 10) or exosome placebo (n = 10)]. The dose level will be determined by the primary researcher based on the findings from Part 1.

Official Title

An Exploratory Study on the Use of Intranasal Administration of Small Extracellular Vesicles for the Treatment of Amyotrophic Lateral Sclerosis

Conditions

Amyotrophic lateral sclerosis

Intervention/Treatment

- Drug: exosomes derived from human umbilical cord blood mesenchymal stem cells for nasal drop
- Drug: a placebo of exosomes derived from human umbilical cord blood mesenchymal stem cells for nasal drop

Other Study ID Numbers

- XMEC-2024-267-002

Study Start (Estimated)
2024-12-01
Primary Completion (Estimated)
2026-05-30
Study Completion (Estimated)
2026-05-30
Enrollment (Estimated)
38
Study Type
Interventional
Phase
Phase 1
Phase 2
Study Contact
Name: Junwei Hao, MD; PhD
Phone Number: 010 8319 8277
Email: haojunwei@vip.163.com
Study Contact Backup
Name: Gaoting Ma, MD
Phone Number: 010 8319 8082
Email: demo_doctor@163.com
This study has 1 location
China
Beijing Locations
Beijing, Beijing, China, 100053
Recruiting

Xuanwu Hospital, Capital Medical University
Contact:
Gaoting Ma, MD01083198082 demo_doctor@163.com
Eligibility Criteria
Description
Inclusion Criteria:

- Age: 18–80 years, inclusion of both genders.
- Disease duration: ≥6 months and ≤2 years (counted from the onset of any ALS symptoms).
- Subjects must meet the El Escorial revised criteria (2000) for the diagnosis of ALS, with a diagnosis of definite ALS, probable ALS, probable laboratory-supported ALS, or possible ALS.
- A score of ≥2 on each item of the revised ALS functional rating scale-revised (ALSFRS-R), with a score of 4 for items related to dyspnea, orthopnea, and respiratory insufficiency.
- BMI: between 18 and 30 kg/m^2.
- Subjects must have a baseline forced vital capacity percentage (%FVC) ≥70%;
- Allowed concomitant treatments: oral administration of riluzole/edaravone at standard doses for ≥30 days; regular intravenous edaravone with planned sequential oral treatment. During the trial and follow-up period, the dosage and type of concomitant medications must remain unchanged.
- Subjects of childbearing potential must use appropriate and effective contraception from 2 weeks prior to trial enrollment until the end of the follow-up period.
- The subject or legal representative must be able to sign an informed consent form and comply with the study requirements for medication administration and follow-up.

Exclusion Criteria:

- Diagnosed as non-ALS based on clinical presentation and available clinical examinations (e.g., neurophysiological tests, MRI, or other imaging, laboratory tests)
- Abnormal nasal anatomy, nasal cavity damage, severe rhinitis, or nasal disease affecting the administration of the study drug
- Requires nasal insertion of a gastric tube
- Peripheral venous hemoglobin (HGB) <100 g/L, absolute neutrophil count (NEUT) <1.5 × 10^9/L, platelet count (PLT) <100 × 10^9/L, white blood cell count (WBC) <4.0 × 10^9/L or ≥ 12 × 10^9/L, serum albumin <30 g/L, alanine aminotransferase (ALT) and aspartate aminotransferase (AST) ≥3× the upper limit of normal (ULN)
- Severe renal insufficiency: glomerular filtration rate (GFR) <30 mL/min (Cockcroft-Gault formula), or other known severe renal diseases
- Positive for hepatitis B surface antigen, e antigen, e antibody, or core antibody combined with positive hepatitis B virus DNA, positive for hepatitis C virus antibody, positive syphilis serum antibody, or positive for HIV antibody

- History of acute myocardial infarction or interventional treatment within the last 6 months, or heart failure (classified as NYHA III-IV)
- Presence of severe localized or systemic infection, immunodeficiency, or currently taking immunosuppressants
- Concurrent severe systemic diseases such as immunodeficiency diseases, coagulation disorders, or malignancies
- Vaccination within 1 month prior to the first administration or during the study until the end of follow-up
- Known allergy to the drugs used in this study or similar drugs
- Participation in another study and administration of an investigational product within the last 3 months
- Contraindications to MRI (e.g., presence of metal implants) or inability to tolerate MRI (e.g., claustrophobia)
- Pregnant or breastfeeding women, or women of childbearing potential who cannot or are unwilling to use appropriate contraception
- Unwillingness or inability to comply with the procedures required by the protocol
- Any other conditions deemed unsuitable for inclusion by the investigators

Ages Eligible for Study
18–80 years (adult, older adult)
Sexes Eligible for Study
All
Accepts Healthy Volunteers
No
Design Details
Primary purpose: treatment
Allocation: randomized
Interventional model: sequential assignment
Masking: quadruple (ParticipantCare ProviderInvestigatorOutcomes Assessor)

Arms and Interventions

Participant group/arm	Intervention/treatment
Experimental: exosome group Patients in this arm will receive exosomes derived from human umbilical cord blood mesenchymal stem cells as a nasal drop, administered once daily, twice a week, for a total of two weeks	Drug: exosomes derived from human umbilical cord blood mesenchymal stem cells for nasal drop Exosomes derived from human umbilical cord blood mesenchymal stem cells for nasal drop (administered once daily, twice a week, for a total of two weeks, based on the recommended dose during the dose-escalation phase) Other names: hUC-MSC-sEV-001

(continued)

Participant group/arm	Intervention/treatment
Placebo comparator: exosome placebo group Patients in this arm will receive a placebo nasal drop mimicking exosomes derived from human umbilical cord blood mesenchymal stem cells, administered once daily, twice a week, for a total of two weeks	Drug: a placebo of exosomes derived from human umbilical cord blood mesenchymal stem cells for nasal drop Exosome placebo Other names: hUC-MSC-sEV-001 placebo

Primary Outcome Measures

Outcome measure	Measure description	Time frame
Number of participants who experienced dose-limiting toxicities (DLTs)	DLTs related to hUC-MSC-sEV-001 include adverse events of grade 3 or higher (including significant clinical laboratory findings) that are possibly, likely, or definitely related to the study drug, accompanied by clinical symptoms and requiring medical treatment within 14 days of administration. Adverse events are graded according to the Common Terminology Criteria for Adverse Events Version 5.0 (CTCAE 5.0)	24 hours, 4±1 weeks

Secondary Outcome Measures

Outcome measure	Measure description	Time frame
Incidence of severe adverse events	The proportion of patients who experienced severe adverse events	4±1 weeks
Change from baseline in ALS functional rating scale – revised	The ALSFRS-R is a rating scale (ratings 0 = cannot do, to 4 = normal ability) used to determine participants' assessment of their capability and independence in 12 functional activities This is a validated scale, both in person and by phone, which provides a total score from four sub-scores which assess speech and swallowing (bulbar function), use of upper extremities (cervical function), gait and turning in bed (lumbar function), and breathing (respiratory function) Total scores range from 0 (most impaired) to 48 (normal ability)	4±1 weeks, 12±1 weeks, 24±1 weeks
Change from baseline in forced vital capacity to predicted value ratio (FVC% pred)	Spirometry is a physiological test that measures how an individual inhales or exhales volumes of air as a function of time. The primary signal measured in spirometry may be volume or flow. The forced vital capacity (FVC) is the maximal volume of air exhaled with maximally forced effort from a maximal inspiration	4±1 weeks, 24±1 weeks
Time to event (death, tracheostomy, and permanent assisted mechanical ventilation)	The number of time-to-event outcomes	Up to 24 weeks

(continued)

Outcome measure	Measure description	Time frame
Change from baseline in the Amyotrophic Lateral Sclerosis Assessment Questionnaire (ALSAQ-40)	ALSAQ-40 score ranges from 0 to 160 points, and higher scores indicate better quality of life	4±1 weeks, 12±1 weeks, 24±1 weeks
Change from baseline in the Edinburgh Cognitive and Behavioral ALS Screen (ECAS)	ECAS determine cognitive and behavioral changes of patients suffering from amyotrophic lateral sclerosis With ECAS, ALS-specific (fluency, executive functions and social cognition, language; minimum score = 0, maximum score = 100) and ALS-nonspecific (memory, visuospatial functions; minimum score = 0, maximum score = 36) functions can be analyzed to enable the distinction from other diseases with cognitive and behavioral impairments	12±1 weeks, 24±1 weeks
Change from baseline in the Neurophysiological Index (NI) and Compound Muscle Action Potential (CMAP) score	The NI is derived from the CMAP, the DML, and the F-wave frequency (CMAP amplitude/DML) x F frequency %), representing aspects of the effects of denervation and reinnervation, of degeneration of the terminal part of the motor axons, and of the excitability of anterior horn cells The negative amplitudes of the CMAP for motor nerve conduction in the median and ulnar nerves in the upper extremities as well as the peroneal and tibial nerves in the lower extremities of ALS patients were recorded (median nerve-wrist, ulnar-wrist, peroneal-ankle, tibial-ankle). These nerves were scored based on the decrease in the amplitudes of each nerve CMAP- 0 (CMAP> = [X-2s]), 1 (50% [X-2s] < CMAP < [X-2s]), 2 (30% [X-2s] < CMAP < 50% [X-2s]), 3 (CMAP < =30% [X-2s]), respectively. The values of X and S for different nerves and different patient age groups, which were applied in the electrophysiology examination room	12±1 weeks
Change from baseline in the Rasch Overall ALS Disability Scale (ROADS)	ROADS score ranges from 0 to 56 points, and higher scores indicate better basic daily function	4±1 weeks, 12±1 weeks, 24±1 weeks
Change from baseline in the Medical Research Council (MRC) Scale	MRC ranges from 0 to V grades, and higher grades indicate higher muscle strength	4±1 weeks, 12±1 weeks, 24±1 weeks
Change from baseline in the Lower Motor Neuro Scale (LMNS)	LMNS was calculated using the score proposed by Devine et al. that assign a separate LMN score for each limb, ranging from 0 (no involvement) to 3 (significant, severe involvement), based on the Medical Research Council and muscle wasting	4±1 weeks, 12±1 weeks, 24±1 weeks

Other Outcome Measures

Outcome measure	Measure description	Time frame
Change from baseline in the neuroimaging indices	Neuroimaging indices include gray matter thickness, gray matter volume, white matter volume, DTI metrics of the corticospinal tract, DTI-ALPS, and QSM of the bilateral motor cortex	24±1 weeks
Change from baseline in the blood markers	A number of blood markers will be examined including C-reactive protein, neurofilament light chain, IL-1β, IL-6, IL-8, IL-10, tumor necrosis factor-alpha	Up to 24 weeks

Sponsor
Xuanwu Hospital, Beijing
Collaborators

- Shengqi Medical Technology (Guangzhou) Co., Ltd.
- Viyun (Xiamen) Biomedical Research Institute Co., Ltd.

Investigators

- Principal Investigator: Junwei Hao, MD; PhD, Xuanwu Hospital, Beijing

Antiaging

Recruiting
Mesenchymal Stem Cells Derived Exosomes in Skin Rejuvenation
ClinicalTrials.gov ID NCT05813379
Sponsor Isfahan University of Medical Sciences
Information provided by Leila Dehghani, Isfahan University of Medical Sciences (Responsible Party)
Last Update Posted 2023-04-14
Study Overview
Brief Summary

Aging is a natural and complex process. The effect of environmental factors and genetics on the body eventually leads to damage in different ways. Exosomes are present in almost all body fluids, such as synovial fluid and blood. Exosomes and microvesicles are very efficient mediators of cell-to-cell communication by transferring their specific cargo to recipient cells; for example, exosomes are involved in the delivery of genetic materials, causing epigenetic modifications in the target cells. The applications of MSC-derived exosomes have more effect in cutaneous regeneration by collagen stimulation. The basic biology of exosomes indicates that MSC exosomes may contain MSC-specific components to exert specific effects on recipient cells, which are somewhat equivalent to the regenerative effects of MSCs. This study aims to slow down the aging process of the skin by using exosome.

Detailed Description

Skin aging is a complex biological process that can be classified into extrinsic or intrinsic aging. Intrinsic aging is an intrinsic degradation process that is caused by a decrease in the proliferation capacity leading to cell senescence. Angiogenesis is essential in various physiological processes, including wound healing and skin tissue regeneration. Literature review shows that exosomes derived from human umbilical cord blood mesenchymal stem cells can cause collagen stimulation and reduction of oxidative stress, and WNT/β-catenin pathway signaling in the initial stages causes the regeneration of skin damage. This study aims to slow down the aging process of the skin by using exosome.

Official Title
Application of Mesenchymal Stem Cell-Derived Exosomes in Skin Rejuvenation
Conditions
Antiaging
Intervention/Treatment

- Combination product: exosome injection

Other Study ID Numbers

- Islamic Azad University

Study Start (Actual)
2022-02-01
Primary Completion (Estimated)
2023-07-29
Study Completion (Estimated)
2023-08-30
Enrollment (Estimated)
20
Study Type
Interventional
Phase
Phase 1
Phase 2
Study Contact
Name: Leila Dehghani, Dr
Phone Number: +983136201250
Email: l_dehghani2002@yahoo.com
This study has 1 location
Iran, Islamic Republic of
Isfahan, Iran, Islamic Republic of, 81745319
Recruiting
Isfahan University of Medical Sciences
Contact:
Leila Dehghani, PhD+983136202020 ext 2146 l_dehghani2002@yahoo.com
Eligibility Criteria
Description

Inclusion Criteria:

- Females
- Ages 35–65 years
- Patients of all racial and ethnic origins
- Patients of all undergoing facial rejuvenation

Exclusion Criteria:

- Female patients in pregnancy or menstrual period
- Patients undergoing facial rejuvenation using other methods including Botox injections, chemical peels, face lifts, and others
- Patients using blood thinners, aspirin, and hormone that cannot be stopped
- Patients suffering from severe organic disease, such as coronary heart disease, hypertension, diabetes, and lung dysfunction
- Patients suffering from mental disease and acute or chronic infectious diseases

Ages Eligible for Study
35–65 years (adult, older adult)
Sexes Eligible for Study
Female
Accepts Healthy Volunteers
Yes
Design Details
Primary purpose: prevention
Allocation: N/A
Interventional model: single group assignment
Masking: none (open label)

Arms and Interventions

Participant group/arm	Intervention/ treatment
Experimental: exosome injection The exosome will be injected into each standardized injection point in a superficial manner. The injection points are along the inferior border of the cheek and mid-cheek and temple, where it will be followed by 10–15 minutes of icing	Combination product: exosome injection Treatment – exosome injection

Primary Outcome Measures

Outcome measure	Measure description	Time frame
Proportion of re-epithelialization	In order to evaluate the treatment effect, to evaluate wrinkles and collagen before the treatment, take a photo/ CT of the face	1 month
Proportion of re-epithelialization	In order to evaluate the treatment effect, to evaluate wrinkles and collagen before the treatment, take a photo/ CT of the face	3 months

Sponsor
Isfahan University of Medical Sciences
Investigators

- Principal investigator: Leila Dehghani, University of Medical Sciences

Autism

Recruiting

Combined Photo-Biomodulation at Acupuncture Points, Autologous PRP, and Umbilical Cord-Derived Exosome Therapy in Autism Spectrum Disorder (Biomodulation)

ClinicalTrials.gov ID NCT06600529

Sponsor Iffat Anwar Medical Complex

Information provided by Iffat Anwar Medical Complex (Responsible Party)

Last Update Posted 2024-09-19

Study Overview

Brief Summary

This randomized controlled trial aims to evaluate the efficacy of a combination of photo-biomodulation at acupuncture points, autologous platelet-rich plasma (PRP), and umbilical cord-derived exosome therapy in children with autism spectrum disorder (ASD). The study will compare these interventions against standard care to determine their impact on the severity of autism symptoms, as measured by the Childhood Autism Rating Scale (CARS) and other related markers.

Detailed Description

The study involves three main interventions:

1. Photo-biomodulation (PBM): PBM will be performed once a week using an 810nm, 210mW laser probe for 20 seconds at each selected acupuncture point.
2. Autologous platelet-rich plasma (PRP): PRP will be administered at 0th day, 15th day, 30th day, and at 45th day ADP-derived autologous PRP.
3. Exosome therapy: exosomes derived from umbilical cord tissue will be injected intravenously at laser acupuncture points. The PRP-exosome sessions will be repeated at 15 days, 6 weeks, 12 weeks, and 24 weeks.

The study will run over a period of 6 months, with follow-ups and assessments at each phase. The primary outcome measure will be the change in CARS score, with secondary outcomes including additional ASD markers.

Official Title

Evaluation of Combined Photo-Biomodulation at Acupuncture Points, Autologous PRP, and Umbilical Cord-Derived Exosome Therapy in Autism Spectrum Disorder: A Randomized Controlled Trial

Conditions

Autism spectrum disorder

Intervention/Treatment

- Device: photo-biomodulation
- Biological: autologous PRP
- Biological: exosome therapy
- Other: standard care (in control arm)

Other Study ID Numbers

- IAMC004

Study Start (Actual)
2024-08-13
Primary Completion (Estimated)
2025-06-10
Study Completion (Estimated)
2025-12-13
Enrollment (Estimated)
100
Study Type
Interventional
Phase
Not applicable
Study Contact
Name: Shahzad Anwar, MBBS, DOM
Phone Number: 0092 0300 9400049
Email: shahzadtirmzi@yahoo.com
This study has 1 location
Pakistan
Punjab Locations
Lahore, Punjab, Pakistan, 54000
Recruiting
Iffat Anwar Medical Complex
Contact:
Shahzad Anwar0092 0300 9400049 shahzadtirmzi@yahoo.com
Contact:
Shahzad Anwar, MBBS, DOM
Contact:
Muhammad Hassan, MBBS, FIPP
Contact:
Sulayman Waquar, M.Phil, PhD (Scholar)
Contact:
Gull a Rukh Shaukat, MS
Eligibility Criteria
Description
Inclusion Criteria:

- Diagnosis of autism spectrum disorder based on DSM-5 criteria
  - Age 3–12 years
  - Stable on current medications for at least 4 weeks prior to study entry
  - Parents or legal guardians willing to provide informed consent

  Exclusion Criteria:

- Severe comorbid medical conditions
  - Prior stem cell or exosome therapy
  - History of hypersensitivity to any component of the interventions
  - Inability to comply with study procedures

  Ages Eligible for Study
  3–12 years (child)
  Sexes Eligible for Study
  All
  Accepts Healthy Volunteers
  No
  Design Details
  Primary purpose: treatment
  Allocation: randomized
  Interventional model: parallel assignment
  Interventional model description:

- Estimated enrollment: 100 patients
- Allocation: randomized
- Intervention model: parallel assignment
- Masking: single (Participant)
- Primary purpose: treatment

  Masking: single (Participant)

Arms and Interventions

Participant group/arm	Intervention/treatment
Experimental: control group Standard care: Procedure: routine conventional applied behavioral analysis (ABA) management and interventions for ASD, as per current clinical guidelines	Other: standard care (in control arm) Routine conventional including applied behavioral analysis (ABA) for autism spectrum disorder (ASD)
Experimental: experimental group The group may be provided with three interventions and then compared with the control group in order to evaluate the effects of the said interventions	Device: photo-biomodulation Application at acupuncture points for 20 seconds each week, using 810nm laser probe Biological: autologous PRP IV injection of autologous plasma-rich platelets (PRP) on days 0, 15, 30, and 45 Biological: exosome therapy IV injection of umbilical cord-derived exosomes at laser acupuncture points

Primary Outcome Measures

Outcome measure	Measure description	Time frame
Change in Childhood Autism Rating Scale (CARS) score (15–60)	Range of CARS score 15–29.5, non-autistic; 30–36.5, mild to moderate autism; 37–60, severe autism	Baseline
Change in Childhood Autism Rating Scale (CARS) score (15–0 60)	Range of CARS score 15–29.5, non-autistic; 30–36.5, mild to moderate autism; 37–60, severe autism	12 weeks
Change in Childhood Autism Rating Scale (CARS) score (15–60)	Range of CARS score 15–29.5, non-autistic; 30–36.5, mild to moderate autism; 37–60, severe autism	6 months
Change in Childhood Autism Rating Scale (CARS) score (15–60)	Range of CARS score 15–29.5, non-autistic; 30–36.5, mild to moderate autism; 37–60, severe autism	1 year

Secondary Outcome Measures

Outcome measure	Measure description	Time frame
Assessment of social interaction using Autism Diagnostic Observation Schedule (ADOS)	It has 4 modules. Each module has 28–30 items. Each item includes a rating of 0–3 (0 being normal, while 3 specifies severe autism)	Baseline
Assessment of social interaction using Autism Diagnostic Observation Schedule (ADOS)	It has 4 modules. Each module has 28–30 items. Each item includes a rating of 0–3 (0 being normal, while 3 specifies severe autism)	12 weeks
Assessment of social interaction using Autism Diagnostic Observation Schedule (ADOS)	It has 4 modules. Each module has 28–30 items. Each item includes a rating of 0–3 (0 being normal, while 3 specifies severe autism)	6 months
Assessment of social interaction using Autism Diagnostic Observation Schedule (ADOS)	It has 4 modules. Each module has 28–30 items. Each item includes a rating of 0–3 (0 being normal, while 3 specifies severe autism)	1 year

Sponsor
Iffat Anwar Medical Complex

Dementia

Recruiting

The Role of Acupuncture-Induced Exosome in Treating Post-Stroke Dementia
ClinicalTrials.gov ID NCT05326724
Sponsor China Medical University Hospital
Information provided by China Medical University Hospital (Responsible Party)
Last Update Posted 2022-04-13
Study Overview
Brief Summary

Stroke is the main cause of disability and the second main cause of dementia. Approximately 21.5% of patients develop dementia within 4 years after stroke. The main clinical manifestation of dementia is memory and cognitive impairment. At present, acetylcholinesterase inhibitors and NMDA glutamate receptor antagonists are used for dementia treatment, but those drugs have limited efficacy. Exosome is an extracellular vesicle from the endosomal, size range from ~40 to 160 nm (average ~100 nm). It contains many cells including DNA, RNA, fat, and metabolites, as well as cytoplasm and cell surface proteins that play a role in regulating intercellular communication. Some studies believe that exosomes in the circulation are an ideal marker to reflect the pathological progress and recovery of stroke and play a key role in the reorganization of tissues and the progress of neurodegeneration after stroke. Our previous studies have shown that acupuncture can increase the long-term potentiation of hippocampal CA1 in rats with ischemic stroke and improve learning-memory and neurological function. Therefore, the purpose of this study is to explore the role of acupuncture-induced exosome in the treatment of post-stroke dementia.

Official Title
The Role of Acupuncture-Induced Exosome in Treating Post-Stroke Dementia
Conditions
Exosome
Post-stroke dementia
Acupuncture
Intervention/Treatment

- Device: acupuncture

Other Study ID Numbers

- CMUH111-REC2-024

Study Start (Estimated)
2022-08-01
Primary Completion (Estimated)
2025-07-31
Study Completion (Estimated)
2025-07-31
Enrollment (Estimated)
30
Study Type
Interventional
Phase
Not applicable
Study Contact
Name: Ching-Liang Hsieh, PhD
Phone Number: +886-4-22053366 ext 3127
Email: clhsieh@mail.cmuh.org.tw
This study has 1 location

Taiwan
North District Locations
Taichung, North District, Taiwan, 40447
Recruiting
China Medical University Hospital
Contact:
Ching-Liang Hsieh, PhD+886-4-22053366 ext 3127 clhsieh@mail.cmuh.org.tw
Eligibility Criteria
Description
Inclusion Criteria:

1. History of stroke
2. MMSE score between 16 and 26

Exclusion Criteria:

1. Those with serious diseases, such as heart failure, chronic failure, or cancer patients
2. Intolerance to acupuncture treatment
3. Allergy to acupuncture needles
4. Refusal to sign the informed consent form

Ages Eligible for Study
50–75 years (adult, older adult)
Sexes Eligible for Study
All
Accepts Healthy Volunteers
No
Design Details
Primary purpose: treatment
Allocation: N/A
Interventional model: single group assignment
Masking: none (open label)

Arms and Interventions

Participant group/ arm	Intervention/treatment
Experimental: acupuncture	Device: acupuncture The stainless steel needles are used to insert into the three points of Sishencong, Baihui, and Dazhui, once a week, once for 20 minutes, for 12 consecutive weeks

Primary Outcome Measures

Outcome measure	Measure description	Time frame
Concentration of exosome		12 weeks
Alzheimer's Disease Assessment Scale-Cognitive Subscale scale	Higher scores indicate greater cognitive impairment	12 weeks
Behavioral and Psychological Symptoms of Dementia scale	The greater cognitive impairment or dementia severity is associated with higher rates of some BPSD (behavioral and psychological symptoms of dementia)	12 weeks

Sponsor
China Medical University Hospital

Epilepsy

Recruiting

1. Induced Pluripotent Stem Cell-Derived Exosome Nasal Drops for the Treatment of Refractory Focal Epilepsy

ClinicalTrials.gov ID NCT05886205
Sponsor Peking Union Medical College Hospital
Information provided by Peking Union Medical College Hospital (Responsible Party)
Last Update Posted 2023-06-07
Study Overview
Brief Summary
Evaluate the safety, tolerability, and preliminary efficacy of GD-iEXo-002 nasal drops in the treatment of focal refractory epilepsy.
Detailed Description
Epilepsy patients can achieve good control after treatment, but still 30% of patients have medically refractory epilepsy, with the vast majority being focal epilepsy. Recurrent seizures seriously affect the normal development, learning, and life of patients. There is an urgent need for effective drugs to treat refractory focal epilepsy in clinical practice.

Exosomes are a kind of vesicle structures secreted by cells, with a diameter of 30–150 nm, carrying proteins, nucleic acids, and other substances. Exosomes have many advantages. As naturally occurring nanoscale secretory membrane vesicles, they have extremely low immunogenicity and good safety and can cross biological barriers such as the blood-brain barrier and the blood-tumor barrier. Exosomes have specific bioactive substances related to source cells, while stem cell exosomes contain TGF-β. Functional factors such as BDNF can inhibit cell apoptosis, inhibit inflammatory response, promote angiogenesis, inhibit fibrosis, and enhance tissue repair potential, with a wide range of potential applications.

Induced pluripotent stem cell (iPSC) originates from single cell amplification, with infinite proliferation ability, good consistency, and stability; MSCs exhibit significant heterogeneity.

The purpose of this single-center, open-label clinical trial is to evaluate the safety, tolerability, and preliminary efficacy of induced pluripotent stem cell-derived exosome (iPSC-Exos) nasal drops in the treatment of focal refractory epilepsy.

Official Title

Exploratory Clinical Study on Induced Pluripotent Stem Cell-Derived Exosome (GD-iEXo-002) Nasal Drops for the Treatment of Refractory Focal Epilepsy

Conditions

Refractory Focal Epilepsy

Intervention/Treatment

- Drug: iPSC-Exos

Other Study ID Numbers

- K2153-K22C1488

Study Start (Estimated)
2023-06-05
Primary Completion (Estimated)
2025-06-13
Study Completion (Estimated)
2025-11-13
Enrollment (Estimated)
34
Study Type
Interventional
Phase
Early Phase 1
Study Contact
Name: Xue Zhao
Phone Number: +8601069154786
Email: zhaoxue_pumch@sina.com
This study has 1 location
China
Beijing Locations
Beijing, Beijing, China, 100730
Recruiting
Peking Union Medical College Hospital
Contact:
Yang Zhang+8601069154126
Eligibility Criteria
Description

Inclusion Criteria:

1. Before conducting this study, understand and sign the informed consent form and comply with the requirements of this study.
2. The subjects are patients with focal epilepsy aged 18 to 70 years (inclusive), regardless of gender.
3. The subjects must comply with the definition of drug-resistant epilepsy (ILAE).
4. Subjects must take 1–6 types of anti-epileptic drugs (AEDs), and before entering the screening period, they must take unadjusted types and stable doses of AEDs for at least 4 weeks.
5. Throughout the entire research process, the subject/legal guardian must be able to accurately record the log of epileptic seizures.
6. Subjects must experience at least 4 countable seizures within 28 days prior to the screening period.
7. The subjects are willing and able to comply with the research requirements.

Exclusion Criteria:

1. Unwilling or unable to follow the procedures stipulated in the agreement.
2. Pregnant or lactating women, or women with reproductive potential who are unable or unwilling to take appropriate contraceptive measures.
3. Other uncontrollable diseases that may interfere with the research results, including but not limited to infection, hypertension, diabetes, and cardiovascular and cerebrovascular diseases.
4. There are situations that may increase the risk of participating in experiments or research product use, such as liver enzyme elevation exceeding twice the normal upper limit and/or GFR<60 mL/min/1.73 m2.
5. Have a history of drug abuse, alcohol dependence, or smoking within one month.
6. Patients with status epilepticus within one month.
7. Have potential progressive nervous system disease, such as encephalitis, brain tumor, multiple sclerosis, or dementia.
8. Patients who plan to undergo epilepsy surgery within six months.
9. Patients with abnormal or diseased nasal structures.
10. Patients with cerebrospinal fluid rhinorrhea.
11. Patients whose family members have not been able to proficiently and correctly master the nasal drip method through standardized training.

Ages Eligible for Study
18–70 years (adult, older adult)
Sexes Eligible for Study
All
Accepts Healthy Volunteers
No
Design Details
Primary purpose: treatment
Allocation: N/A
Interventional model: single group assignment
Masking: none (open label)

Arms and Interventions

Participant group/arm	Intervention/ treatment
Experimental: iPSC-exosome treatment Group 1, low-dose group, 8 patients are treated with 2 μg iPSC-Exos in 200 μL. Group 2, mid-dose group, 8 patients are treated with 6 μg iPSC-Exos in 200 μL. Group 3, mid-dose group, 8 patients are treated with 18 μg iPSC-Exos in 200 μL. Group 4, dose expansion, 10 patients are treated with iPSC-Exos in 200 μL. iPSC-Exos were administered for nasal drip, bid for 12 weeks	Drug: iPSC-Exos iPSC-Exos were administered for nasal drip, bid for 12 weeks

Primary Outcome Measures

Outcome measure	Measure description	Time frame
Adverse events as assessed by CTCAE	All potentially treated subjects to assess the safety	24 weeks from post-administration

Secondary Outcome Measures

Outcome measure	Measure description	Time frame
Number of participants with abnormal vital signs and abnormal physical examination findings		Screening, after the first administration 1 week, 2 weeks, 4 weeks, 8 weeks, 12 weeks, 16 weeks, 24 weeks
Number of participants with abnormal neurological examination	Evaluate general neurological status, muscle strength and tension, sensory ataxia, and pathological signs	Screening, after the first administration 1 week, 2 weeks, 4 weeks, 8 weeks, 12 weeks, 16 weeks, 24 weeks
Number of participants with abnormal laboratory test results	Blood routine test, blood biochemistry test, and electrolyte test	Screening, after the first administration 1 week, 2 weeks, 4 weeks, 8 weeks, 12 weeks, 16 weeks, 24 weeks
Number of participants with abnormal urine analysis	Urine routine examination	Screening, after the first administration 1 week, 2 weeks, 4 weeks, 8 weeks, 12 weeks, 16 weeks, 24 weeks

(continued)

Outcome measure	Measure description	Time frame
Seizure frequency	Seizure frequency: i. No seizures: any type of seizure disappeared after 28 days of observation. ii. Significantly effective: 75–99% reduction in seizure frequency compared with baseline. iii. Effective: 50–75% reduction in seizure frequency compared with baseline. iv. Improvement: 25–50% reduction in the number of seizures compared with baseline, or prolongation, reduction in degree, and shortening of duration between episodes. v. Ineffectiveness and exacerbation: ineffectiveness refers to a decrease or increase of <25% in the number of seizures compared with baseline, and exacerbation refers to an increase in the frequency of seizures from baseline ≥25%	Before administration; administration; after the first administration 1 week, 2 weeks, 4 weeks, 8 weeks, 12 weeks, 16 weeks, 24 weeks
Scalp electroencephalogram monitoring		Screening, after the first administration 12 weeks
Head magnetic resonance imaging (MRI) examination		Screening, after the first administration 12 weeks

Other Outcome Measures

Outcome measure	Measure description	Time frame
Exploratory research-1	The protein concentration of GFAP, IL-1 β, IL-, IL-1, IL-17, TGF- β, MCP-1, and TNF-α in blood	Screening, after the first administration 1 week, 2 weeks, 4 weeks, 8 weeks, 12 weeks, 16 weeks, 24 weeks
Exploratory research-2	T cell, B cell, NK cell subpopulation analysis	Screening, after the first administration 1 week, 2 weeks, 4 weeks, 8 weeks, 12 weeks, 16 weeks, 24 weeks

Sponsor
Peking Union Medical College Hospital
Collaborators

- Guidon Pharmaceutics Ltd.

Investigators

- Principal Investigator: Xiaohong Han, Peking Union Medical College Hospital

Erectile Dysfunction

Not Yet Recruiting

Regenerative Injection of Stem Cells or Stem Cell-Derived Exosomes for Erectile Dysfunction (RISE)

ClinicalTrials.gov ID NCT06605508

Sponsor Jumeirah American Clinic

Information provided by Ranjith Ramasamy, Jumeirah American Clinic (Responsible Party)

Last Update Posted 2024-12-05

Study Overview

Brief Summary

The goal of this prospective observational study is to evaluate whether injections of stem cells derived from the patient's own fat tissue (adipose tissue) can improve erectile function in men aged 30 to 75 years who have erectile dysfunction (ED) and have not responded well to standard treatments like phosphodiesterase type 5 (PDE-5) inhibitors (e.g., Viagra).

The main questions the study aims to answer are:

Will the stem cell injections improve erectile function, as measured by the International Index of Erectile Function (IIEF) score? Are there any changes in blood flow to the penis, which will be measured using a Doppler ultrasound?

Participants will:

Receive injections of their own stem cells (obtained from a biopsy of fat) directly into the penis.

Undergo assessments to check erectile function before and after treatment. Have follow-up visits at 3, 6, 9, and 12 months to monitor long-term effects. The study will also look for any possible side effects or complications and evaluate biological markers in the penis that may indicate the effectiveness of the treatment.

Participants will be recruited from a clinic where they are already receiving care for ED. To take part, they must be in good overall health, with no severe heart disease, uncontrolled diabetes, cancer, or other conditions that could make stem cell therapy unsafe for them.

Detailed Description:

This prospective observational study is designed to evaluate the safety and preliminary efficacy of intracavernosal injections of autologous adipose tissue-derived stem cells (ADSCs) or stem cell-derived exosomes for treating erectile dysfunction (ED) in men unresponsive to conventional therapies, such as phosphodiesterase type 5 (PDE-5) inhibitors. The primary focus will be on improvements in erectile function, as measured by changes in the International Index of Erectile Function (IIEF) score. Additionally, the study will assess penile hemodynamics, monitor adverse events, and explore biomarkers that may predict therapeutic outcomes.

Background and Rationale:

Erectile dysfunction affects a significant proportion of the male population, particularly with advancing age, and can result from various causes, including vascular, neurogenic, and psychogenic factors. Current standard treatments, such as PDE-5 inhibitors, are effective for many, but a substantial subset of patients, especially those with underlying vascular or nerve-related pathologies, experience inadequate therapeutic responses.

Regenerative medicine has emerged as a promising approach for addressing ED through tissue repair and vascular regeneration. Both ADSCs and stem cell-derived exosomes are potential therapies due to their ability to promote angiogenesis, tissue regeneration, and anti-inflammatory effects. ADSCs can be harvested from the patient's adipose tissue, minimizing the risk of immunogenicity or rejection. Exosomes derived from stem cells, on the other hand, offer a cell-free approach, delivering growth factors and signaling molecules to the target tissues. Preclinical studies have demonstrated the potential of these therapies to restore erectile function through tissue remodeling and enhanced penile blood flow following intracavernosal injection.

Primary Objective:

To evaluate the safety and efficacy of intracavernosal ADSC or stem cell-derived exosome injections in improving erectile function, as determined by changes in the IIEF score from baseline through subsequent follow-ups. The IIEF is a validated, comprehensive questionnaire used to assess erectile function and sexual satisfaction.

Secondary Objectives:

Penile hemodynamics: Doppler ultrasound will evaluate changes in penile blood flow post-treatment, providing insight into the vascular effects of the therapies.

Long-term effects: follow-up visits at 3, 6, 9, and 12 months will include IIEF scoring, Doppler ultrasound assessments, and patient-reported outcomes to evaluate the durability of treatment effects.

Safety and adverse events: all potential adverse events, including injection-site reactions and systemic complications, will be closely monitored and documented throughout the study.

Biomarker exploration: exploratory analyses will aim to identify biomarkers, including vascular and tissue-specific markers, which may predict patient response to the treatment.

Study Design:

This open-label, single-arm, pilot observational study will serve as a preliminary investigation of ADSC or stem cell-derived exosome therapy in ED, providing foundational data on their feasibility and safety. As a prospective observational study, the emphasis will be on safety and gathering initial efficacy data rather than delivering definitive conclusions.

Study Population:

The study will enroll 30 men aged 30 to 75 years with a diagnosis of mild to moderate erectile dysfunction who have failed or experienced suboptimal responses to PDE-5 inhibitors. Participants will be recruited from Dr. Ranjith Ramasamy's clinic, where they are receiving care for ED. Inclusion and exclusion criteria have been carefully designed to select participants who are most likely to benefit from these therapies and ensure patient safety.

Sample Size Rationale:

A sample size of 30 was chosen based on the exploratory nature of the study. The primary goal is to assess feasibility, safety, and preliminary efficacy while providing sufficient data to inform the design of future, more extensive studies. Recruitment of 30 participants is feasible within the clinic's patient population over the planned two-year period.

Study Procedures:

Informed consent: participants will be fully informed about the study, including its risks and benefits, and will provide written consent prior to enrollment.

Baseline assessments: baseline data, including IIEF scores, penile Doppler ultrasound, and blood tests, will be collected to assess pre-treatment erectile function and overall health.

Therapeutic Administration:

For ADSCs: ADSCs will be isolated from autologous adipose tissue harvested via minimally invasive liposuction. The cells will be processed and prepared for direct injection into the corpus cavernosum. A tourniquet will be placed for 15 minutes around the base of the penis after the injection to minimize systemic dispersion.

For exosomes: exosomes derived from stem cells will be isolated and purified and then injected intracavernosally using a similar protocol.

Follow-up monitoring: participants will be monitored for immediate post-injection reactions and at regular intervals (3, 6, 9, and 12 months) for changes in erectile function (IIEF), penile hemodynamics (Doppler ultrasound), and adverse events. Exploratory biomarker analysis will also be conducted.

Data Collection and Analysis:

Data will be analyzed to evaluate primary and secondary outcomes. IIEF score changes will be the primary efficacy measure, while penile hemodynamics and adverse event rates will be assessed for safety. Exploratory analyses will investigate the correlation between biomarkers and clinical outcomes, providing insights into potential predictors of treatment response.

Ethical Considerations:

This study will adhere to ethical standards for clinical research. Informed consent will be obtained from all participants, and the protocol will be reviewed and approved by an ethics committee. Participants will have the right to withdraw at any point, and their standard medical care will not be affected by their participation.

Expected Outcomes:

The study aims to provide early evidence on the safety and potential efficacy of ADSC or stem cell-derived exosome therapy for ED. If successful, participants are expected to show improvements in erectile function with minimal adverse events. The findings from this study will inform larger, more definitive trials and contribute to the development of novel regenerative therapies for erectile dysfunction.

Official Title

Prospective Observational Study on Intracavernosal Injection of Autologous Adipose Tissue-Derived Stem Cells (ADSCs) or Stem Cell-Derived Exosomes for the Treatment of Erectile Dysfunction

Conditions

Erectile dysfunction
Erectile dysfunction associated with type 2 diabetes mellitus
Erectile dysfunction following radical prostatectomy
Intervention/Treatment

- Procedure: autologous adipose tissue-derived stem cell injection for erectile dysfunction
- Procedure: stem cell-derived exosome injection for erectile dysfunction

Other Study ID Numbers

- 001

Study Start (Estimated)
2025-01-01
Primary Completion (Estimated)
2028-12-31
Study Completion (Estimated)
2029-12-31
Enrollment (Estimated)
30
Study Type
Observational
Study Contact
Name: Ranjith Ramasamy, MD
Phone Number: +971 800 522823
Email: ranjith.ramasamy@jac.ae
Study Contact Backup
Name: Jessie Bagolor, RN
Email: jessie.bagolor@jac.ae
This study has 1 location
United Arab Emirates
Dubai, United Arab Emirates
Jumeirah American Clinic
Contact:
Ranjith Ramasamy, MD+971 800 522823 ranjith.ramasamy@jac.ae
Contact:
Jessie Magoncia Bagolor, RN+971 50 869 8497 jessie.bagolor@jac.ae
Eligibility Criteria
Description
Inclusion Criteria:

- Age: adult males aged 30 to 75 years
- Diagnosis: confirmed diagnosis of erectile dysfunction (ED) of mild to moderate severity, as defined by an International Index of Erectile Function (IIEF) score
- Treatment response: failure or suboptimal response to conventional ED treatments, such as PDE-5 inhibitors

- General health: overall good health without contraindications to stem cell therapy
- Informed consent: ability and willingness to provide written informed consent to participate in the study

Exclusion Criteria:

- Severe cardiovascular disease: presence of severe cardiovascular conditions, including uncontrolled hypertension or significant heart disease
- Active infections: ongoing infections that could interfere with treatment or pose a risk to the participant
- Malignancies: history of or current cancer, including malignancies that could affect safety or treatment outcomes
- Contraindications to stem cell therapy: any medical conditions or treatments that contraindicate the use of stem cell therapy
- Uncontrolled diabetes: poorly controlled diabetes or other metabolic disorders that could impact treatment efficacy or safety
- Psychiatric or cognitive impairments: significant psychiatric or cognitive disorders that may affect the participant's ability to comply with study protocols or provide informed consent
- Recent surgery or trauma: recent major surgeries or physical trauma that could impact the study or interfere with the intervention
- Participation in other studies: participation in other clinical trials or studies that may affect the outcomes or safety of this study.

Study Population

The study population will consist of men aged 30 to 75 years with a clinical diagnosis of mild to moderate erectile dysfunction (ED). Eligible participants are those who have experienced suboptimal or no response to standard therapies, including phosphodiesterase type 5 (PDE-5) inhibitors. The inclusion criteria are designed to focus on individuals most likely to benefit from regenerative therapy while ensuring safety.

Participants will be recruited from Dr. Ranjith Ramasamy's clinic, where they are actively seeking care for erectile dysfunction. This population is expected to represent a diverse group of patients with varying etiologies of ED, including vascular, neurogenic, and idiopathic causes.

Ages Eligible for Study

30–75 years (adult, older adult)

Sexes Eligible for Study

Male

Accepts Healthy Volunteers

No

Sampling Method

Non-probability Sample

Design Details

Observational model: cohort

Time perspective: prospective

Groups and Interventions

Groups/cohorts	Intervention/treatment
Intracavernosal injection of autologous adipose stem cells for erectile dysfunction treatment In this arm of the study, participants will receive intracavernosal injections of autologous adipose tissue-derived stem cells (ADSCs). The ADSCs are collected from the participant's own body fat through a minimally invasive liposuction procedure. After processing, the stem cells will be injected directly into the erectile tissue of the penis. This treatment aims to improve erectile function by stimulating tissue regeneration and enhancing blood flow. Participants will be monitored for safety and efficacy, including erectile function assessments using the International Index of Erectile Function (IIEF) and penile hemodynamics measured by Doppler ultrasound. Follow-up evaluations will occur at 3, 6, 9, and 12 months post-treatment	Procedure: autologous adipose tissue-derived stem cell injection for erectile dysfunction This intervention involves the use of autologous adipose tissue-derived stem cells (ADSCs) to treat erectile dysfunction. The process begins with a minimally invasive liposuction procedure to harvest fat tissue from the participant's own body. The harvested fat is then processed to isolate stem cells, which are subsequently injected directly into the erectile tissue of the penis. This approach aims to enhance erectile function by promoting tissue regeneration and improving blood flow. Unlike other treatments for erectile dysfunction, this intervention uses stem cells derived from the participant's own fat, which may reduce the risk of immune rejection and offer a novel regenerative therapy option. The treatment is designed to address ED in patients who have not responded adequately to conventional therapies like PDE-5 inhibitors Other names: ADSC injection for ED Fat-derived stem cell therapy for erectile dysfunction Autologous fat stem cell injection
Intracavernosal injection of stem cell-derived exosomes In this arm of the study, participants will receive intracavernosal injections of stem cell-derived exosomes. These exosomes, which are nano-sized extracellular vesicles obtained from cultured stem cells, are rich in growth factors and bioactive molecules that facilitate tissue repair and regeneration. Unlike stem cell therapy, this cell-free approach minimizes potential risks associated with live cell transplantation while still delivering therapeutic benefits. Participants will be monitored for safety and efficacy, including erectile function assessments using the International Index of Erectile Function (IIEF) and penile hemodynamics measured by Doppler ultrasound. Follow-up evaluations will occur at 3, 6, 9, and 12 months post-treatment	Procedure: stem cell-derived exosome injection for erectile dysfunction This intervention involves the use of stem cell-derived exosomes to treat erectile dysfunction. Exosomes are nano-sized extracellular vesicles secreted by stem cells, containing bioactive molecules such as growth factors and signaling proteins that promote tissue repair and regeneration. Unlike therapies requiring the transplantation of live cells, this cell-free approach eliminates the need for invasive harvesting procedures. The exosomes are carefully purified from cultured stem cells and prepared for direct injection into the erectile tissue of the penis. This approach aims to enhance erectile function by stimulating tissue regeneration, reducing inflammation, and improving blood flow. Unlike other treatments for erectile dysfunction, exosome therapy offers a novel regenerative option, potentially benefiting patients who have not responded adequately to conventional therapies such as PDE-5 inhibitors. Other names: Extracellular vesicle therapy Cell-free regenerative therapy for ED

Primary Outcome Measures

Outcome measure	Measure description	Time frame
Change in erectile function as measured by the International Index of Erectile Function (IIEF) score	The primary outcome measure for this study is the change in erectile function as assessed by the International Index of Erectile Function (IIEF) score. The IIEF is a validated questionnaire designed to evaluate various aspects of sexual health, including erectile function, sexual satisfaction, and overall sexual performance. Participants will complete the IIEF questionnaire at baseline and at follow-up visits to track changes in erectile function over time. The goal is to determine whether the intracavernosal injection of autologous adipose tissue-derived stem cells leads to significant improvements in erectile function compared to pre-treatment levels. The IIEF score will provide a comprehensive measure of treatment effectiveness and help assess the impact of the intervention on participants' sexual health and quality of life	12 months

Secondary Outcome Measures

Outcome measure	Measure description	Time frame
Penile hemodynamics as measured by Doppler ultrasound	The secondary outcome measure for this study is penile hemodynamics assessed by Doppler ultrasound. Doppler ultrasound is a noninvasive imaging technique used to evaluate blood flow and vascular function in the penis. This assessment will be conducted at baseline and during follow-up visits to determine changes in penile blood flow and vascular characteristics following the intracavernosal injection of autologous adipose tissue-derived stem cells. Improvements in penile hemodynamics, such as increased blood flow and better vascular function, will be used to gauge the effectiveness of the stem cell therapy in enhancing erectile function. This measure will complement changes in the International Index of Erectile Function (IIEF) score and provide a detailed understanding of the physiological effects of the treatment	12 months

Sponsor
Jumeirah American Clinic
Publications

- Narasimman M, Sandler M, Bernstein A, Loloi J, Saltzman RG, Bernie H, Ramasamy R. A primer on the restorative therapies for erectile dysfunction: a narrative review. Sex Med Rev. 2024 Jun 26;12(3):505-512. doi: 10.1093/sxmrev/qeae012.
- Israeli JM, Lokeshwar SD, Efimenko IV, Masterson TA, Ramasamy R. The potential of platelet-rich plasma injections and stem cell therapy for penile rejuvenation. Int J Impot Res. 2022 May;34(4):375-382. doi: 10.1038/s41443-021-00482-z. Epub 2021 Nov 6.

- Lokeshwar SD, Patel P, Shah SM, Ramasamy R. A Systematic Review of Human Trials Using Stem Cell Therapy for Erectile Dysfunction. Sex Med Rev. 2020 Jan;8(1):122-130. doi: 10.1016/j.sxmr.2019.08.003. Epub 2019 Oct 19.
- Khodamoradi K, Golan R, Dullea A, Ramasamy R. Exosomes as Potential Biomarkers for Erectile Dysfunction, Varicocele, and Testicular Injury. Sex Med Rev. 2022 Apr;10(2):311-322. doi: 10.1016/j.sxmr.2021.10.001. Epub 2021 Nov 24.

Jaundice

Not Yet Recruiting

The Role of Breastmilk and Serum Exosomes in Neonatal Jaundice Due to ABO Incompatibility

ClinicalTrials.gov ID NCT06502847

Sponsor Kanuni Sultan Suleyman Training and Research Hospital

Information provided by Seda Yilmaz Semerci, Kanuni Sultan Suleyman Training and Research Hospital (Responsible Party)

Last Update Posted 2024-07-17

Study Overview

Brief Summary

Neonatal jaundice is a major global health issue that can lead to serious complications and even death if not promptly treated. ABO incompatibility is a common cause of pathological neonatal jaundice, but there are currently no specific tests to predict its severity or progression. This project aims to study the role of exosomes in the diagnosis and treatment of newborn jaundice, focusing on their impact on infants with ABO incompatibility. The study will take place at a reference neonatal intensive care unit, involving 45 infants. Serum and breast milk samples will be collected and analyzed to determine any relationships and possible correlations.

Official Title

The Role of Breast Milk and Serum Exosome Profile in Prediction of the Severity and Treatment Requirement of Neonatal Jaundice Due to ABO Incompatibility

Conditions

Neonatal jaundice from other specified causes

ABO incompatibility

ABO hemolytic disease

Intervention/Treatment

- Other: exosome profile study

Other Study ID Numbers

- 43057

Study Start (Estimated)

2024-08-01

Primary Completion (Estimated)
2025-06-01
Study Completion (Estimated)
2025-08-01
Enrollment (Estimated)
45
Study Type
Observational
Study Contact
Name: Seda Yilmaz Semerci
Phone Number: 05337180683
Email: sedayilmazsemerci@gmail.com
No location data
Eligibility Criteria
Description
Inclusion Criteria:

- Newborns who are needed treatment for neonatal jaundice due to ABO incompatibility
- Newborns who are admitted to the study center due to ABO hemolytic disease
- Newborns with ABO incompatibility
- Healthy newborns
- Healthy mothers

Exclusion Criteria:

- Lack of informed consent
- Congenital abnormalities
- Maternal liver diseases
- Neonatal liver diseases
- Sepsis
- Neonatal jaundice due to the causes other than ABO incompatibility
- Acute or chronic disease state in newborn
- Maternal acute or chronic disease
- Medication or substance use affecting liver functions

Study Population
It is planned to include a total of 45 babies in the study, including healthy babies (n = 15) in the first group, babies who developed jaundice due to ABO incompatibility but did not need treatment (n = 15) in the second group, and babies who developed jaundice due to ABO incompatibility and needed treatment (n = 15) in the third group.
Ages Eligible for Study
Up to 28 days (child)
Sexes Eligible for Study
All
Sampling Method

Non-probability Sample
Design Details
Observational model: case-control
Time perspective: prospective

Groups and Interventions

Groups/cohorts	Intervention/treatment
Case ABO1 Newborns who receive treatment due to the ABO Incompatibility will be included in this group	Other: exosome profile study Neonatal serum and maternal exosome profiles will be studied in all groups
Case ABO2 Newborns who have the ABO incompatibility, but do not require treatment will be included in this group	Other: exosome profile study Neonatal serum and maternal exosome profiles will be studied in all groups
Control Healthy newborns without any disease or health condition will be included in this group	Other: exosome profile study Neonatal serum and maternal exosome profiles will be studied in all groups

Primary Outcome Measures

Outcome measure	Measure description	Time frame
Number of participants who need for treatment	Association between the serum and breast milk exosome and need for treatment due to ABO incompatibility	12 months

Sponsor
Kanuni Sultan Suleyman Training and Research Hospital

Hair

Not Yet Recruiting

Study Evaluating the Efficacy and Safety of BENEV Exosome Regenerative Complex+ for Self-Perceived Thinning Hair

ClinicalTrials.gov ID NCT06571799

Sponsor Ablon Skin Institute Research Center

Information provided by Ablon Skin Institute Research Center (Responsible Party)

Last Update Posted 2024-08-26

Study Overview

Brief Summary

The goal of this clinical trial is to further substantiate the effectiveness and safety of BENEV Exosome Regenerative Complex+ post SylFirmX® RF microneedling procedure for self-perceived thinning hair in healthy men and women ages 18–65 years over the course of four months. Participants will be asked to have treatments monthly for 4 sessions, attend a follow-up appointment 4 weeks after the 4th session, have photos taken of their hair, and answer questionnaires related to their thinning hair.

Detailed Description

Exosomes represent promising new regenerative medicine treatments for facial rejuvenation and to enhance other cosmetic procedures. Exosomes can provide effective treatment for skin rejuvenation, scar reduction, hyperpigmentation, and hair growth. This new technology can be used alone but is often combined with other older existing aesthetic treatments. Specifically, the use of exosomes in hair loss has been anecdotally observed, but treatment protocols remain elusive and not universally accepted. Since hair loss has a multifactorial etiology, and traditional treatments have limitations, we explore the use of adipose tissue stem cell-derived lyophilized exosomes for novel addition to the armamentarium of options to reverse hair thinning or shedding.

Exosome is defined as a 30–200 nm endoplasmic reticulum that is secreted for cell-to-cell communication and plays an important role in influencing the microenvironment around cells. ExoSCRT™ is an innovative technology to separate and refine 0.1% pure exosomes from stem cells and helps the virtualization of natural skin energy by affecting skin cells effectively. BENEV Exosome Regenerative Complex+® is an intensive dual-action complex formulated to absorb quickly into the skin and scalp delivering the concentrated power of stem cell-derived lyophilized exosomes, potent growth factors, peptides, coenzymes, minerals, amino acids, and vitamins.

The purpose of this clinical research study is to further evaluate the efficacy and safety of BENEV Exosome Regenerative Complex+® post SylFirmX® RF microneedling procedure of the scalp for self-perceived thinning hair in thirty (30) healthy male and female subjects, ages 18–65 years over the course of four (4) months.

Official Title

A 4-Month, Single-Arm Study Evaluating the Efficacy and Safety of BENEV Exosome Regenerative Complex+® Post SylfirmX® RF Microneedling to Promote Hair Growth in Healthy Men and Women with Self-Perceived Thinning Hair

Conditions

Thinning hair

Intervention/Treatment

- Other: BENEV Exosome Regenerative Complex+

Other Study ID Numbers

- BNV-EXO-HAIR-01

Study Start (Estimated)

2024-09

Primary Completion (Estimated)

2025-09

Study Completion (Estimated)

2025-09
Enrollment (Estimated)
30
Study Type
Interventional
Phase
Not applicable
Study Contact
Name: Shelley Joyce, RN, BSN
Phone Number: 310-727-3376
Email: shelley@abloninstitute.com
This study has 1 location
United States
California Locations
Manhattan Beach, California, United States, 90266
Ablon Skin Institute & Research Center
Eligibility Criteria
Description
Inclusion Criteria
Subjects meeting all of the following criteria will be eligible for study entry:

1. Healthy males and females of all Fitzpatrick skin types between 18 and 65 years of age.
2. Subjects must be willing to provide verbal understanding and sign an informed consent form, HIPAA form, and photography release form approved by the Institutional Review Board.
3. Subjects must be in general good health, as determined by the investigator.
4. Subjects with self-perceived hair thinning as determined on initial study assessment by the investigator (excluding patients with medically diagnosed telogen effluvium).
5. Subjects willing to undergo a brief physical exam to include height, weight, blood pressure, pulse, physical scalp exam, and basic systems evaluation (skin, respiratory, cardiovascular, gastrointestinal, endocrine, neurological, and musculoskeletal systems) by the investigator.
6. Subjects willing to not substantially change their current diet, medications, or exercise routines for the duration of the study. If a subject receives physician guidance during the study to change diet, medications, or exercise routine, the subject will need to notify the clinic as soon as possible.
7. Females of childbearing potential (FOCBP) must be willing to have a urine pregnancy test and practice effective contraception for the duration of the study. (Effective contraception is defined as stabilized on oral contraceptive for at least 3 months as of the start of the study, intrauterine device, condom with spermicide, diaphragm with spermicide, implant, NuvaRing®, injection, transdermal patch, or abstinence.) Females on birth control pills must have taken the same type of pill for at least 3 months prior to entering the study and must not

change type during the study. Those who have used birth control pills in the past must have discontinued usage at least 3 months prior to the start of the study. The initiation of birth control should not have been associated with the initiation of hair loss/thinning.

8. FOCBP must have a negative urine pregnancy test at the baseline visit.
9. Subjects willing to give a blood sample collected for routine laboratory analysis (complete blood count and comprehensive metabolic panel).
10. Subjects willing to have 2D digital photography of the entire head/hair region for overall evaluation of general hair growth and quality by the investigator.
11. Subjects willing to have digital trichoscopy photography of the target site areas on the scalp for analysis of hair counts and other hair measurements.
12. Subjects willing to have RF microneedling procedure of the scalp region followed by application of IP.
13. Subjects must be willing and able to complete and understand the rating questionnaires.
14. Subjects must maintain a consistent length, cut, style, and color throughout the four (4)-month study period.
15. Subjects who have color-treated hair must be willing to have the color treatment performed at the same time interval prior to visits.
16. Subjects willing to maintain their normal hair-shampooing frequency, use a mild non-medicated shampoo and conditioner for the duration of the study, and attend visits with clean and dry hair (shampoo must be done 24 hours or more prior to the visit).
17. Subjects must be willing and able to attend all study visits and comply with the post-procedure and lifestyle instructions.

Exclusion Criteria

Subjects meeting any of the following criteria will be excluded from the study:

1. Subjects who are pregnant, nursing mothers, planning a pregnancy during the course of the study, or become pregnant during the study.
2. Subjects who have had a hair transplant.
3. Subjects with any known allergy or sensitivity to any shampoo and/or conditioner.
4. Subjects with known stressful incident within the last six months (e.g., death in family, miscarriage).
5. Subjects who have recently (within the last 3 months) started the use of hormones for birth control or hormone replacement therapy (HRT). Women currently using hormones for birth control or HRT must have been on a stable dose (3 months or longer) in order to be eligible for the study.
6. Subjects using low-level laser therapy (LLLT) or other light therapy to treat thinning hair in the last 3 months.
7. Subjects who have regularly used Rogaine (minoxidil), Nioxin, and/or Finasteride or undergone any other hair or scalp treatments within the last 3 months.

8. Subjects who have used prescription drugs known to affect the hair growth cycle within the last 3 months (e.g., hormone-based birth control for less than 3 months, cyproterone acetate, Aldactone/spironolactone, or any 5-alpha-reductase inhibitor).
9. Subjects who have regularly used anti-androgenic therapies (i.e., spironolactone, flutamide, cyproterone acetate, progesterone, and/or bicalutamide) or undergone any other hair or scalp treatments within the last 3 months.
10. Subjects suffering from other hair loss disorders, such as alopecia areata, scarring alopecia, androgenetic alopecia, and telogen effluvium as determined during initial study assessment and physical exam by the investigator.
11. Subjects with self-reported uncontrolled diseases (i.e., diabetes, hypertension, hyperthyroidism, hypothyroidism). Whether medical conditions are under control with or without treatment will be assessed on an individual basis by the investigator based on her medical and clinical expertise.
12. Subjects with self-reported active hepatitis, immune deficiency, HIV, or autoimmune disease.
13. Subjects having a known active dermatologic condition of the scalp that may place the subject at a greater risk or interfere with clinical evaluations (i.e., seborrheic dermatitis, psoriasis, atopic dermatitis, advanced skin cancer) as determined by the investigator based on her medical and clinical expertise.
14. Subjects who are unable to communicate or cooperate with the investigator due to language problems, poor mental development, or impaired cerebral function.
15. Subjects with any underlying disease that the investigator deems uncontrolled and poses a concern for the subject's safety while participating in the study.
16. Subjects with use of any medications that are known to potentially cause hair loss or affect hair growth as determined by the investigator based on her medical and clinical expertise.

Ages Eligible for Study
18–65 years (adult, older adult)
Sexes Eligible for Study
All
Accepts Healthy Volunteers
Yes
Design Details
Primary purpose: treatment
Allocation: N/A
Interventional model: single group assignment
Interventional model description: open-label study evaluating the efficacy and safety
Masking: none (open label)
Masking description: open-label study evaluating the efficacy and safety

Arms and Interventions

Participant group/arm	Intervention/treatment
Other: BENEV Exosome Regenerative Complex+ BENEV Exosome Regenerative Complex+® post SylFirmX® RF microneedling procedure applied to the scalp monthly for 4 sessions	Other: BENEV Exosome Regenerative Complex+ BENEV Exosome Regenerative Complex+® is an intensive dual-action complex formulated to absorb quickly into the skin and scalp delivering the concentrated power of stem cell-derived lyophilized exosomes, potent growth factors, peptides, coenzymes, minerals, amino acids, and vitamins

Primary Outcome Measures

Outcome measure	Measure description	Time frame
Change in terminal hair counts	Terminal hair is defined as coarse hair, short or long, found on the scalp with minimum cross-sectional diameter of 40 micrometers. This is calculated by the Canfield HairMetrix System	Baseline to day 120 or end of study visit
Change in vellus hair counts	Vellus hair is defined as fine, short hairs found on the scalp with maximum cross-sectional diameter of 40 micrometers. This is calculated by the Canfield HairMetrix System	Baseline to day 120 or end of study visit
Change in total hair counts	Total hairs equal the sum of terminal and vellus hairs in the target area. This is calculated by the Canfield HairMetrix System	Baseline to day 120 or end of study visit

Secondary Outcome Measures

Outcome measure	Measure description	Time frame
Change in terminal to vellus hair count ratio	Terminal hair is defined as coarse hair, short or long, found on the scalp with minimum cross-sectional diameter of 40 micrometers. Vellus hair is defined as fine, short hairs found on the scalp with maximum cross-sectional diameter of 40 micrometers. This ratio is calculated by the Canfield HairMetrix System	Baseline to day 120 or end of study visit
Change in average hairs per follicular unit	This is the average number of hairs measured in each follicular unit. This is calculated by the Canfield HairMetrix System	Baseline to day 120 or end of study visit
Change in average hair width	This is the average hair width calculated in micrometers by the Canfield HairMetrix System	Baseline to day 120 or end of study visit
Change in follicular hair units per cm2	This is the number of follicles per cm2 measured by the Canfield HairMetrix System	Baseline to day 120 or end of study visit

(continued)

Outcome measure	Measure description	Time frame
Change in interfollicular hair mean distance	This is the distance between hair follicles measured in millimeters by the Canfield HairMetrix System	Baseline to day 120 or end of study visit
Change in Investigator Hair Growth Global Improvement Scale	The treating investigator will complete this assessment by circling the number on the scale that corresponds to the description that best fits the current global growth improvement at delineated visits as indicated in the schedule of events, compared to baseline. The investigator will complete this assessment during the study at visits 2, 3, 4, and 5. The investigator must complete this assessment using global photographs obtained compared to baseline. In addition, the investigator may use their clinical judgment from the in-person visit. 3 greatly worsened 2 moderately worsened 1 slightly worsened. 0 no change 1 slightly improved 2 moderately improved 3 greatly improved	Baseline to day 120 or end of study visit
Change in Investigator Hair Quality Global Improvement Scale	The treating investigator will complete this assessment by circling the number on the scale that corresponds to the description that best fits the current hair quality at delineated visits as indicated in the schedule of events, as compared to the subject's hair quality at baseline. Assessment grading is to be based upon the Investigator's appraisal of hair brittleness, dryness, texture, shine, scalp coverage, and overall appearance. The investigator will complete this assessment during the study at visits 2, 3, 4, and 5. The investigator must complete this assessment using global photographs obtained compared to baseline. In addition, the investigator may use their clinical judgment from the in-person visit. 3 greatly worsened 2 moderately worsened 1 slightly worsened 0 no change 1 slightly improved 2 moderately improved 3 greatly improved	Baseline to day 120 or end of study visit
Change in Hair Shedding Pull Test scores	The hair pull test will be performed by the investigator to evaluate hair shedding. In the hair pull test, gentle traction will be applied on a group of hairs (approximately 60 hairs) from proximal to distal end, in the vertex area, both parietal and occipital areas of the scalp. The grasp is made with the help of the thumb, index finger, and middle finger, ensuring consistent pressure with each pull. If more than 10% (~6 or more) hairs come out with every pull, the test is considered positive. Subjects will be Instructed not to shampoo or wash their hair 24 hours prior to the test for accurate results	Baseline to day 120 or end of study visit

(continued)

Outcome measure	Measure description	Time frame
Change in Subject Hair Self-Assessment Questionnaire scores	This scale is used to rate the qualities listed below: 1. Greatly decreased/worsened 2. Moderately decreased/worsened 3. Slightly decreased/worsened 4. No change 5. Slightly increased/improved 6. Moderately increased/improved 7. Greatly increased/improved Overall hair growth. Overall hair volume. Scalp coverage. Hair thickness. Hair fullness. Hair quality. Hair shine. Hair strength. Hair softness. Amount of noticeable new. Hair growth rate. Hair growth on top of your head (scalp coverage). Hair growth of the hairline (at the front of your head or hairline coverage). Hair length (ability to grow longer than usual) Ease of styling. Overall hair appearance. Nail strength. Nail growth rate. Growth of eyebrow. Hair growth of eyelashes. Skin smoothness. Overall skin health	Baseline to day 120 or end of study visit
Change in Hair Treatment Subject Satisfaction Questionnaire scores	1. How satisfied are you with this treatment for your thinning hair? 5 = very satisfied, 4 = satisfied, 3 = neutral, 2 = dissatisfied, 1 = very dissatisfied 2. How satisfied are you with the overall health of your hair after this treatment? 5 = very satisfied, 4 = satisfied, 3 = neutral, 2 = dissatisfied, 1 = very dissatisfied 3. Overall, how satisfied are you with the ease of this treatment? 5 = very satisfied, 4 = satisfied, 3 = neutral, 2 = dissatisfied, 1 = very dissatisfied 4. Overall, now that you have tried this treatment and completed the study, how likely are you to continue the treatment in the future? 5 = very likely, 4 = somewhat likely, 3 = neutral, 2 = somewhat unlikely, 1 = very unlikely 5. Overall, how likely are you to recommend this treatment to a family member or friend? 5 = very likely, 4 = somewhat likely, 3 = neutral, 2 = somewhat unlikely, 1 = very unlikely	Baseline to day 120 or end of study visit

Other outcome measures

Outcome measure	Measure description	Time frame
Frequency of both local and systemic adverse events	An adverse event is any adverse change from the subject's baseline condition, i.e., any subjective signs and symptoms, or change in a concomitant disease present at the screening visit. This includes intercurrent signs, symptoms, illness, and significant deviations from baseline which may occur during the course of the clinical study, whether considered related to treatment or not	Baseline to day 120 or end of study visit

(continued)

Outcome measure	Measure description	Time frame
Changes in clinical laboratory analyses of complete blood count without differential and with platelets	Number of participants with abnormal clinical laboratory analyses of complete blood count with differential and with platelets panel (this is a single blood panel). The analyses will be conducted on blood samples collected from subjects at baseline and day 120 visits. All results will be reported, including results that are abnormal. The complete blood count with differential and with platelets panel (single blood panel) contains the following tests: WBC, RBC, hemoglobin, hematocrit, MCV, MCH, MCHC, RDW, platelets	Baseline to day 120 or end of study visit
Change in clinical laboratory analyses of complete metabolic panel	Number of participants with abnormal clinical laboratory analyses of complete metabolic panel (this is a single blood panel). The analyses will be conducted on blood samples collected from subjects at baseline and day 120 visits. All results will be reported, including results that are abnormal. The complete metabolic panel includes the following tests: alkaline phosphatase(ALP), alanine aminotransferase (ALT), aspartate aminotransferase (AST), bilirubin, blood urea nitrogen (BUN), creatinine, sodium, potassium, carbon dioxide, chloride, albumin, total protein, glucose, and calcium	Baseline to day 120 or end of study visit

Sponsor
Ablon Skin Institute Research Center
Collaborators

- Benev Company, Inc.

Not Yet Recruiting

2. Efficacy and Safety of AGE ZERO™ EXOSOMES to Treat Men and Women with Androgenetic Alopecia

ClinicalTrials.gov ID NCT06482541
Sponsor Levit Dermatology
Information provided by Levit Dermatology (Responsible Party)
Last Update Posted 2024-07-16
Study Overview
Brief Summary

The purpose of this study is to determine whether Wharton's Jelly mesenchymal stem cell-derived exosome microneedling on the scalp is an effective treatment for androgenetic alopecia (pattern hair loss).

Detailed Description

After being informed about the study and potential risks, all participants who give written consent and meet the later discussed inclusion criteria and don't fall under the exclusion criteria will be enrolled in the study.

The investigators will conduct a double-blinded placebo-controlled study to test whether Wharton's jelly mesenchymal stem cell-derived exosome (WJMSC-exosome) application with microneedling is an effective treatment for androgenetic alopecia. Participants will be broken down into a 5 billion exosome group versus saline group and a 50 billion exosome versus saline group.

Treatment will be applied to the following treatment area: two rectangles on the scalp vertex each measuring 4cm on the sagittal plane by 2cm on the coronal plane. One rectangle will be 2.0 mm left of the midline of the scalp, and another will be 2.0 mm right of the midline of the scalp. Each treatment area will be divided into an anterior and posterior half with 1 permanent microdot tattoo in the middle (4 tattoos in total). The microdot tattoo (composed of iron oxide, glycerol, alcohol, and distilled water and red, D&C Red #30, glycerol, alcohol, and distilled water) will allow HairMetrix® by Canfield, an AI-driven hair consultation device, to accurately and reproducibly access changes in hair growth in the treatment areas.

Participants in the 5 billion exosome group will receive topical applications of 5 billion WJMSC exosomes on one side of the treatment area and an equal volume of placebo (an identically looking saline solution) application on the opposite side of the treatment area.

The 50 billion exosome group will receive topical applications of 50 billion WJMSC exosomes on one side of the treatment area and an equal volume of placebo application on the opposite side of the treatment area.

Immediately after topical application, all participants will receive microneedling at a depth of .5 mm on the entire treatment area.

Treatment will be administered in 4 sessions, monthly for the first three months and for a 4th time 4 months after the third session.

The study will go on for 12 months from the date of the first treatment. Participant's changes in hair growth (hair count, hair thickness, and hair color) and adverse events will be evaluated and recorded.

Official Title

1-Year Double-Blinded Placebo-Controlled Study to Evaluate the Effect of AGE ZERO™ EXOSOMES on Hair Regrowth in Healthy Men and Women with Androgenetic Alopecia

Conditions

Androgenetic alopecia

Intervention/Treatment

- Combination product: 5 billion exosomes and saline solution microneedling
- Combination product: 50 billion exosomes and saline solution microneedling

Other Study ID Numbers

- 2023-06-001

Study Start (Estimated)

2024-07

Primary Completion (Estimated)

2025-07

Study Completion (Estimated)

2025-08

Enrollment (Estimated)

100

Study Type

Interventional
Phase
Phase 1
Study Contact
Name: Eyal K Levit, M.D.
Phone Number: 917-868-5112
Email: eyallevit@gmail.com
Study Contact Backup
Name: Nicholas L Gitsin
Phone Number: 347-932-9894
Email: nicholasgitsin8a@gmail.com
This study has 1 location
United States
New York Locations
Brooklyn, New York, United States, 11235
Levit Dermatology
Contact:
Eyal K Levit, MD917-868-5112 eyallevit@gmail.com
Contact:
Nicholas L Gitsin347-932-9894 nicholasgitsin8a@gmail.com
Principal Investigator:
Eyal K Levit, M.D.
Eligibility Criteria
Description
Inclusion Criteria:

- Participant is experiencing hair loss and is diagnosed with androgenetic alopecia.

Exclusion Criteria:

- Patients cannot have taken any medications, therapies, or treatment modalities of any kind to treat hair loss in the last six months.
- Patients cannot have open wounds, eczema, or psoriatic plaques on the treatment area of the scalp.
- Patients who are undergoing or have undergone chemotherapy and/or radiation therapy within the past 6 months.
- Patients with a history of an autoimmune bullous disorder (having autoantibodies to Dsg-1 or Dsg-3).
- Patients who are currently immunocompromised or have a low white count making patients prone to infections.

Ages Eligible for Study
18 years and older (adult, older adult)
Sexes Eligible for Study
All
Accepts Healthy Volunteers
Yes

Design Details

Primary purpose: treatment

Allocation: randomized

Interventional model: single group assignment

Interventional Model Description: Participants will act as their own control. Each participant will get exosome treatment on one half of the treatment area and placebo on the other half of the treatment area. The treatment area will be two rectangles each measuring 4cm on the sagittal plane by 2cm on the coronal plane on the scalp vertex. One rectangle will be 2.0 mm left of the midline of the scalp, and another will be 2.0 mm right of the midline of the scalp. Participants in the 5 billion exosome group will receive 5 billion WJMSC-exosome treatment on one side of the treatment area and an equivalent volume of saline on the other side of the treatment area. Participants in the 50 billion exosome group will receive 5 billion WJMSC-exosome treatment on one side of the treatment area and an equivalent volume of placebo on the other side of the treatment area.

Masking: quadruple (Participants, Care Provider, Investigator Outcomes, Assessor)

Arms and Interventions

Participant group/arm	Intervention/treatment
Experimental: 5 billion exosome group This arm receives 5 billion WJMSC-exosome treatment on one side of the aforementioned treatment area and an equivalent volume of placebo on the contralateral half of the treatment area	Combination product: 5 billion exosomes and saline solution microneedling Participants will receive 5 billion WJMSC-exosome topical application on one half of the treatment area and an equivalent volume of saline solution on the contralateral half of the treatment area. Microneedling at a depth of .5mm on the entire treatment area will immediately follow the exosome and saline application. Participants will also receive 4 permanent microdot tattoos on the aforementioned locations
Experimental: 50 billion exosome group This arm receives 50 billion WJMSC-exosome treatment on one half of the aforementioned treatment area and an equivalent volume of placebo on the contralateral half of the treatment area	Combination product: 50 billion exosomes and saline solution microneedling Participants will receive 50 billion WJMSC-exosome topical application on one half of the treatment area and an equivalent volume of saline solution on the contralateral half of the treatment area. Microneedling at a depth of .5mm on the entire treatment area will immediately follow the exosome and saline application. Participants will also receive 4 permanent microdot tattoos on the aforementioned locations

Primary Outcome Measures

Outcome measure	Measure description	Time frame
Hair count	Evaluated by HairMetrix® by Canfield, an AI-driven hair consultation device	Evaluated on monthly visits for a year

(continued)

Outcome measure	Measure description	Time frame
Hair thickness	Evaluated by HairMetrix® by Canfield, an AI-driven hair consultation device	Evaluated on monthly visits for a year
Hair color	Evaluated by HairMetrix® by Canfield, an AI-driven hair consultation device	Evaluated on monthly visits for a year

Secondary Outcome Measures

Outcome measure	Measure description	Time frame
Adverse events	Patients will self-report adverse events on a questionnaire on a scale of 1–10, with 1 being minimal discomfort and 10 being worst discomfort ever experienced	Participants will self-report adverse events during monthly visits for the entire 1-year duration
Self-reported hair changes	Patients will self-report impressions of hair growth changes on each treatment area on a scale of -10 to 10, with -10 being extreme worsening of hair loss and 10 being extreme regrowth. Patients will scale impressions of hair thickness, hair density, hair color, hair growth speed, hair texture, and overall satisfaction with therapy applied to each treatment area	Patients will self-report on questionnaire during monthly visits for the entire 1-year duration

Sponsor
Levit Dermatology
Collaborators

- ResilielleTM Age ZeroTM Exosomes
- Dorisca Research Consulting, LLC

Investigators

- Principal Investigator: Eyal K Levit, M.D., Owner and chief physician

Active, Not Recruiting

3. Umbilical Cord-Derived Mesenchymal Stem Cell Exosomes on Hair Growth in Patients with Androgenetic Alopecia

ClinicalTrials.gov ID NCT06697080
Sponsor Nanfang Hospital, Southern Medical University
Information provided by Nanfang Hospital, Southern Medical University (Responsible Party)
Last Update Posted 2024-11-20
Study Overview
Brief Summary
A total of 50 patients with androgenetic alopecia were selected for the study. Patients who met the inclusion/exclusion criteria were randomly assigned to groups A and B in a 1:1 ratio to receive treatment, with the enrollment date designated as Day 1. Group A visited the clinic once each in the first, second, and third months for

treatment with exosomes, while Group B visited the clinic twice each in the first, second, and third months for treatment with exosomes. At the time points of 1, 2, 3, and 6 months after the start of the treatment period, dermatoscopic examinations were conducted on patients in both groups. The differences in hair growth density, hair shaft thickness, and follicle counts within a 1 cm diameter area were compared between the two groups. Additionally, the data differences for each subject at baseline and at the end of the experiment were also assessed.

Official Title

A Randomized Controlled Clinical Trial to Treat Chinese Advanced AGA with Umbilical Cord-Derived Mesenchymal Stem Cell Exosomes

Conditions

Androgenic alopecia

Intervention/Treatment

- Drug: human umbilical cord mesenchymal stem cells

Other Study ID Numbers

- NFEC-2024-323

Study Start (Actual)

2024-06-28

Primary Completion (Actual)

2024-09-28

Study Completion (Estimated)

2024-12-28

Enrollment (Actual)

50

Study Type

Interventional

Phase

Not Applicable

This study has 1 location

China

Guangdong Locations

Guangzhou, Guangdong, China

Department of Plastic and Aesthetic Surgery, Nanfang Hospital Southern Medical University

Eligibility Criteria

Description

Inclusion Criteria: clinical diagnosis of androgenic alopecia. AGA classification: the no grade for male hair loss was II–V and the Ludwig grade for female hair loss was I–III.

Exclusion Criteria: (1) using medications or supplements, including finasteride, dutasteride, minoxidil, or any other hormonal products, which can affect hair growth; (2) patients with severe diseases, immune diseases, endocrine diseases, and nervous system diseases; and (3) patients with infection, allergic disease, and malignant tumor

Ages Eligible for Study
18–50 years (adult)
Sexes Eligible for Study
All
Accepts Healthy Volunteers
Yes
Study Plan
Design Details
Primary purpose: diagnostic
Allocation: randomized
Interventional model: parallel assignment
Masking: triple (ParticipantCare ProviderInvestigator)

Arms and Interventions

Participant group/arm	Intervention/treatment
Experimental: group A Group A visited the clinic once each in the first, second, and third months for treatment with exosomes	Drug: human umbilical cord mesenchymal stem cells Human umbilical cord mesenchymal stem cells
Experimental: group B Group B visited the clinic twice each in the first, second, and third months for treatment with exosomes	Drug: human umbilical cord mesenchymal stem cells Human umbilical cord mesenchymal stem cells

Primary Outcome Measures

Outcome measure	Measure description	Time frame
Hair diameters changed over time	Hair diameters changed over time	0 days, 1 month, 3 months, 6 months

Sponsor
Nanfang Hospital, Southern Medical University

Healthy

Active, Not Recruiting
Effect of Acute Exercise on Exosome-Associated Biomarkers
ClinicalTrials.gov ID NCT05541133
Sponsor Mayo Clinic
Information provided by K. Sreekumaran Nair, Mayo Clinic (Responsible Party)
Last Update Posted 2024-07-24
Study Overview

Brief Summary

This research study is being done to understand the underlying mechanism by which exercise affects the body on the cellular level, in an acute aerobic endurance setting. This may help to better understand the overall benefits of endurance exercise.

Official Title

Effect of Acute Exercise on Exosome-Associated Biomarkers

Conditions

Healthy

Other Study ID Numbers

- 22-000001

Study Start (Actual)

2022-06-21

Primary Completion (Actual)

2022-07-09

Study Completion (Estimated)

2024-12-31

Enrollment (Estimated)

12

Study Type

Observational

This study has 1 location

United States

Minnesota Locations

Rochester, Minnesota, United States, 55905

Mayo Clinic in Rochester

Eligibility Criteria

Description

Inclusion Criteria:

- Ages: 18–45 years

Exclusion Criteria:

- BMI >32 kg/m2. Cardiovascular, metabolic (type 2 diabetes, fasting plasma glucose at or above 110 mg/dL, and untreated hypo- or hyperthyroidism), or renal disease
- Orthopedic problems that would keep them from being able to perform an exercise
- Medications that are known to affect mitochondrial function: corticosteroids, opiates, benzodiazepines, tricyclic antidepressants, beta-blockers, sulfonylureas, insulin, anticoagulants, barbiturates, insulin sensitizers, fibrates (PPAR gamma agonist)
- Smoking
- Pregnancy

Study Population

Generally healthy individuals around the Rochester MN area.
Ages Eligible for Study
18–45 years (adult)
Sexes Eligible for Study
All
Accepts Healthy Volunteers
Yes
Sampling Method
Non-probability sample
Design Details
Observational model: cohort
Time perspective: prospective
Biospecimen retention: samples without DNA
Biospecimen description: blood samples collected before, during, and after acute exercise

Primary Outcome Measures

Outcome measure	Measure description	Time frame
List of biomarkers	Exosome proteomes and MiRNA from blood samples	Baseline

Sponsor
Mayo Clinic
Investigators

- Principal investigator: K. Sreekumaran Nair, MD, PhD, Mayo Clinic

Hypercholesterolemia

Not Yet Recruiting
Exosome-Based Nanoplatform for Ldlr mRNA Delivery in FH (ENDFH)
ClinicalTrials.gov ID NCT05043181
Sponsor Tang-Du Hospital
Information provided by Lijun Yuan, MD, PhD, Tang-Du Hospital (Responsible Party)
Last Update Posted 2021-09-14
Study Overview
Brief Summary
mRNA therapy is a highly promising gene therapeutic strategy in the treatment of homozygous familial hypercholesterolemia (HoFH). Exosomes are safe and efficient carriers for mRNA drug delivery, due to their biocompatibility and bioavailability. This first-in-human study is aimed to evaluate the safety and preliminary effectiveness of exosome-based ldlr mRNA nanoplatform for gene therapy in HoFH.

Detailed Description

Familial hypercholesterolemia (FH) is an autosomal dominant genetic disease characterized by severely elevated plasma low-density lipoprotein (LDL) cholesterol (LDL-C) and premature coronary heart disease. Most of FH patients (about 95% of cases) are attributed to functional loss mutation of the LDL receptor (LDLR) gene. The prevalence of the heterozygous mutations in LDLR has been estimated at 1 in 200 to 1 in 500 in the population and the homozygous form in 1 in 100000 individuals. As a key lipoprotein receptor on the surface of hepatocyte, the LDLR is critical for liver clearing LDL-C from the circulation. By endocytosis and further processing of the LDL-C, LDLR is responsible for removing most excess LDL-C from the serum, and there are no substitutes in vivo. These heterozygotes (HeFH) typically have twice the normal plasma LDL levels and cardiovascular diseases at an earlier age. Homozygous individuals (HoFH) face much higher LDL-C levels and often die before the age of 20 years if untreated. Although existing therapeutics, such as statins, ezetimibe, and PCSK9 inhibitors, have some beneficial effects on HeFH, few drugs have therapeutic effects on HoFH even at high doses. Lipid apheresis and liver transplantation are the current clinical managements to reduce the LDL-C level, while gene therapy holds the promise.

Exosomes are small intracellular vesicles ranging in 30–150 nm size and have an important role in cell-cell communication. Many studies show that exosome can efficiently deliver cargos, such as mRNA, miRNA, and even plasmid DNA, to target cells, emerging as a promising therapeutic carrier for gene therapy. Compared with virus, exosomes, as "natural nanoparticles," are easy to handle, non-cytotoxic, and non-immunogenic. It is thus promising to develop exosome-based LDLR-gene delivery strategy and explore the therapeutic effects on HoFH.

In this study, an Ldlr-expressing virus vector will be constructed to generate Ldlr mRNA-enriched exosomes. To meet the standards of clinical trials, we will use the GMP-grade compliant normal donor bone marrow-derived MSCs to produce exosomes. Exosomes will be enriched by filtration and ultracentrifugation and then normalized by Nanosight, electron microscopy, and key exosome biomarkers. In order to ensure the safety of patients, we plan to inject exosomes through abdominal puncture under ultrasound guidance and purchase medical insurance for patients. This first-in-human study is aimed to evaluate the safety of this exosome product for gene therapy and preliminary evidence of efficacy using plasma LDL-C levels as a surrogate biomarker. The study is promising to provide a new therapeutic approach for the treatment of homozygous familial hypercholesterolemia patients.

Official Title

Exosome-Based Nanoplatform for Ldlr mRNA Delivery in Familial Hypercholesterolemia

Conditions

Familial hypercholesterolemia

Intervention/Treatment

- Biological: low-density lipoprotein receptor mRNA exosomes

Other Study ID Numbers

- 20210817V2.0

  Study Start (Estimated)
  2021-12
  Primary Completion (Estimated)
  2026-12
  Study Completion (Estimated)
  2026-12
  Enrollment (Estimated)
  30
  Study Type
  Interventional
  Phase
  Phase 1
  Study Contact
  Name: Zhelong Li
  Phone Number: 13319189556
  Email: lzlfmmu@foxmail.com
  Study Contact Backup
  Name: Changyang Xing
  Phone Number: 13571864787
  Email: xingcy712@163.com
  This study has 1 location
  China
  Shannxi Locations
  Xi'an, Shannxi, China, 710038
  Tangdu Hospital, Air Force Medical University
  Eligibility Criteria
  Description
  Inclusion Criteria:

1. Age 18–45 years, no gender limitation
2. Patients with homozygous familial hypercholesterolemia diagnosed by genetic testing
3. Understand the study and be willing to participate in the study with the informed consent signed

Exclusion Criteria:

1. Those who have severe comorbidities, including any of the following: A) unstable angina pectoris and/or congestive heart failure requiring hospitalization; B) myocardial infarction or cerebrovascular accident within the last 6 months; C) chronic obstructive pulmonary disease worsening or requiring hospitalization; D) serious diseases of vascular, nervous system, blood, gastrointestinal and endocrine systems, or metabolic disorders; E) autoimmune/immune deficiency diseases such as rheumatoid arthritis, acquired immune and deficiency syndrome; and F) malignant tumor or other chronic infection.

2. Those who previously received targeted drug therapy, cell therapy, gene therapy, or other immunotherapy.
3. Those who had organ transplants in the past.
4. Any of the following abnormalities are found in the laboratory examination: A) blood routine examination, absolute neutrophil count (ANC) <1.5×109/L, or platelet (PLT) <50×109/L, or hemoglobin (HGB) <80 g/dL; B) coagulation function, prothrombin time (PT), or activated partial thrombin time (APTT), or INR >1.5×ULN; C) liver function, total bilirubin (TBIL) >2×ULN (upper limit of normal value), or alanine transferase (ALT), aspartate transferase (AST), or alkaline phosphatase (ALP) >5×ULN; D) renal function, serum creatinine (Cr) ≥1.5×ULN or glomerular filtration rate (GFR) <60 mL/min·1.73m2; E) cardiac ultrasound. left ventricular ejection fraction (LVEF) <50%.
5. Those who are known or expected to have an allergic reaction to or have a history of allergic reaction to any of the ingredients treated by this test.
6. Those who have a history of contrast agent allergic.
7. Those who have a clear history of mental disorders in the past.
8. Those who have a history of drug abuse or drug use.
9. Pregnant or lactating women.
10. Women of childbearing age and fertile men cannot take effective and adequate contraceptive measures (such as intrauterine device (IUD), condom, spermicidal gel plus condom, uterine cap) during the period of receiving the study drug and 3 months after the end of the study.
11. Those who participated in the clinical study of other drugs within 3 months before joining the group.
12. Subjects that are not suitable to participate in this study for other reasons judged by the investigators.

Ages Eligible for Study
18–45 years (adult)
Sexes Eligible for Study
All
Accepts Healthy Volunteers
No
Design Details
Primary purpose: treatment
Allocation: N/A
Interventional model: single group assignment
Masking: none (open label)

Arms and Interventions

Participant group/arm	Intervention/treatment
Experimental: homozygous familial hypercholesterolemia	Biological: low-density lipoprotein receptor mRNA exosomes The study consists of two phases: dose-escalation phase and extension phase. Dose-escalation phase: for the intervention of low-density lipoprotein receptor mRNA (LDLR mRNA) exosomes. A total of six dose groups are planned, with a single dose of 0.044 mg/kg, 0.088 mg/kg, 0.145 mg/kg, 0.220 mg/kg, 0.295 mg/kg, and 0.394 mg/kg, respectively. About 3 subjects are enrolled in each dose group. In the 0.044 mg/kg group, the second and third subjects are required to start exosome infusion treatment after the treatment of the previous subjects, and the other dose groups are not required to do this. There are three treatments in total, and the interval between each exosome treatment is 7±1 d Extension phase: about 12 subjects are further enrolled. The subjects will receive 3 intravenous/peritoneal infusion treatment of LDLR mRNA exosomes once a week for three weeks, whose single dose is determined in the dose-escalation phase

Primary Outcome Measures

Outcome measure	Measure description	Time frame
Changes of total cholesterol	mmol/L	Changes from baseline total cholesterol at day 19
Changes of low-density lipoprotein cholesterol	mmol/L	Changes from baseline low-density lipoprotein cholesterol at day 19
Changes of high-density lipoprotein cholesterol	mmol/L	Changes from baseline high-density lipoprotein cholesterol at day 19
Changes of triglyceride	mmol/L	Changes from baseline triglyceride at day 19

Secondary Outcome Measures

Outcome measure	Measure description	Time frame
Changes of degree of coronary stenosis	% determined by coronary CT	Changes from baseline degree of coronary stenosis at day 28
Changes of volume of carotid artery plaques	cm3 determined by ultrasound	Changes from baseline volume of carotid artery plaques at day 28
Changes of stability of carotid artery plaques	Grade I, II, III determined by ultrasound	Changes from baseline stability of carotid artery plaques at day 28

Sponsor
Tang-Du Hospital
Collaborators

- Air Force Military Medical University, China

  Investigators

- Principal investigator: Lijun Yuan, Tangdu Hospital, Air Force Medical University

Metabolism

Active, Not Recruiting

Training-Induced Muscle Exosome Release (TIMER)

ClinicalTrials.gov ID NCT04500769

Sponsor Yuan Wen

Information provided by Yuan Wen, University of Kentucky (Responsible Party)

Last Update Posted 2024-12-10

Study Overview

Brief Summary

The primary objective of this study is to quantify miR-1 release from muscle in extracellular vesicles following an acute resistance exercise bout and potential delivery to subcutaneous adipose tissue in young healthy and obese adults.

Detailed Description

Numerous studies in humans and animals have shown that aerobic exercise is beneficial to adipose tissue function and whole-body metabolism. Both acute and chronic aerobic exercises enhance adipocyte catecholamine sensitivity in humans and animals. Although relatively few studies have investigated whether adipose adrenergic signaling is affected by resistance exercise (RE), it is known that a single bout of RE can increase circulating NEFA and resting energy expenditure and decrease respiratory quotient for up to 24 hours, indicative of increased adipocyte lipolysis and muscle fatty acid oxidation. Furthermore, the lipolytic response to RE is impaired in obese men. Using synergist ablation, a model of RE in mice, the investigators show that adipose transcriptional responses are exosome dependent and that serum exosomes enhance adipocyte catecholamine sensitivity and lipolysis for at least 24 hours. To the investigator's knowledge, this is the first demonstration of a potential mechanism whereby RE imparts metabolic adaptations in adipose. Since adipose metabolic function is crucial for determining whole-body metabolic outcomes, the ability of RE-induced exosomes to improve adipose metabolism has significant clinical implications.

Official Title

Muscle-Derived Extracellular Vesicles and Their Interactions with Adipocytes in Human Metabolic Dysfunction

Conditions

Metabolism

Intervention/Treatment

- Behavioral: acute resistance exercise

Other Study ID Numbers

- 43910
- 3R01DK119619-02S1 (U.S. NIH Grant/Contract)

Study Start (Actual)
2019-03-14
Primary Completion (Estimated)
2025-11-30
Study Completion (Estimated)
2026-11-30
Enrollment (Actual)
38
Study Type
Interventional
Phase
Not Applicable
This study has 1 location
United States
Kentucky Locations
Lexington, Kentucky, United States, 40536
University of Kentucky
Eligibility Criteria
Description
Inclusion Criteria:

- 18–30 years of age
- Either BMI <25 or >30
- Relatively sedentary, reporting no participation in regular (>1 day per week) exercise for at least the past 3 months
- Non-smoker

Exclusion Criteria:

- BMI between 25 and 30
- Evidence or signs and symptoms for cardiovascular disease (previous heart attack, arrhythmias, angina, shortness of breath, extreme fatigue, unusual pain in neck, jaw, throat, upper abdomen, or back, swelling in feet, legs, or ankles)
- Evidence or signs and symptoms of metabolic syndrome or disorder (diagnosis of diabetes or insulin resistance, elevated BP, high fasting blood sugar, abnormal cholesterol or triglyceride levels)
- Chronic aspirin or NSAID use (unless it can be safely stopped prior to the biopsies), and any other use of an anticoagulant (e.g., Coumadin) or history of bleeding including history of hypo- or hypercoagulation disorders
- Neurological, musculoskeletal, or other disorder that would preclude safe participation in the weight lifting tasks and all performance tests

- Any other medical condition that would interfere with testing or increase one's risk of complications during exercise, as judged by the study physician
- Any other condition or events considered exclusionary by the PI and/or physician, such as noncompliance
- Lidocaine allergy (1% lidocaine is the local anesthetic used during the muscle biopsy procedure)
- Pregnancy

Ages Eligible for Study
18–30 years (adult)
Sexes Eligible for Study
All
Accepts Healthy Volunteers
Yes
Study Plan
Design Details
Primary purpose: supportive care
Allocation: N/A
Interventional model: single group assignment
Masking: none (open label)

Arms and Interventions

Participant group/arm	Intervention/treatment
Experimental: acute resistance exercise Participants will perform four exercises: squat, knee extension, leg press, and lat pulldown at 80% of 1-RM determined during a previous visit	Behavioral: acute resistance exercise Participants will perform three sets of eight repetitions, with a 90–120 second rest between sets, with a fourth set performed to failure. All resistance exercise will be performed on pneumatic resistance devices (Keiser Sports Health Equipment, Fresno, CA). Other names: Strength training

Primary Outcome Measures

Outcome measure	Measure description	Time frame
miR-1 abundance	Exosomal, muscle, and adipose miR-1 abundance will be quantified at baseline and following an acute bout of resistance exercise by qPCR	90 minutes

Sponsor
Yuan Wen
Collaborators

- National Institute of Diabetes and Digestive and Kidney Diseases (NIDDK)

Investigators

- Principal investigator: John McCarthy, Ph.D., University of Kentucky
- Principal investigator: Yuan Wen, Ph.D., University of Kentucky

Neurodevelopmental

Not Yet Recruiting

The Pilot Experimental Study of the Neuroprotective Effects of Exosomes in Extremely Low Birth Weight Infants

ClinicalTrials.gov ID NCT05490173

Sponsor Federal State Budget Institution Research Center for Obstetrics, Gynecology and Perinatology Ministry of Healthcare

Information provided by Federal State Budget Institution Research Center for Obstetrics, Gynecology and Perinatology Ministry of Healthcare (Responsible Party)

Last Update Posted 2022-09-28

Study Overview

Brief Summary

To study the safety and efficacy of intranasal administration of exosomes derived from mesenchymal stromal cells on long-term neurodevelopmental outcome in extremely low birth weight infants born at gestational age 25/0–27/6 weeks.

Detailed Description

Surviving extremely low birth weight (ELBW) infants are at risk of severe neurodevelopmental disability. Exosomes or extracellular vesicles (EVs) derived from mesenchymal stromal cells (MSCs) can mediate a variety of different effects, including synaptic plasticity, nutritional metabolic support, nerve regeneration, inflammatory response, anti-stress effect, cellular waste disposal, treating neurological injury, preventing hemorrhagic and ischemic brain lesions, playing an important role in health, and neuroprotection in extremely premature newborns during neonatal intensive care.

The proposed blinded randomized controlled trial was designed to compare the effect of intranasal administration of exosomes on long-term neurodevelopmental outcome in ELBW infants.

ELBW infants will be randomized to receive (group 1) and not receive exosomes (control group).

Group 1: Neonates will receive exosomes (1 dose will be obtained from a daily conditioned culture medium of 120 million MSCs) suspended in 500 μl of phosphate buffer in each nostril at 50 μl with an interval of 2–3 minutes. The therapeutic course will consist of 5 instillations with an interval of 1 days.

The primary outcome measure is the incidence of death, the incidence of survival with any of either severe intraventricular hemorrhage (IVH), cystic periventricular leukomalacia (PVL), or brain injury on cranial ultrasound and MRI or major neurodevelopmental impairment determined at 36 months of age corrected for prematurity (where major neurodevelopmental impairment is defined as any of the following: cognitive deficit, cerebral palsy, or severe visual or hearing impairment. Cognitive delay is defined as mental developmental index (MDI) score on the Griffiths-II and Bayley Scales of Infant Development (2nd edition) < 85, cerebral palsy, or severe visual or hearing impairment.

To investigate these outcomes and the mechanisms by which extracellular vesicles (EVs) might affect, we will analyze the biomarkers of perinatal brain injury (S-100, NSE, EPO) and mRNA.

Key secondary outcomes are incidences of short-term outcomes: individual components of the composite primary outcome, survival with and without major neonatal morbidity including severe retinopathy of prematurity (ROP), bronchopulmonary dysplasia (BPD), and necrotizing enterocolitis (NEC).

Safety analyses will assess the injures or damages of the nasal mucosa, allergic reaction to EVs, and any adverse events after intranasal administration of EVs.

The results of this trial may help to improve the quality of life of ELBW infants and reduce long-term healthcare costs.

Official Title

The Pilot Experimental Study of the Neuroprotective Effects of Exosomes in Extremely Low Birth Weight Infants

Conditions

Premature birth

Extreme prematurity

Preterm intraventricular hemorrhage

Hypoxia-ischemia, cerebral

Neurodevelopmental disorders

Intervention/Treatment

- Other: exosomes derived from mesenchymal stromal cells (MSCs)

Other Study ID Numbers

- ncagp4382277

Study Start (Estimated)

2022-10-05

Primary Completion (Estimated)

2026-05-22

Study Completion (Estimated)

2026-12-28

Enrollment (Estimated)

10

Study Type

Interventional

Phase

Not applicable

Study Contact

Name: Oleg Ionov, PhD, MD

Phone Number: +74954382277
Email: dr.ionov@hotmail.com
Study Contact Backup
Name: Diiana Sharafutdinova
Phone Number: +79859865567
Email: dikarush@gmail.com
This study has 1 location
Russian Federation
Moscow, Russian Federation, 117997
Federal State Budget Institution Research Center for Obstetrics, Gynecology and Perinatology Ministry of Healthcare
Contact:
Elena A Gorodnova, PhD+7 (495) 531-44-44 e_gorodnova@oparina4.ru
Contact:
Diiana Sharafutdinova+79859865567 dikarush@gmail.com
Principal Investigator:
Diiana RASHIDOVNA SHARAFUTDINOVA
Eligibility Criteria
Description
Inclusion Criteria:

- Premature newborns of gestational age (GA) 25/0–27/6 weeks

Exclusion Criteria:

- Missing written parental consent
- Damages to the nasal mucosa
- Maxillofacial defects
- Major congenital anomalies (including chromosomal aberrations, cyanotic congenital heart defects, syndromes likely affecting long-term outcome, and major congenital malformations requiring surgical correction during newborn period)
- Infants who died before 48 hours, infants in whom the clinical decision to withhold intensive care was made, and infants who were not considered viable
- Infants with edematous hemolytic disease of newborns and nonimmune fetal dropsy
- Multifetal gestations
- Participation in another study with ongoing use of an unlicensed investigational product from 28 days before study enrollment until the end of the study

Ages Eligible for Study
1–3 days (child)
Sexes Eligible for Study
All
Accepts Healthy Volunteers
No
Design Details
Primary purpose: prevention

Allocation: randomized

Interventional model: parallel assignment

Interventional Model Description: Participants (ELBW infants GA 25/0–27/6 weeks) are randomized to one of two groups in parallel for the duration of the study. The first group (exosome treatment group) will receive intranasal administration of exosomes, and the second (control group) will not receive exosomes. Patients in both groups will receive standard basic therapy.

Masking: single (participant)

Arms and Interventions

Participant group/arm	Intervention/treatment
Experimental: intranasal exosome administration ELWB newborns who will receive intranasal exosomes	Other: exosomes derived from mesenchymal stromal cells (MSCs) Exosomes derived from mesenchymal stromal cells (MSCs) will be administered intranasally in ELBW infants
No intervention: control ELWB newborns who will not receive intranasal exosomes	

Primary Outcome Measures

Outcome measure	Measure description	Time frame
Occurrence and rate of dose-limiting toxicity	Dose-limiting toxicity consists of the following events: Death occurring within 24 hours after intranasal administration of EVs. Hypersensitivity/anaphylactic to EVs defined as any severe systemic inflammatory response syndrome with negative blood culture not consistent with the overall clinical course of the infant occurring within 72 hours after intranasal administration of EVs. Any other serious adverse event not expected in this patient population for which there is no alternative explanation but the administration of EVs, occurring within 1 week of injection	Up to 1 week following after intranasal administration of EVs

Secondary Outcome Measures

Outcome measure	Measure description	Time frame
Rate of death	Rate of death until discharge or 40 weeks corrected gestational age, whichever comes first	From enrollment until discharge or 40 weeks corrected gestational age (whichever occurs first)

(continued)

Outcome measure	Measure description	Time frame
Occurrence of other severe complications of prematurity	Blood culture-proven sepsis Patent ductus arteriosus (treated medically or surgically) Necrotizing enterocolitis Isolated intestinal perforation Retinopathy of prematurity requiring treatment Severe intraventricular hemorrhage (≥ grade 3) Cystic periventricular leukomalacia Incidence and severity of BPD, measured as mild, moderate, or severe	From enrollment until discharge or 40 weeks corrected gestational age (whichever occurs first)
Need for ventilatory support	Time to extubation Duration of mechanical ventilation Duration of noninvasive positive pressure respiratory support Duration of supplemental oxygen	From enrollment until discharge, 40 weeks corrected gestational age, or death (whichever occurs first)
Changes in hemodynamics	Targeted neonatal echocardiography to assess	Time frame: at enrollment, 48 hours following intranasal administration of EVs, 28 days of life, and 36 weeks corrected gestational age
Feasibility: administration	Successful recruitment and administration of extracellular vesicles to 10 patients in 18 months	Day of life 1–10
Feasibility: recruitment efficiency	Proportion of potentially eligible patients that are successfully screened Proportion of participants successfully screened who do not enroll (reason for failure to enroll will be recorded)	Day of life 1–10
Feasibility: recruitment timing	Median time from screening to enrollment Median time from screening to extracellular vesicles	Day of life 1–10
Feasibility: participant retainment	Proportion of patients that do not complete administration of extracellular vesicles Proportion of patients enrolled that do not undergo scheduled follow-up	From enrollment until follow-up at 18–36 months of age
Griffiths-II and Bayley Scales of Infant Development (2nd edition)	Assessment of cognitive, language, and motor development. Cognitive delay defined as mental developmental index (MDI) score on the Griffiths-II and Bayley Scales of Infant Development (2nd edition) <85, cerebral palsy, or severe visual or hearing impairment	18–36 months of age
Long-term safety follow-up	Participant's overall health will be assessed through a questionnaire administered over the phone, once a year for 3 years	3 years following follow-up visit

Sponsor

Federal State Budget Institution Research Center for Obstetrics, Gynecology and Perinatology Ministry of Healthcare

Investigators

- Principal Investigator: Oleg Ionov, PhD, MD, National Medical Research Center For Obstetrics, Gynecology and Perinatology Named After Academician V.I. Kulakov
- Principal Investigator: Ekaterina Balashova, PhD, MD, National Medical Research Center For Obstetrics, Gynecology and Perinatology Named After Academician V.I. Kulakov
- Principal Investigator: Denis Silachev, PhD, MD, National Medical Research Center For Obstetrics, Gynecology and Perinatology Named After Academician V.I. Kulakov
- Principal Investigator: Anna Kirtbaya, PhD, MD, National Medical Research Center For Obstetrics, Gynecology and Perinatology Named After Academician V.I. Kulakov
- Principal Investigator: Victor Zubkov, PhD, MD, National Medical Research Center For Obstetrics, Gynecology and Perinatology Named After Academician V.I. Kulakov
- Principal Investigator: Dmitriy Degtyarev, PhD, MD, National Medical Research Center For Obstetrics, Gynecology and Perinatology Named After Academician V.I. Kulakov

Publications

- Ophelders DR, Wolfs TG, Jellema RK, Zwanenburg A, Andriessen P, Delhaas T, Ludwig AK, Radtke S, Peters V, Janssen L, Giebel B, Kramer BW. Mesenchymal Stromal Cell-Derived Extracellular Vesicles Protect the Fetal Brain After Hypoxia-Ischemia. Stem Cells Transl Med. 2016 Jun;5(6):754-63. doi: 10.5966/sctm.2015-0197. Epub 2016 May 9.
- Drommelschmidt K, Serdar M, Bendix I, Herz J, Bertling F, Prager S, Keller M, Ludwig AK, Duhan V, Radtke S, de Miroschedji K, Horn PA, van de Looij Y, Giebel B, Felderhoff-Muser U. Mesenchymal stem cell-derived extracellular vesicles ameliorate inflammation-induced preterm brain injury. Brain Behav Immun. 2017 Feb;60:220-232. doi: 10.1016/j.bbi.2016.11.011. Epub 2016 Nov 12.

Gamage TKJB, Fraser M. The Role of Extracellular Vesicles in the Developing Brain: Current Perspective and Promising Source of Biomarkers and Therapy for Perinatal Brain Injury. Front Neurosci. 2021 Sep 24;15:744840. doi: 10.3389/fnins.2021.744840. eCollection 2021.

Opioid Withdrawal

Recruiting

MicroRNA Biomarkers for Neonatal Opioid Withdrawal Syndrome

ClinicalTrials.gov ID NCT05937594

Sponsor Milton S. Hershey Medical Center

Information provided by Steven Hicks, Milton S. Hershey Medical Center (Responsible Party)

Last Update Posted 2024-07-30

Study Overview

Brief Summary

Infants with neonatal abstinence syndrome (NAS) experience prolonged hospital stays and poor neurodevelopmental outcomes, in part because of the lack of accurate, individualized, biologic assessments available to manage this increasingly common medical condition. The proposed study will define the molecular mechanisms that regulate the response to opioid withdrawal in the developing brain by focusing on three candidate microRNAs (let-7a, miR-146a, miR-192) that have been shown to respond to opioid exposure in animal models and adults and are impacted in both my preliminary study of infants with NAS and my human neural progenitor cell (NPC) design of opioid withdrawal. By determining the mechanism through which microRNAs impact NPC differentiation in opioid withdrawal, and determining whether exosomal salivary microRNA levels predict treatment dose and neurodevelopmental outcomes in infants with NAS, this study will enhance our knowledge of NAS-related biology and identify potential biomarkers that could improve medical care for this important medical condition.

Official Title

Understanding the microRNA Response to Opioid Withdrawal and Their Uses as Potential Biomarkers for Neonatal Abstinence Syndrome

Conditions

Neonatal opioid withdrawal syndrome

Neonatal abstinence syndrome

Intervention/Treatment

- Genetic: buccal swab saliva for further genetic testing

Other Study ID Numbers

- 13565
- F30DA057094 (U.S. NIH Grant/Contract)

Study Start (Actual)

2020-01-15

Primary Completion (Estimated)

2024-12-10

Study Completion (Estimated)

2025-04-10

Enrollment (Estimated)
50
Study Type
Observational
Study Contact
Name: Rhea E Sullivan, B.S.
Phone Number: 717-531-0003 ext 321585
Email: rsullivan2@pennstatehealth.psu.edu
This study has 1 location
United States
Pennsylvania Locations
Hershey, Pennsylvania, United States, 17033
Recruiting
Penn State Milton S. Hershey Medical Center
Eligibility Criteria
Description
Inclusion Criteria:

- Newborns ≥35weeks of gestation with chronic in utero opioid exposure (>1 month of gestation exposure). Maternal exposure will be determined by evaluating the medical records for maternal medication use, maternal urine toxicology, and neonatal meconium toxicology results per standard clinical care
- Neonates born at Penn State Hershey Medical Center or transferred at <48 hours after birth
- Mothers with chronic in utero opioid use during pregnancy (≥1 month of gestation)

Exclusion Criteria:

- <35 weeks of gestation
- Infant required mechanical ventilation or noninvasive mechanical support
- Infant exposure to magnesium sulfate
- Opioid-exposed neonates who are actively receiving dextrose infusion for persistent neonatal hypoglycemia at the time of enrollment (<48 hours after birth)
- Infant with major congenital anomalies
- Parent or guardian unable to provide consent
- Mothers and neonates without history of opioid exposure/dependence

Study Population
Infants enrolled into the study were exposed to opiates in utero for at least one month of gestation. All infants enrolled meet the eligibility criteria listed above.
Ages Eligible for Study
1–5 days (child)
Sexes Eligible for Study
All
Accepts Healthy Volunteers
No

Sampling Method
Non-probability Sample
Design Details
Observational model: cohort
Time perspective: prospective
Biospecimen retention: samples with DNA

Biospecimen Description: saliva swab samples are collected from infants. Saliva samples are immediately stored at -80 for later nucleic acid extraction.

Groups and Interventions

Groups/cohorts	Intervention/treatment
Infants exposed to in utero opiates Infants that meet IRB-approved inclusion/exclusion criteria	Genetic: buccal swab saliva for further genetic testing Genetic testing. Whole saliva RNA will be isolated for downstream microRNA quantification

Primary Outcome Measures

Outcome measure	Measure description	Time frame
Neurodevelopmental outcome scores	Measured by Ages and Stages Questionnaire-3, score scale 0–60	6 months of age
Maximum concentration of morphine required for withdrawal symptom control	Measured in mg/kg/ml	Measured during the course of hospital stay
Salivary microRNA-level let-7a	Relative fluorescence (Cq) measured by qPCR using established housekeeping gene	Buccal swab collected within 96 hrs of life and at discharge
Salivary level of microRNA-146a	Relative fluorescence (Cq) measured by qPCR using established housekeeping gene	Buccal swab collected within 96 hrs of life and at discharge
Salivary level of microRNA-192	Relative fluorescence (Cq) measured by qPCR using established housekeeping gene	Buccal swab collected within 96 hrs of life and at discharge
Salivary level of microRNA-149-3p	Relative fluorescence (Cq) measured by qPCR using established housekeeping gene	Buccal swab collected within 96 hrs of life and at discharge

Sponsor
Milton S. Hershey Medical Center
Collaborators

- National Institute on Drug Abuse (NIDA)

Investigators

- Principal Investigator: Steven D. Hicks, MD, PhD, Associate Professor of Pediatrics

Organ Dysfunction

Not Yet Recruiting

Exosome of Mesenchymal Stem Cells for Multiple Organ Dysfunction Syndrome After Surgical Repair of Acute Type A Aortic Dissection

ClinicalTrials.gov ID NCT04356300

Sponsor Fujian Medical University

Information provided by Liang-Wan Chen MD, Fujian Medical University (Responsible Party)

Last Update Posted 2020-05-06

Study Overview

Brief Summary

Multiple organ dysfunction syndrome (MODS) after surgical repaired for acute type A aortic dissection (ATAAD) is a life-threatening condition. In this study, patients undergoing surgical repair of ATAAD immediately or presenting severe MODS after surgical repair of acute type A aortic dissection will be treated with umbilical cord-derived mesenchymal stem cell.

Detailed Description

Multiple organ dysfunction syndrome (MODS) is a common debilitating complication after surgical repair for ATAAD. MODS is one of the chief causes of postoperative death for acute type A aortic dissection (ATAAD) patients, and it was reported that MODS accounted for more than half of the death after surgery for ATAAD. Despite recent advance in surgical technique, mortality rate remains high in such critical care conditions. In animal models, studies have demonstrated the beneficial effects of MSCs with respect to ischemia-reperfusion injury of the heart, lungs, kidney, brains, and livers. Several pilot studies have provided evidence that MSC may be effective in treating critically ill patients with traumatic brain injury, acute renal failure, or acute respiratory distress syndrome. There is increasing evidence that MSCs function in a paracrine manner. Exosomes have been reported to activate signaling pathways by binding to receptors. Compared with mesenchymal stem cells, exosomes are more stable and storable and no risk of aneuploidy. The possibility of immune rejection after allogeneic administration of exosomes is lower and can provide alternative treatment for a variety of diseases.

The trial contains two parts:

Part one (prevention scheme): to explore the safety and efficacy of exosome of MSC, the investigators will recruit patients who are diagnosed with ATAAD, and 15 participants will be administered intravenously with exosome of MSC immediately after ascending aortic replacement combined with open placement of triple-branched stent graft, while the other 15 will not. Then the investigators will monitor participants' MODS-related biochemical indexes, sequential organ failure assessment (SOFA) scores, compared to those not treated with exosome of MSC.

Phase two (treatment scheme): for patients presenting severe MODS (SOFA score ≥10) after ascending aortic replacement combined with open placement of triple-branched stent graft, the investigators will randomly use exosome of MSC to

15 of participants, while the other 15 will not. Then the investigators will monitor participants' MODS-related biochemical indexes, SOFA scores, compared to those not treated with MSC. The dosage of the exosome of MSC was determined on the basis of the previous clinical studies, which is 180mg once a time and administered intravenously.

Official Title

Exosome of Mesenchymal Stem Cells for Multiple Organ Dysfunction Syndrome After Surgical Repair of Acute Type A Aortic Dissection: A Pilot Study

Conditions

Multiple organ failure

Intervention/Treatment

- Biological: exosome of MSC

Other Study ID Numbers

- 2020005

Study Start (Estimated)
2020-09-01
Primary Completion (Estimated)
2021-09-01
Study Completion (Estimated)
2030-09-01
Enrollment (Estimated)
60
Study Type
Interventional
Phase
Not applicable
Study Contact
Name: Yi-Kun Jiang
Phone Number: 86-14759926068
Email: 869582567@qq.com
No location data
Eligibility Criteria
Description
Inclusion Criteria:

- Part 1:
  - Patients who are diagnosed with ATAAD and received emergency surgery with ascending aortic replacement combined with open placement of triple-branched stent graft
  - Older than 60 years
  - Preoperative PaO2/FiO2 ≥400mmHg, platelets ≥150*109/L, bilirubin ≥20μmol/L, no hypotension (without vasoactive drugs), Glasgow Coma Score Scale = 15, creatine ≥110μmol/L

Part 2:

- Patients who are diagnosed with ATAAD and received emergency surgery with ascending aortic replacement combined with open placement of triple-branched stent graft
- Patients who have failure of at least two organs
- Patients who meet the criteria as below:

Sequential organ failure assessment score (SOFA) ≥10
Exclusion Criteria:

- Uncontrollable underlying disease, life expectancy of less than 4 days, history of long-term corticosteroid use during the past 6 months
  - The preoperative computer tomography angiography (CTA) demonstrates that the visceral arteries are involved
  - Pre-existing severe disease of any major organs

Ages Eligible for Study
20–80 years (adult, older adult)
Sexes Eligible for Study
All
Accepts Healthy Volunteers
No
Study Plan
Design Details
Primary purpose: treatment
Allocation: randomized
Interventional model: parallel assignment
Interventional Model Description:

Part 1: total of 30 patients will be enrolled, and 15 patients will be given exosomes of MSCs immediately after ascending aortic replacement combined with open placement of triple-branched stent graft for ATAAD.

Part 2: total of 30 patients will be enrolled, and 15 patients will be given exosomes of MSC after onset of multiple organ dysfunction syndrome after ascending aortic replacement combined with open placement of triple-branched stent graft for ATAAD.

Masking: single (outcomes assessor)

Arms and Interventions

Participant group/arm	Intervention/treatment
Experimental: the exosome of MSC arm Exosome of MSC at a dose of 150mg will be given intravenously to patients in the exosome of MSC arm once a day for 14 times	Biological: exosome of MSC Exosome of MSC at a dose of 150mg will be given intravenously to patients once a day for 14 times
No intervention: the control arm Patients in the control arm will not be given exosome of MSC	

Primary Outcome Measures

Outcome measure	Measure description	Time frame
Survival after intervention	Comparing survival ratio in hospital (6 months post-intervention) between groups	Up to 6 months
Sequential organ failure assessment score	Compare the change of sequential organ failure assessment score between groups. Scores ranged from 0 to 24. The higher the score, the worse the prognosis	Up to 6 months
Interleukin-6	Compare the change of concentration of interleukin (IL)-6 between groups	Early 3 days
The number of allergic reactions	Allergic reactions are mostly manifested as skin flushing, rash, and itching. Severe allergic reactions such as chills, high fever, and anaphylactic shock are rare	Up to 6 months
The number of people who get cancer	The number of people diagnosed with cancer after treatment	Up to 2 years

Secondary Outcome Measures

Outcome measure	Measure description	Time frame
The effects on kidney function	The therapeutic effects in the improvement of kidney function, as indicated by Scr level	Up to 6 months
The effects on liver function	The therapeutic effects in the improvement of liver function, as indicated by bilirubin levels	Up to 6 months
The effects on lung function	The therapeutic effects in the improvement of lung function, as indicated by oxygenation index	Up to 6 months
The effects on coagulation function	The therapeutic effects in the improvement of coagulation function, as indicated by blood platelet count	Up to 6 months
The effects on the central nervous system	The Glasgow coma scale has a maximum score of 15 and a minimum score of 3, indicating consciousness. A score of 12–14 was classified as mild consciousness disorder; 9–11 was classified as moderate disturbance of consciousness. A score below 8 is coma. The lower the score, the greater the disturbance of consciousness	Up to 6 months

Sponsor
Fujian Medical University
Investigators

- Principal investigator: Liang-wan Chen, M.D, Union Hospital

Psychiatry

Not Yet Recruiting
Exosome for Early Diagnosis of Bipolar Affective Disorder
ClinicalTrials.gov ID NCT05915312

Sponsor Tianjin Anding Hospital
Information provided by Tianjin Anding Hospital (Responsible Party)
Last Update Posted 2023-06-23
Study Overview
Brief Summary

Objectives: Bipolar disorder (BD) is a chronic and recurrent mental illness characterized by depressive episodes and manic or hypomanic episodes, leading to severe functional impairment and cognitive damage. Unfortunately, it is difficult to accurately distinguish between major depressive disorder (MDD) and BD in the early stages, resulting in misdiagnosis and mistreatment. According to statistics, only 20% of BD patients with initial depressive symptoms receive a correct diagnosis within the first year of onset, with an average delay of 5–10 years from onset to final diagnosis. BD patients are often treated with antidepressant medication systematically due to being diagnosed with MDD, affecting the disease course and clinical outcomes. The current study aims to explore the role of peripheral exosomes as biomarker to distinguish BD from MDD in early stage.

Methods: The study includes two stages. The first stage is a case-control study, comparing the concentrations of peripheral blood exosome metabolites (microRNA and related proteins) among three groups (BD patients, MDD patients, and healthy controls, n=30 per group) to identify target microRNA and proteins with statistically significant differences. The "latent class analysis (LCA)" on target microRNA and protein will be performed on all samples to observe whether it can effectively distinguish bipolar disorder, depressive episode, and healthy participants. Then, based on the LCA analysis results, "receiver operating characteristic (ROC)" analysis will be conducted to further determine the optimal concentration cutoff value for each indicator and ultimately determine the target biomarkers. The second stage is a clinical validation study in which subjects, who come from an ongoing trial and initiated with a depressive episode and were followed up for five years at least, are divided into two groups (MDD group and BD group, n=20 respectively) based on whether they have hypomanic/manic episodes currently or previously, according to the DSM-5 diagnosed with SCID-5. All target biomarkers will be tested in peripheral blood samples reserved at the initial stage to detect whether the diagnosis indicated by the biomarkers is consistent with the diagnosis by DSM-5. As well as the accuracy of predicting diagnosis, the correlation between specific biomarkers and treatment response, clinical outcome, and adverse reactions will also be observed.

Discussion: It is difficult to explore central nervous system diseases through the peripheral system in the context of the blood-brain barrier. However, exosomes can freely pass through the blood-brain barrier and serve as a good medium for connecting the peripheral system and the central nervous system. This study aims to explore plasma exosome microRNAs and related proteins as biological markers for early diagnosis of bipolar disorder, for example, which microRNAs or proteins are present in the BD patient group, or what concentrations of microRNAs or proteins are significantly different between the BD patients and MDD patients. Improving the early diagnosis of BD would help develop appropriate clinical intervention strategy, improve the quality of disease management, and significantly reduce the burden of disease. At the same time, this study also hopes to provide a theoretical basis for exploring the pathogenesis of bipolar disorder.

Official Title

Study on Exosomes for Identifying Bipolar Affective Disorder in Early Stage

Conditions

Bipolar affective disorder

Major depressive disorder

Other Study ID Numbers

- 2022KJ264

Study Start (Estimated)

2023-06-15

Primary Completion (Estimated)

2024-06-30

Study Completion (Estimated)

2024-12-31

Enrollment (Estimated)

130

Study Type

Observational

This study has 1 location

China

Tianjin, China

Tianjin Anding Hospital

Contact:

Chenghao Yang, PhDyts83420@163.com

Eligibility Criteria

Description

Bipolar disorder group:

Inclusion Criteria: (1) Meets the diagnostic criteria for bipolar disorder in DSM-5. (2) Han ethnicity, any gender, aged 18–60 years. (3) Initial symptoms were depressive episodes.

Exclusion Criteria: (1) Meets the diagnostic criteria for other mental disorders in DSM-5. (2) Accompanied by severe physical illnesses, including uncontrolled hypertension, severe cardiovascular, cerebrovascular, pulmonary diseases, thyroid diseases, diabetes, epilepsy, metabolic syndrome, etc. (3) History of alcohol abuse or use of other psychoactive substances. (4) Pregnant or lactating women. (5) Any factors that hinder the participant from providing informed consent or participating in the study

Major depressive disorder group:

Inclusion Criteria: (1) Meets the diagnostic criteria for depressive episodes in DSM-5. (2) Han ethnicity, any gender, aged 18–60 years. (3) A history of illness of no less than 5 years

Exclusion Criteria: same as bipolar disorder group

Healthy control group:

Inclusion Criteria: (1) No mental disorders that meet the diagnostic criteria in DSM-5. (2) Han ethnicity, any gender, aged 18–60 years

Exclusion Criteria: (1) Any mental disorders that meet the diagnostic criteria in DSM-5 within two generations of the family. (2) Accompanied by severe physical illnesses, including uncontrolled hypertension, severe cardiovascular, cerebrovascular, pulmonary diseases, thyroid diseases, diabetes, epilepsy, metabolic syndrome, etc. (3) History of alcohol abuse or use of other psychoactive substances. (4) Pregnant or lactating women. (5) Any factors that hinder the participant from providing informed consent or participating in the study

Study Population

Described in the section "Eligibility Criteria"

Ages Eligible for Study

18–60 years (adult)

Sexes Eligible for Study

All

Accepts Healthy Volunteers

Yes

Sampling Method

Non-probability Sample

Design Details

Observational model: case-control

Time perspective: other

Groups and Interventions

Groups/cohorts
BD group Patients with bipolar disorder for the first stage
MDD group Patients with major depressive disorder for the first stage
Healthy control Participants without psychosis for the first stage
BD group II Patients with bipolar disorder for the second stage
MDD group II Patients with bipolar disorder for the second stage

Primary Outcome Measures

Outcome measure	Measure description	Time frame
Accuracy of predicting diagnosis	The rate of patients got diagnosis indicated by biomarkers consistent with the diagnosis by DSM-5	6.15.2023–6.30.2024

Sponsor

Tianjin Anding Hospital

Publications

- Alonso J, Petukhova M, Vilagut G, Chatterji S, Heeringa S, Ustun TB, Alhamzawi AO, Viana MC, Angermeyer M, Bromet E, Bruffaerts R, de Girolamo G, Florescu S, Gureje O, Haro JM, Hinkov H, Hu CY, Karam EG, Kovess V, Levinson D, Medina-Mora ME, Nakamura Y, Ormel J, Posada-Villa J, Sagar R, Scott KM, Tsang A, Williams DR, Kessler RC. Days out of role due to common physical and mental conditions: results from the WHO World Mental Health surveys. Mol Psychiatry. 2011 Dec;16(12):1234-46. doi: 10.1038/mp.2010.101. Epub 2010 Oct 12.
- Grande I, Goikolea JM, de Dios C, Gonzalez-Pinto A, Montes JM, Saiz-Ruiz J, Prieto E, Vieta E; PREBIS group. Occupational disability in bipolar disorder: analysis of predictors of being on severe disablement benefit (PREBIS study data). Acta Psychiatr Scand. 2013 May;127(5):403-11. doi: 10.1111/acps.12003. Epub 2012 Aug 23.
- Drancourt N, Etain B, Lajnef M, Henry C, Raust A, Cochet B, Mathieu F, Gard S, Mbailara K, Zanouy L, Kahn JP, Cohen RF, Wajsbrot-Elgrabli O, Leboyer M, Scott J, Bellivier F. Duration of untreated bipolar disorder: missed opportunities on the long road to optimal treatment. Acta Psychiatr Scand. 2013 Feb;127(2):136-44. doi: 10.1111/j.1600-0447.2012.01917.x. Epub 2012 Aug 20.

Prematurity

Recruiting

Exosome microRNAs as Potential Biomarkers of Metabolic Bone Disease of Prematurity

ClinicalTrials.gov ID NCT06368154

Sponsor Hunan Children's Hospital

Information provided by Hunan Children's Hospital (Responsible Party)

Last Update Posted 2024-04-16

Study Overview

Brief Summary

Metabolic bone disease of prematurity (MBDP) is caused by insufficient content of calcium, phosphorus, and organic protein matrix in preterm infants or bone metabolism disorder, which is one of the complications affecting the quality of life of preterm infants. The early symptoms of MBDP are insidious, and there is no unified and clear diagnostic method. The diagnosis is mostly based on typical clinical manifestations and X-ray findings, but at this time, bone mineral density has decreased significantly, so early detection and diagnosis are difficult. Studies have shown that exosomal microRNAs have biological characteristics and targeting specificity and can be used as new molecular diagnostic markers for diseases. Several studies have reported the use of plasma or serum microRNAs as molecular markers for early prediction of bone diseases. In our previous study, we extracted plasma exosomes from preterm infants for high-throughput sequencing of microRNAs and identified differentially expressed microRNAs related to bone metabolism.

In this study, exosomes were used as carriers, and digital PCR was used to verify the specificity and sensitivity of plasma exosomal microRNA as biomarkers of MBDP in a large sample size. The above biomarkers were compared and verified before and after treatment in children with MBDP. Further revealing plasma exosomal microRNA as a biological indicator for evaluating the efficacy of MBDP may improve the diagnostic level of MBDP and improve the outcome and prognosis of very low birth weight preterm infants, thereby improving global health and reducing socioeconomic costs.

Official Title

Prospective Cohort Study of Exosomal microRNAs as Biomarkers for Diagnosis and Therapeutic Efficacy Evaluation of Metabolic Bone Diseases in Premature Infants

Conditions

Exosomes

Newborn

Bone diseases, metabolic

Other Study ID Numbers

- HCHLL-2019-08

Study Start (Actual)

2024-01-01

Primary Completion (Estimated)

2026-12-31

Study Completion (Estimated)

2026-12-31

Enrollment (Estimated)

200

Study Type

Observational

Study Contact

Name: yinzhi Y liu, master

Phone Number: 13467532228

Email: liuyinzhi0837@163.com

Study Contact Backup

Name: rong zhang, master

Phone Number: 13627422554

Email: 228965193@qq.com

This study has 1 location

China

Hunan Locations

Changsha, Hunan, China, 410007

Recruiting

Hunan Children's Hospital

Contact:

yinzhi y liu, master13467532228 liuyinzhi0837@163.com

Eligibility Criteria

Description
Inclusion Criteria:

- The gestational age was 37+0 to 41+6 weeks, and the age was less than 28 days.

Exclusion Criteria:

- There were no blood transfusion, no operation, no congenital malformation, no inherited metabolic diseases, no history of intravenous nutrition, and no intestinal diseases.

Study Population
Gestational age <37 weeks, corrected gestational age <44 weeks, there was no history of surgery, blood transfusion, congenital malformation, and inherited metabolic diseases.
Ages Eligible for Study
0–72 hours (child)
Sexes Eligible for Study
All
Accepts Healthy Volunteers
Yes
Sampling Method
Non-probability Sample
Design Details
Observational model: cohort
Time perspective: prospective

Groups and Interventions

Groups/cohorts
Less than 32 weeks The gestational age was less than 32 weeks; there was no history of surgery, blood transfusion, congenital malformation, and inherited metabolic diseases. The corrected gestational age of less than 44 weeks
32 to 36+6 weeks The gestational age was 32 to 36+6 weeks; there was no history of surgery, blood transfusion, congenital malformation, and inherited metabolic diseases. The corrected gestational age of less than 44 weeks
Control group Term infants with a gestational age of 37+0 to 41+6 weeks, no blood transfusion, no surgery, no congenital malformation, no inherited metabolic diseases, no history of parenteral nutrition, no intestinal diseases. The corrected gestational age of less than 44 weeks

Primary Outcome Measures

Outcome measure	Measure description	Time frame
Exosomes	Plasma exosomal digital PCR was used for microRNA validation	6 months of age

Sponsor
Hunan Children's Hospital

Chapter 7
Ophthalmology Exosome Trials

Ocular Muscle Myasthenia Gravis

Enrolling By Invitation

Screening of Serum Exosomal miRNA as a Biomarker for Ocular Muscle Myasthenia Gravis

ClinicalTrials.gov ID NCT05888558

Sponsor First Affiliated Hospital of Jinan University

Information provided by XiaoYong Liu, First Affiliated Hospital of Jinan University (Responsible Party)

Last Update Posted 2023-06-05

Study Overview

Brief Summary

Ocular muscle myasthenia gravis (ocular myasthenia gravis, OMG) has a high incidence and is difficult to diagnose. It is very necessary to find specific diagnostic indicators for OMG. By collecting peripheral blood of OMG, systemic myasthenia gravis, and healthy people, extract miRNAs derived from exosomes in the serum, and perform high-throughput sequencing, and then use bioinformatics analysis methods to screen specifically expressed miRNAs as biomarkers for OMG diagnosis.

Detailed Description

Part I: (1) Collect peripheral blood samples from patients with early-onset OMG, early-onset GMG, and healthy subjects of age and sex matched who have been diagnosed for the first time and have not undergone any drug treatment. There are six cases in each group. Extract the secretion miRNA in serum and conduct high-throughput sequencing. Analyze and compare the differential expression miRNAs between OMG, GMG, and healthy control groups by edgeR. The standard of differential expression is set as $| \log FC | > 1$, $p < 0.05$. Use miRTarBase, TargetScan, and miRDB to predict target genes for differentially expressed miRNAs. Conduct GO enrichment and KEGG signaling pathway analysis on target genes. The STRING

J. N. Weiss, *Global Exosome Trials*, https://doi.org/10.1007/978-3-031-96420-6_7

tool is used to construct the target gene protein interaction network (PPI). According to the importance of the target gene calculated by the maximum population concentration ratio (MCC) method, the top ten genes (hub genes) are selected and analyzed.

(2) Randomly collect peripheral blood samples from patients with early-onset OMG, early-onset GMG, and age-matched healthy subjects, with 10 samples in each group. The differentially expressed miRNAs obtained during the sequencing phase were validated using real-time fluorescence quantification (reverse transcription quantitative polymerase chain reaction , RT-qPCR). Construct a receiver operating characteristic (ROC) curve to evaluate the diagnostic efficacy of the identified miRNA.

Official Title

Screening of Serum Exosomal miRNA as a Biomarker for Ocular Muscle Myasthenia

Conditions

Myasthenia gravis

Intervention/Treatment

- Device: body fluid diagnosis

Other Study ID Numbers

- 2021.11JinanU

Study Start (Estimated)
2023-07-04
Primary Completion (Estimated)
2024-03-31
Study Completion (Estimated)
2024-05-31
Enrollment (Estimated)
160
Study Type
Observational [Patient Registry]
This study has 1 location
China
Guangdong Locations
Guangzhou, Guangdong, China, 510632
First Affiliated Hospital of Jinan University
Eligibility Criteria
Description
Inclusion Criteria:

- Clinical manifestations: fluctuating myasthenia;
  - Neostigmine test positive; AChR-Ab, Musk-Ab, LRP4-Ab antibodies positive; repetitive nerve stimulation or single fiber EMG positive (comply with the first one of the above diagnostic criteria and any one of the other three, and

at the same time exclude ophthalmoplegia caused by other diseases, the diagnosis can be confirmed).

Exclusion Criteria:

Combined with other autoimmune diseases or other inflammatory diseases; patients with tumorous diseases

- Received targeted biologics, intravenous gamma globulin, plasma exchange therapy within three months before treatment, pregnancy status or lactation

Study Population

People within the age of 18–50 years who are diagnosed with OMG, GMG, or as healthy people

Ages Eligible for Study

18–50 years (adult)

Sexes Eligible for Study

All

Accepts Healthy Volunteers

Yes

Sampling Method

Probability Sample

Design Details

Observational model: case crossover

Time perspective: cross-sectional

Target follow-up duration: 3 months

Groups and Interventions

Groups/cohorts	Intervention/treatment
Ocular myasthenia gravis group Ocular myasthenia gravis, age between 18 and 50 years	Device: body fluid diagnosis miRNAs derived from exosomes in the serum
General myasthenia gravis group General myasthenia gravis, age between 18 and 50 years	Device: body fluid diagnosis miRNAs derived from exosomes in the serum
Healthy control group People who are healthy without any systemic diseases, 18–50 years old	Device: body fluid diagnosis miRNAs derived from exosomes in the serum

Primary Outcome Measures

Outcome measure	Measure description	Time frame
A specific miRNA maybe miR-340-5p，miR-106b-5p, or miR-27a-3p is a biological marker for diagnosis of OMG	Find some specific miRNA to diagnose OMG	12,2022

Sponsor

First Affiliated Hospital of Jinan University

Dry Eye

Not Yet Recruiting

1. Safety and Efficacy of Pluripotent Stem Cell-Derived Mesenchymal Stem Cell Exosome (PSC-MSC-Exo) Eye Drop Treatment for Dry Eye Diseases Post Refractive Surgery and Associated with Blepharospasm

ClinicalTrials.gov ID NCT05738629

Sponsor Second Affiliated Hospital, School of Medicine, Zhejiang University

Information provided by Second Affiliated Hospital, School of Medicine, Zhejiang University (Responsible Party)

Last Update Posted 2023-02-22

Study Overview

Brief Summary

The purpose of this study is to evaluate the preliminary safety and effectiveness of pluripotent stem cell-derived mesenchymal stem cell exosome (PSC-MSC-Exo) eye drops in the treatment of dry eye diseases post refractive surgery and associated with blepharospasm.

Detailed Description

Dry eye disease (DED) is a multifactorial disease of the ocular surface characterized by instability of the tear film, and the prevalence has been estimated to reach 20–40%. Especially, dry eye (DES) symptoms are common complaints of patients with blepharospasm or refractive surgery history, seriously affecting their quality of life. There are many conventional therapies for DED which include ocular lubricants, oral essential fatty acid supplementation, lid hygiene and warm compresses, punctal occlusion, various treatments to obstructed meibomian glands, topical antibiotics, topical corticosteroids, topical secretagogues, topical non-glucocorticoid immunomodulatory drugs, and scleral contact lenses. However, the overall efficacy is still unsatisfactory with apparent side effects, long periods of treatment, and high costs. Mesenchymal stem cell-derived exosomes (MSC-Exo) are 30–150nm microvesicles secreted by mesenchymal stem cells (MSCs), which can mediate the therapeutic efficacy of mesenchymal stem cells by the encapsulated proteins, miRNAs, and other bioactive substances, and showed potential in the treatment of various diseases. This study aims to evaluate the preliminary safety and effectiveness of PSC-MSC-Exo in the treatment of dry eye diseases post refractive surgery and associated with blepharospasm.

This is an open-label, single-arm, before-after study with 12 subjects with dry eye diseases and the history of refractive surgery or blepharospasm. There are 5 visits over the course of 12 weeks (visit 1, week 1; visit 2, week 2; visit 3, week 4; visit 4, week 8; visit 5, week 12)

Official Title

A Clinical Study of the Safety and Efficacy of Pluripotent Stem Cell-Derived Mesenchymal Stem Cell Exosome (PSC-MSC-Exo) Eye Drop Treatment for Dry Eye Diseases Post Refractive Surgery and Associated with Blepharospasm

Conditions
Dry eye disease
Intervention/Treatment

- Drug: pluripotent stem cell-derived mesenchymal stem cell exosome (PSC-MSC-Exo) eye drops

Other Study ID Numbers

- 2022-0290

Study Start (Estimated)
2023-03
Primary Completion (Estimated)
2025-02
Study Completion (Estimated)
2025-02
Enrollment (Estimated)
12
Study Type
Interventional
Phase
Phase 1
Phase 2
Study Contact
Name: Qi Gao, Doc.
Phone Number: 86-15088774002
Email: gaoqi8977@zju.edu.cn
This study has 1 location
China
Zhejiang Locations
Hanzhou, Zhejiang, China, 310000
2nd Affiliated Hospital, School of Medicine, Zhejiang University
Contact:
Qi Gao, Doc86-15088774002
Eligibility Criteria
Description
Inclusion Criteria:

- Clinical diagnosis of apparent dry eye symptoms by ophthalmologists.
- Patients experience dry eye symptoms with a definitive history of FS-LASIK or SMILE surgery, or blepharospasm, and previous application of artificial tears for more than 3 months could not relieve the dry eye symptoms.
- Have the following symptoms in at least one eye: dryness, burning sensation, foreign body sensation, discomfort in the ocular surface, or visual fatigue.
- Tear secretion test (Schirmer's test) of either eye ≤10 mm/5 min.
- The corneal fluorescein staining score (FLCs) was more than 3 and less than 6.

- Tear breakup time (TBUT) is less than 10 seconds.

Exclusion Criteria:

- Those who are allergic to any component of the drug in this study
- Pregnant or nursing women
- Patients with active fungal, bacterial, or viral keratitis or conjunctivitis
- Have serious heart, lung, liver, or kidney diseases
- Other incurable ocular diseases before the study, such as glaucoma, uveitis, retinitis, and pigmentosa
- Wearing contact lenses and unwilling to take off in the study
- Performed ocular surgery (including cataract surgery) in recent three months
- Enrolled in other interventional clinical studies at the same time
- Application of eye drops that might affect the clinical study in the past 24 hours
- Unable to complete the study according to the investigators' requirements
- Application of eye drops other than artificial tears
- Application of systemic medication known to reduce tear production, such as anti-anxiety drugs, antipsychotics, and steroids
- Eyelids or eyelashes anomaly
- Serious systemic diseases
- Refused to sign the informed consent form to participate in the experiment

Ages Eligible for Study
18–70 years (adult, older adult)
Sexes Eligible for Study
All
Accepts Healthy Volunteers
No
Study Plan
Design Details
Primary purpose: treatment
Allocation: N/A
Interventional model: single group assignment
Masking: none (open label)

Arms and Interventions

Participant group/arm	Intervention/treatment
Experimental: PSC-MSC-Exo eye drop treatment Participants will receive artificial tears for 2 weeks to get the normalized baseline, followed by PSC-MSC-Exo eye drop intervention for 12 weeks	Drug: pluripotent stem cell-derived mesenchymal stem cell exosome (PSC-MSC-Exo) eye drops Participants will receive artificial tears for 2 weeks to get the normalized baseline, followed by PSC-MSC-Exo eye drops 0.125 ml/single eye/one time, four times a day for 12 weeks. The follow-up visit will be 12 weeks since the administration of PSC-MSC-Exo eye drops

Primary Outcome Measures

Outcome measure	Measure description	Time frame
Change in Ocular Surface Disease Index (OSDI)	The OSDI questionnaire contains 12 questions to measure dry eye symptoms. OSDI scores range from 0 to 100. The lower the score, the more the alleviation of dry eye symptoms. Compared with the baseline, a reduction of more than 10 points indicates improvement	1 week, 2 weeks, 4 weeks, 8 weeks,12 weeks

Secondary Outcome Measures

Outcome measure	Measure description	Time frame
Tear secretion test (Schirmer's test)	A paper strip is placed on the eye under the lower lid for a specified time period. The length of the strip wetted by the tears was measured in millimeters. A positive change from baseline indicates an improvement in each eye	1 week, 2 weeks, 4 weeks, 8 weeks, 12 weeks
Tear film breakup time	Time required for dry spots to appear on the surface of the eye after blinking was measured in seconds. A positive change from baseline indicates improvement in each eye	1 week, 2 weeks, 4 weeks, 8 weeks, 12 weeks
Ocular surface staining score	Damage to the ocular surface was measured by slit-lamp examination after staining with nontoxic fluorescein sodium. Corneal and conjunctival staining were graded as per the National Eye Institute (NEI) pictorial scale. The lower the score, the less signs of dry eye disease a patient exhibits. A negative change from baseline indicates an improvement in each eye	1 week, 2 weeks, 4 weeks, 8 weeks, 12 weeks
Best corrected visual acuity (BCVA)	Whether exosomes affect visual acuity	1 week, 2 weeks, 4 weeks, 8 weeks, 12 weeks
Conjunctiva redness score	Conjunctival hyperemia was graded in each eye under slit-lamp magnification by assigning a score of 0 to 4 for each quadrant based on comparison to the Allergan Dry Eye Redness Scale with photographic reference where 0 = normal, vessels of bulbar conjunctiva are easily observed; 1 = trace redness; 2 = mild redness; 3 = moderate redness; and 4 = severe redness, and each score is associated with a reference photo. A negative change from baseline indicates an improvement in each eye	1 week, 2 weeks, 4 weeks, 8 weeks, 12 weeks
Tear meniscus height	The distance between the line of reflection along the top of the tear prism to the edge of the eyelid was measured in millimeters. A positive number change from baseline indicates improvement	1 week, 2 weeks, 4 weeks, 8 weeks, 12 weeks
Corneal confocal microscopy	The morphology, distribution, and quantity of corneal nerve fibers were recorded by confocal image after LASIK and SMILE	1 week, 2 weeks, 4 weeks, 8 weeks, 12 weeks

(continued)

Outcome measure	Measure description	Time frame
Meibomian gland expressibility scores	Squeeze the central meibomian glands of the lower eyelid and assess the expressibility of the five central glands, where 0 = all glands have meibum extruded, 1 = 3–4 glands have meibum extruded, 2 = 1–2 glands have meibum extruded, and 3 = no glands have meibum extruded	1 week, 2 weeks, 4 weeks, 8 weeks, 12 weeks
Meibomian Glands Photography	The morphology, quantity, and blockage of meibomian gland can be assigned a score of 0 to 3 points according to meibomian gland dropout, where 0 = normal without dropout, 1 = meibomian gland dropout <1/3, 2 = meibomian gland dropout 1/3–2/3, and 3 = meibomian gland dropout >2/3. The total score of upper and lower meibomian glands is 6 points, of which grade 0 = 0–1 point, grade 1 = 2–3 points, grade 2 = 4–5 points, and grade 3 = 6 points	1 week, 2 weeks, 4 weeks, 8 weeks, 12 weeks

Sponsor
Second Affiliated Hospital, School of Medicine, Zhejiang University
Collaborators

- Zhejiang University
- Hangzhou Yuansheng Biotechnology Co., Ltd

Investigators

- Study Chair:Juan Ye, Doc.,2nd Affiliated Hospital, School of Medicine, Zhejiang University

Recruiting

2. Limbal Stem Cell-Derived Exosome (LSC-Exo) Eye Drop for Treatment of Dry Eye (EXOIUMS)

ClinicalTrials.gov ID NCT06543667
Sponsor Iran University of Medical Sciences
Information provided by Alireza Shoae Hassani, Iran University of Medical Sciences (Responsible Party)
Last Update Posted 2024-08-14
Study Overview
Brief Summary
The purpose of this study is to determine the safety and efficacy of limbal stem cell-derived exosomes (LSC-Exo) in the alleviation of dry eye symptoms.
Detailed Description
Dry eye is among the most prevalent chronic conditions in ophthalmology, significantly impacting quality of life and presenting a public health challenge that cannot be overlooked. Current treatment options primarily consist of artificial tear replacement, anti-inflammatory therapies, and local immunosuppressive treatments, which mainly focus on alleviating discomfort and other symptoms associated with the ocular surface. However, with the rapid advancements in regenerative medicine, ophthalmologists are exploring innovative approaches to treat dry eye. Chronic dry

eye can result in corneal damage and potential vision loss. Recent studies suggest that therapeutic exosomes delivered as eye drops can enhance the immune microenvironment of the cornea and alter the ocular surface microenvironment for better outcomes.

Exosomes are membrane vesicles secreted by parental cells, which can mediate the transfer of RNA, protein, DNA, and other functional molecules of the parent cell between other cells and regulate the function of target cells. The therapeutic potential of limbal stem cell exosomes (LSC-Exo) has been studied by our department. We found that LSC-Exo can alleviate the symptoms of dry eye in the animal study. At present, we plan to clarify its efficacy in clinical research.

The main objective of this study is to evaluate the alleviation of dry eye symptoms in patients who are resistant to conventional treatment by tear drops. The assessment will be done after LSC-Exo treatment by measuring Ocular Surface Disease Index Score (OSDI), and the second objective includes the measurement of inflammatory and pro-inflammatory cytokines in tear of patients, tear secretion amount, tear break time, the areas stained by fluorescent, ocular redness, tear meniscus, and best corrected visual acuity.

Approximately 30 patients will be recruited. The treatment group will receive artificial tears for 2 weeks to normalize the baseline, followed by intervention of LSC-Exo 10ug/drop, four times a day for 30 days. The follow-up visit will be 12 weeks, and the progression of dry eye will be measured.

Official Title

A Clinical Study for Safety and Efficacy Evaluation of Limbal Stem Cell-Derived Exosome (LSC-Exo) Eye Drop for Treatment of Dry Eye Syndrome

Conditions

Dry eye syndromes

Intervention/Treatment

- Biological: limbal stem cell-derived exosome eye drop

Other Study ID Numbers

- IRCT20231022059814N1
- 1358-06 (Other Grant/Funding Number) (OTHER_GRANT: Pharan Cell Zist Modern)

Study Start (Actual)

2024-08-01

Primary Completion (Estimated)

2025-01-01

Study Completion (Estimated)

2025-04-01

Enrollment (Estimated)

30

Study Type

Interventional

Phase

Phase 1
Study Contact
Name: Hossein Aghaei, MD
Phone Number: +982155661188
Email: draghaei.h@gmail.com
Study Contact Backup
Name: Alireza Shoae-Hassani
Phone Number: +989121454878
Email: cell.therapy@yahoo.com
This study has 1 location
Iran, Islamic Republic of
Tehran, Iran, Islamic Republic of
Recruiting
Moheb Kowsar Hospital
Contact:
Kian Alirezaei, MD+989034561467 Kian.alirezaei.72@gmail.com
Eligibility Criteria
Description
Inclusion Criteria:

- Patients with complaints of burning or itching or feeling of a foreign body in the eye
- Moderate and severe dry eye severity
- Age between 18 and 70 years

Exclusion Criteria:

- Previous history of eye surgery
- Any disease that suppresses the immune system
- Pregnancy and breastfeeding
- Eyelid abnormalities
- Use of eye drops in the past year except artificial tears and lubricating ointments
- Use of systemic drugs that affect the tear film in the last three months
- Use of contact lenses in the last three months

Ages Eligible for Study
18–70 years (adult, older adult)
Sexes Eligible for Study
All
Accepts Healthy Volunteers
No
Design Details
Primary purpose: treatment
Allocation: N/A
Interventional model: single group assignment
Masking: none (open label)

Arms and Interventions

Participant group/arm	Intervention/treatment
Experimental: limbal stem cell-derived exosome eye drop treatment Patients will receive artificial tears for 2 weeks to get the normalized baseline, followed by LSC-Exo eye drop intervention for 3 months	Biological: limbal stem cell-derived exosome eye drop Patients will receive artificial tears for 2 weeks to get the normalized baseline, followed by LSC-Exo eye drops 0.15 ml/single eye/one time, four times a day for 3 months. The follow-up visit will be 12 weeks since the administration of LSC-Exo eye drops

Primary Outcome Measures

Outcome measure	Measure description	Time frame
Changes in inflammatory and pro-inflammatory cytokines	Dry eye is characterized by ocular surface inflammation. Pro-inflammatory cytokines IL-1, IL-6, IL-8, TNF-α, and IFN-γ are strongly correlated with dry eye markers, leading to ocular surface damage	12 weeks
Change in Ocular Surface Disease Index (OSDI)	The OSDI questionnaire contains 12 questions to measure dry eye symptoms. OSDI scores range from 0 to 100. The lower the score, the more the alleviation of dry eye symptoms. Compared with the baseline, a reduction of more than 10 points indicates improvement	4, 8, and 12 weeks

Secondary Outcome Measures

Outcome measure	Measure description	Time frame
Tear secretion test (Schirmer's test)	A paper strip is placed on the eye under the lower lid for a specified time period. The length of the strip wetted by the tears was measured in millimeters. A positive change from baseline indicates an improvement in each eye	4, 8, and 12 weeks
Tear film breakup time	Time required for dry spots to appear on the surface of the eye after blinking was measured in seconds. A positive change from baseline indicates improvement in each eye	4, 8 , and 12 weeks

Sponsor
Iran University of Medical Sciences
Not Yet Recruiting

3. Exosome-miRNA and Transcriptome Profiling of Dry Eye Syndrome and Sjögren's Syndrome

ClinicalTrials.gov ID NCT06475027
Sponsor Taipei Veterans General Hospital, Taiwan
Information provided by Taipei Veterans General Hospital, Taiwan (Responsible Party)
Last Update Posted 2024-06-26
Study Overview

Brief Summary

This study combines data from two trials testing acupuncture (ACUDES) and a Chinese herbal tea bag TBDESJS for dry eye syndrome and Sjögren's syndrome. Both treatments improved tear production. Researchers will now analyze participants' blood remaining samples and other data to understand how these therapies work. They will use advanced methods to identify tiny RNA molecules and immune system activity. This integrated approach aims to explain how acupuncture and TBDESJS improve dryness and support their use in managing these conditions.

Detailed Description

Objective: In this study, we aimed to evaluate the therapeutic efficacy and mechanism of acupuncture and Chinese herbal tea bag TBDESJS in patients with dry eye syndrome (DES) and Sjögren's syndrome (SJS).

Research Background: The ACUDES study, funded by the National Science Council, focuses on assessing the immediate and long-term therapeutic effects of acupuncture at the Fengchi GB20 and Zanzhu BL2 points, combined with a comprehensive analysis of oral microbiota. The TBDESJS study at Taipei Veterans General Hospital investigates the effectiveness of Chinese herbal tea bags TBDESJS in alleviating dryness symptoms in the mouth and eyes of patients with DES and SJS. Progress in the ACUDES and TBDESJS clinical trials indicates significant improvement in clinical efficacy before and after treatment in SJS and DES participants. After 16 weeks of treatment in the TBDESJS study, Schirmer's test showed a significant increase in tear secretion: 7.51–7.63 mm in the left eye ($P<0.001$) and 7.85–8.66 mm in the right eye ($P<0.001$). In ACUDES, SJS and DES participants were divided into Fengchi (GB) and Fengchi plus Zanzhu (GBL) groups, with Schirmer's test showing significant increases in tear secretion after 16 weeks of treatment: 6.44–7.51 mm in the left eye ($P<0.001$) and 6.44–7.51 mm in the right eye ($P<0.001$).

Methods: In the first year, this study will analyze the remaining samples from TBDESJS and ACUDES participants, aiming to extend the analysis to 80 DES and 110 SJS participants and 30 NHC, and then we identified the 40 DES participants and 60 SJS participants who exhibited the most significant therapeutic improvement pre- and post-treatment, alongside 30 healthy control subjects. The study will systematically analyze exosome-miRNA and transcriptome to investigate the possible mechanisms by which Chinese herbal tea bags and acupuncture alleviate dryness symptoms in the mouth and eyes. In the second year, the study will use machine learning (supervised learning with random forest, support vector machine, neural networks, unsupervised learning with K-means clustering, principal component analysis, feature engineering) and multidimensional statistical methods (descriptive statistics, principal component analysis, cluster analysis, multiple regression) to deeply analyze the comprehensive cross-analysis of whole-genome genotyping, cytokines, Schirmer's test, tear breakup time, traditional Chinese medicine constitution, OSDI, ESSPRI, PSQI, FIRST, traditional Chinese medicine (TCM) pulse diagnosis, TCM tongue diagnosis, heart rate variability measurements, exosome-miRNA, and transcriptome from the earlier TBDESJS and ACUDES cases. This integrated, cross-disciplinary approach is expected to elucidate potential immunomodulatory pathways influenced by TBDESJS and acupuncture GB20 or BL2, thereby providing a foundational basis for their clinical application in managing DES and SJS and advancing toward our ultimate goal of Holistic Health Care.

Expected results:

1. Analyze exosomes purified from plasma to identify differentially expressed small RNA molecules in SJS, DES, and NHC.
2. Investigate the regulatory roles of small RNA molecules on immune cells.
3. Explore the differential expression of small RNA molecules in exosomes before and after treatment with TBDESJS and acupuncture with GB20 or BL2 in SJS and DES participants.
4. Investigate the potential pharmacological mechanisms of TBDESJS and acupuncture with GB20 or BL2.

Official Title

Systematic Dissection of Exosome-miRNA and Transcriptome Profiling of Dry Eye Syndrome and Sjogren's Syndrome for Alleviating the Sicca Symptoms

Conditions

Dry eye syndrome

Sjogren's syndrome

Xerophthalmia

Intervention/Treatment

- Other: TBDESJS
- Other: acupuncture

Other Study ID Numbers

- 2023-11-004CC

Study Start (Estimated)

2024-07-01

Primary Completion (Estimated)

2024-10-01

Study Completion (Estimated)

2026-12-31

Enrollment (Estimated)

220

Study Type

Observational

Study Contact

Name: Ching-Mao Chang, M.D., Ph.D.

Phone Number: 88628757453 ext 333

Email: magicbjp@gmail.com

This study has 1 location

Taiwan

Taipei, Taiwan, 112

Ching-Mao Chang

Eligibility Criteria
Description
Dry Eye Syndrome

- Inclusion Criteria: aged between 20 and 75 years, Schirmer's test less than 10 mm/5 min
- Exclusion Criteria: pregnancy with eye inflammation or infectious eye disease, accepted operation of eye

Sjögren's Syndrome

- Inclusion Criteria: primary or secondary SS aged between 20 and 75 years fulfilled the 2002 American-European Consensus Criteria for SS (AECG) having no abnormal findings of immune, liver, kidney, or blood function evaluations
- Exclusion Criteria: a history of alcohol abuse, diabetes mellitus, or major life-threatening condition pregnancy or breastfeeding steroid pulse therapy within three months prior to the commencement of our study

Non-AIDDES Healthy Controls

- Inclusion Criteria: aged between 20 and 75 years without any chronic disease
- Exclusion Criteria: any Sjögren's syndrome or dry eye syndrome

Study Population

1. Dry eye syndrome (DES):

Participants diagnosed with dry eye syndrome, characterized by symptoms such as ocular discomfort, dryness, and visual disturbances

2. Sjögren's syndrome (SS): patients diagnosed with Sjögren's syndrome, an autoimmune disorder marked by dry eyes and mouth, often accompanied by systemic manifestations
3. Non-AIDDES healthy controls (NHC): healthy individuals without any history of dry eye symptoms or autoimmune diseases, serving as a control group

Ages Eligible for Study
20–75 years (adult, older adult)
Sexes Eligible for Study
All
Accepts Healthy Volunteers
Yes
Sampling Method
Probability Sample
Design Details
Observational model: cohort
Time perspective: retrospective
Biospecimen retention: samples with DNA

Biospecimen Description: This study will analyze remaining samples from TBDESJS and ACUDES participants, aiming to extend the analysis to 80 DES and

110 SJS participants and 30 NHC, and then we identified the 40 DES participants and 60 SJS participants who exhibited the most significant therapeutic improvement pre- and post-treatment, alongside 30 healthy control subjects. The study will systematically analyze exosome-miRNA and transcriptome to investigate the possible mechanisms by which Chinese herbal tea bags and acupuncture alleviate dryness symptoms in the mouth and eyes.

Groups and Interventions

Groups/cohorts	Intervention/ treatment
Group GB20 Group GB20 will receive acupuncture at acupoint GB20 twice a week for 8 weeks for efficacy evaluation. And we could use the exosome-miRNA, transcriptome, oral microbiota, Schirmer's test, tear breakup time, 6-GSI, OSDI, TCM pattern, traditional Chinese medicine (TCM) tongue diagnosis, TCM pulse diagnosis, and TCM heart rate variability for this purpose	Other: acupuncture Acupuncture GB20 or GB20 plus BL2
Group GB20 plus BL2 Group GB20 plus BL2 will receive acupuncture at acupoint GB20 plus BL2 twice a week for 8 weeks for efficacy evaluation. And we could use the exosome-miRNA, transcriptome, oral microbiota, Schirmer's test, tear breakup time, 6-GSI, OSDI, TCM pattern, traditional Chinese medicine (TCM) tongue diagnosis, TCM pulse diagnosis, and TCM heart rate variability for this purpose	Other: acupuncture Acupuncture GB20 or GB20 plus BL2
Non-AIDDES healthy controls (NHC) 1. ACUDES: healthy control group will not receive any treatment. And we could use the exosome-miRNA, transcriptome, oral microbiota, TCM pattern, traditional Chinese medicine (TCM) tongue diagnosis, TCM pulse diagnosis, and TCM heart rate variability to find the difference with the comparison between the dry eye syndrome and healthy control 2. TBDESJS: non-DES SJS healthy controls (NHC) will receive Chinese herbal tea TBDESJS for 8 weeks on nourishing yin and moistening dryness. And we could use Schirmer's test, tear breakup time, Ocular Surface Disease Index (OSDI), EULAR Sjogren's Syndrome Patient Reported Index (ESSPRI), Pittsburgh Sleep Quality Index (PSQI), Ford Insomnia Response to Stress Test (FIRST), cytokine markers, whole-genome genotyping, TCM pattern, traditional Chinese medicine (TCM) tongue diagnosis, TCM pulse diagnosis, and TCM heart rate variability for this purpose	Other: acupuncture Acupuncture GB20 or GB20 plus BL2
Waiting list Group waiting list will not receive any treatment at acupoint GB20 plus BL2 twice a week for 8 weeks for efficacy evaluation. And we could use the exosome-miRNA, transcriptome, oral microbiota, Schirmer's test, Tear breakup time, 6-GSI, OSDI, TCM pattern, traditional Chinese medicine (TCM) tongue diagnosis, TCM pulse diagnosis, and TCM heart rate variability for this purpose	Other: acupuncture Acupuncture GB20 or GB20 plus BL2

(continued)

Groups/cohorts	Intervention/ treatment
Dry eye syndrome (DES) Dry eye syndrome (DES) will receive Chinese herbal tea TBDESJS for 8 weeks on nourishing yin and moistening. And we could use the exosome-miRNA, transcriptome, Schirmer's test, tear breakup time, Ocular Surface Disease Index (OSDI), EULAR Sjogren's Syndrome Patient Reported Index (ESSPRI), Pittsburgh Sleep Quality Index (PSQI), Ford Insomnia Response to Stress Test (FIRST), cytokine markers, whole-genome genotyping, TCM pattern, traditional Chinese medicine (TCM) tongue diagnosis, TCM pulse diagnosis, and TCM heart rate variability for this purpose	Other: TBDESJS Chinese herbal tea TBDESJS
Sjögren's syndrome (SJS) Sjögren's syndrome (SJS) will receive Chinese herbal tea TBDESJS for 8 weeks on nourishing yin and moistening dryness the ocular dryness evaluation. And we could use the exosome-miRNA, transcriptome, Schirmer's test, tear breakup time, Ocular Surface Disease Index (OSDI), EULAR Sjogren's Syndrome Patient Reported Index (ESSPRI), Pittsburgh Sleep Quality Index (PSQI), Ford Insomnia Response to Stress Test (FIRST), cytokine markers, whole-genome genotyping, TCM pattern, traditional Chinese medicine (TCM) tongue diagnosis, TCM pulse diagnosis, and TCM heart rate variability for this purpose	Other: TBDESJS Chinese herbal tea TBDESJS

Primary Outcome Measures

Outcome measure	Measure description	Time frame
Schirmer's test	Dry eye syndrome (DES) and Sjögren's syndrome (SJS) take the Schirmer's test	8 weeks
Ocular Surface Disease Index (OSDI)	Dry eye syndrome (DES) and Sjögren's syndrome (SJS) take the OSDI (Ocular Surface Disease Index)	8 weeks

Secondary Outcome Measures

Outcome measure	Measure description	Time frame
TCM pattern	Dry eye syndrome (DES), Sjögren's syndrome (SJS), and non-DES SJS healthy controls (NHC) take the TCM pattern to differentiate the nine types of TCM constitutions	8 weeks
TCM tongue diagnosis	Dry eye syndrome (DES), Sjögren's syndrome (SJS), and non-DES SJS healthy controls (NHC) take the TCM tongue diagnosis with camera photo to differentiate the TCM tongue feature factors about tongue body, tongue coating, red spot, tooth marks, and ecchymosis. TCM tongue feature factors would present the status of inflammation, blood stasis, heat, and dampness with TCM theory	8 weeks

(continued)

Outcome measure	Measure description	Time frame
TCM pulse diagnosis	Dry eye syndrome (DES), Sjögren's syndrome (SJS), and non-DES SJS healthy controls (NHC) take the TCM pulse diagnosis with blood pressure monitors to differentiate the TCM pulse feature factors about floating, deep, slow, rapid, deficient, excessive, slippery, rough, string-like, soggy, fine, and weak. TCM tongue feature factors would present the status of inflammation, blood stasis, heat, and dampness with TCM theory	8 weeks
TCM heart rate variability	Dry eye syndrome (DES), Sjögren's syndrome (SJS), and non-DES SJS healthy controls (NHC) take the TCM heart rate variability	8 weeks
Whole-genome genotyping (TWBv2.0)	Dry eye syndrome (DES), Sjögren's syndrome (SJS), and non-DES SJS healthy controls (NHC) take the whole-genome genotyping (TWBv2.0)	8 weeks
Cytokine markers	Dry eye syndrome (DES), Sjögren's syndrome (SJS), and non-DES SJS healthy controls (NHC) take the cytokine markers (IL-17, MMP-9, BAFF, BCMA) analysis	8 weeks
Pittsburgh Sleep Quality Index	Dry eye syndrome (DES), Sjögren's syndrome (SJS), and non-DES SJS healthy controls (NHC) take the Pittsburgh Sleep Quality Index	8 weeks
Ford Insomnia Response to Stress Test	Dry eye syndrome (DES), Sjögren's syndrome (SJS), and non-DES SJS healthy controls (NHC) take the Ford Insomnia Response to Stress Test	8 weeks
EULAR Sjogren's Syndrome Patient Reported Index (ESSPRI)	Dry eye syndrome (DES), Sjögren's syndrome (SJS), and non-DES SJS healthy controls (NHC) take the EULAR Sjögren's Syndrome Patient Reported Index (ESSPRI)	8 weeks
Tear breakup time (TBUT)	Tear breakup time (TBUT) is a clinical test used to assess for evaporative dry eye disease	8 weeks
Exosome-miRNA, transcriptome	Exosome-miRNA and transcriptome can be used to assess for dry eye syndrome (DES), Sjögren's syndrome (SJS), and non-DES SJS healthy controls (NHC)	8 weeks

Sponsor
Taipei Veterans General Hospital, Taiwan
Investigators

- Principal investigator: Ching-Mao Chang, M.D., Ph.D., Taipei Veterans General Hospital, Taiwan

Diabetic Retinopathy

Not Yet Recruiting

1. Proteomic Study of Plasma Exosomes in Patients with Diabetic Retinopathy

   ClinicalTrials.gov ID NCT06188013

Sponsor Xuanwu Hospital, Beijing
Information provided by Xuanwu Hospital, Beijing (Responsible Party)
Last Update Posted 2024-01-03
Study Overview
Brief Summary

Objective: Explore the biomarkers related to proliferative diabetic retinopathy by analyzing the protein expression profile changes of plasma exosomes in patients with different phases of diabetic retinopathy, and investigate potential molecular mechanisms and therapeutic targets. Methods: Enrich exosomes from plasma by a column extraction method. NTA, WB, and TEM were used to characterize the obtained exosomes, and exosome proteomics was performed by chromatography-mass spectrometry. Cohorts: The study was divided into four groups—a healthy control group, a diabetic without diabetic retinopathy group, a non-proliferative diabetic retinopathy group, and a proliferative diabetic retinopathy group, with six cases in each group.

Official Title
Proteomic Study of Plasma Exosomes in Patients with Diabetic Retinopathy
Conditions
Diabetic retinopathy
Other Study ID Numbers

- wuhang2317

Study Start (Estimated)
2024-01-02
Primary Completion (Estimated)
2024-03-31
Study Completion (Estimated)
2024-06-30
Enrollment (Estimated)
24
Study Type
Observational
Study Contact
Name: Hang Wu, Master
Phone Number: +86-13911993866
Email: wuhang2317@163.com
Study Contact Backup
Name: Zhen Li, Doctor
Phone Number: +86-13581646689
Email: zhenli_xwyy@163.com
No location data
Eligibility Criteria
Description
Inclusion Criteria:

- Healthy volunteers without diabetes/senile cataract patients without diabetes
- Patients with diabetes who are diagnosed without DR, NPDR, and PDR by mydriatic fundus photography (or FFA)

Exclusion Criteria:

- Patients with systemic diseases such as cancer, immune diseases, infectious diseases, and blood diseases
- Patients with cerebral infarction, myocardial infarction, and other cardiovascular and cerebrovascular diseases

Study Population

Plasma exosomal proteomics studies in patients with diabetic retinopathy should include healthy volunteers without diabetes mellitus and elderly cataract patients without diabetes mellitus; patients with systemic diseases such as cancer, immune disorders, infectious diseases, and hematological disorders, as well as patients suffering from cerebral infarcts, cardiac infarcts, and other cardiovascular diseases, are not eligible for enrollment.

Ages Eligible for Study

18 years and older (adult, older adult)

Sexes Eligible for Study

All

Accepts Healthy Volunteers

Yes

Sampling Method

Non-probability Sample

Study Plan

Design Details

Observational model: case-control

Time perspective: prospective

Groups and Interventions

Groups/cohorts
Proliferative diabetic retinopathy Age ≥18 years; patients diagnosed with PDR by FFA
Non-proliferative diabetic retinopathy Age ≥18 years; patients diagnosed with NPDR by FFA
Diabetes mellitus without retinopathy Age ≥18 years; patients diagnosed with diabetes mellitus; patients were not diagnosed with diabetic retinopathy
Healthy control Age ≥18 years; patients were not diagnosed with diabetes mellitus

Primary Outcome Measures

Outcome measure	Measure description	Time frame
Differential proteins of exosomes	Exosomes were extracted and isolated from plasma, proteomics analysis of proteins in exosomes was performed to compare the number of types of changes in exosomal proteins of the four groups and to identify proteins that were upregulated and/or downregulated, and the relationship between the proteins and diabetic retinopathy was then analyzed to look for possible mechanisms and therapeutic targets for diabetic retinopathy	December 2023–June 2024

Sponsor
Xuanwu Hospital, Beijing
Not Yet Recruiting

2. Study on Exosome Changes in Patients with Proliferative Diabetic Retinopathy

ClinicalTrials.gov ID NCT06198543
Sponsor Xuanwu Hospital, Beijing
Information provided by Xuanwu Hospital, Beijing (Responsible Party)
Last Update Posted 2024-01-10
Study Overview
Brief Summary

Diabetic retinopathy is a common complication of diabetes and one of the leading causes of low vision and blindness in adults. In recent years, the prevalence of diabetes and the incidence of diabetic retinopathy have increased significantly in our country. Epidemiological studies show that the prevalence rate of diabetes in China is 12.8%, and the prevalence rate of DR in adult diabetic patients is 24.7–37.5%, that is, there are about 3200–48 million DR patients in China, and the patients have a trend of younger people. DR has become a serious public health problem threatening people's lives and health.

At present, it is known that the pathogenesis of DR is related to hypoxia, oxidative stress, inflammation, abnormal expression of cytokines, and gene methylation, but the specific pathogenesis has not been fully clarified. Due to the hidden early symptoms of DR, the lack of basic screening conditions in primary medical and health institutions, and the lack of awareness of DR by patients themselves, many DR patients have already developed serious retinopathy when they seek medical treatment, resulting in irreversible visual function impairment. In addition, the current clinical treatment methods for DR mainly include retinal photocoagulation therapy, intraocular anti-VEGF drug injection, and vitrectomy surgery. These methods are aimed at relatively severe diabetic retinopathy, and there is no effective treatment method for early diabetic retinopathy that can prevent or slow down the occurrence and development of DR. Therefore, to further explore the pathogenesis of DR and develop new therapeutic methods has become an urgent problem.

Exosomes are extracellular vesicles secreted by living cells with a diameter of 40–150nm. With a bilayer lipid membrane structure, exosomes contain a variety of biomolecules, such as lipids, proteins, nucleic acids, cytokines, and autoantigens, and are important mediators for the transmission of biological information between cells. Almost all cells can secrete exosomes, and exosomes from different cells have different functions. Exosomes transfer their contents to nearby or distant cells and participate in cell growth, angiogenesis, immune regulation, and other processes. Previous studies have shown that exosomes secreted by various cells in the retina are present in the vitreous and aqueous humor of patients and play an important role in the pathogenesis of DR. At the same time, exosomes in the systemic circulation of diabetic patients can also reach the retina through the blood circulation, participate in the initiation process of DR, and play an important role. At the same time, due to the double-layer lipid membrane structure, exosomes can also target the coated components to specific cells and tissues through biological barriers such as blood-brain and blood-eye, which is expected to become a highly efficient drug delivery route. Therefore, the role of exosomes in DR treatment has also attracted much attention.

Detailed Description

Research Purpose

1. Compared the changes of exosomes in intraocular fluid and blood of patients with proliferative diabetic retinopathy and non-diabetic patients
2. Analyzed differentially expressed proteins in the exosomes of the two groups of patients using proteomic techniques, laying the foundation for screening possible biomarkers and potential therapeutic targets for the early diagnosis of diabetic retinopathy

Design

1. Subject population: patients with proliferative diabetic retinopathy and non-diabetic macular epiretinal membrane/macular hole requiring vitrectomy were admitted to the Ophthalmology Department of Xuanwu Hospital, Capital Medical University.
2. Sample size: a total of 60 patients were included in the study.
3. Grouping of subjects: experimental group, proliferative diabetic retinopathy; control group, patients with macular epiretinal membranes and macular holes without diabetes.

Official Title

Study on Exosome Changes in Patients with Proliferative Diabetic Retinopathy

Conditions

Diabetic retinopathy

Other Study ID Numbers

- Wuhang

Study Start (Estimated)

2024-01

Primary Completion (Estimated)

2025-01

Study Completion (Estimated)

2025-04
Enrollment (Estimated)
60
Study Type
Observational
Study Contact
Name: Hang Wu, Master
Phone Number: +8613911993866
Email: wuhang2317@163.com
Study Contact Backup
Name: Zhen Li, Doctor
Phone Number: +8613581646689
Email: zhenli_xwyy@163.com
No location data
Eligibility Criteria
Description
Inclusion Criteria:

1. Age ≥18 years
2. Patients diagnosed with PDR by FFA and requiring vitrectomy for treatment
3. Patients with no history of diabetes and diagnosed with macular anterior membrane or macular hiatus by color fundus photography and OCT
4. Sign the informed consent form

Exclusion Criteria:

1. Suffering from cancer, immune diseases, infectious diseases, and other systemic diseases.
2. Patients with retinal arteriovenous obstruction.
3. Intraocular infection.
4. Patients with uveitis.
5. In patients with high myopia, the equivalent spherical lens was >-9.0D.
6. Recent history of cerebral infarction, myocardial infarction, and other thrombi.
7. Patients with contraindications to surgery.

Study Population

All subjects enrolled in this study were patients over 18 years of age who signed an informed consent form requiring vitrectomy treatment. Subjects in the experimental group were patients with proliferative diabetic retinopathy, and those in the control group were patients who did not have diabetes but had macular holes or epiretinal membranes. Those with the following conditions could not be enrolled in the study: (1) suffering from cancer, immune diseases, infectious diseases and other systemic diseases; (2) patients with retinal arteriovenous obstruction; (3) intraocular infection; (4) patients with uveitis; (5) in patients with high myopia, the equivalent spherical lens was >-9.0D; (6) recent history of cerebral infarction, myocardial infarction, and other thrombi; and (7) patients with contraindications to surgery.

Ages Eligible for Study

18 years and older (adult, older adult)
Sexes Eligible for Study
All
Accepts Healthy Volunteers
No
Sampling Method
Non-probability Sample
Design Details
Observational model: case-control
Time perspective: cross-sectional

Groups and Interventions

Groups/Cohorts
Experimental group Proliferative diabetic retinopathy
Control group Patients with macular epiretinal membranes and macular holes without diabetes

Primary Outcome Measures

Outcome measure	Measure description	Time frame
Differential proteins of exosomes	Exosomes from plasma, atrial fluid, and vitreous fluid were isolated and extracted, and proteomic analysis of proteins in exosomes was performed to analyze the number of differentially expressed protein species in the test and control groups, and bioinformatics analysis of upregulated or downregulated expressed proteins was performed	January 2024–January 2025

Sponsor
Xuanwu Hospital, Beijing

Chapter 8
Orthopedic Exosome Trials

Recruiting

Mesenchymal Stem Cell-Derived Exosomes in Osteoarthritis Patients

ClinicalTrials.gov ID NCT06466850

Sponsor Isfahan University of Medical Sciences

Information provided by Leila Dehghani, Isfahan University of Medical Sciences (Responsible Party)

Last Update Posted 2024-06-20

Study Overview

Brief Summary

Present research focuses on the potential of exosomes, which are small vesicles secreted by mesenchymal stem cells (MSCs), as a therapeutic approach for osteoarthritis (OA).

OA is a degenerative joint disorder characterized by the destruction of cartilage and loss of extracellular matrix. It is associated with pro-inflammatory cytokines and increased expression of matrix metalloproteinase (MMP) and "a disintegrin and metalloproteinase with thrombospondin motifs" (ADAMTS).

MSCs have been explored as a new treatment for OA over the last decade. It is suggested that the paracrine secretion of trophic factors, in which exosomes play a crucial role, contributes to the mechanism of MSC-based treatment of OA.

Exosomes derived from MSCs may suppress OA development. They carry bioactive molecules of the parental cells, including non-coding RNAs (ncRNAs) and proteins and anti-inflammatory factors. These exosomes have shown a significant impact on the modulation of various physiological behaviors of cells in the joint cavity.

J. N. Weiss, *Global Exosome Trials*, https://doi.org/10.1007/978-3-031-96420-6_8

This research provides hope for developing more effective and predictable methods of using MSC-derived exosomes for OA treatment.

Official Title

The Efficacy of Allogenic Mesenchymal Stem Cell-Derived Exosomes in Osteoarthritis Patients

Conditions

Osteoarthritis, knee

Intervention/Treatment

- Biological: exosome

Other Study ID Numbers

- Isfahan med

Study Start (Actual)
2024-01-01
Primary Completion (Estimated)
2024-12-25
Study Completion (Estimated)
2025-01-25
Enrollment (Estimated)
20
Study Type
Interventional
Phase
Not applicable
Study Contact
Name: Leila Dehghani, Dr
Phone Number: 36202020 ext 031
Email: l_dehghani2002@yahoo.com
Study Contact Backup
Name: Masoud Soleimani, Prof
Phone Number: 03136202020 ext 031
Email: a70.leiladehghani@gmail.com
This study has 1 location
Iran, Islamic Republic of
Isfahan, Iran, Islamic Republic of
Recruiting
Leila Dehghani
Contact:
Leila Dehghani, Assisstant Prof
36202020 ext 031 l_dehghani2002@yahoo.com
Contact:
Masoud Soleimani, Prof
36202020 ext 031 a70.leiladehghani@gmail.com
Eligibility Criteria

Description
Inclusion Criteria:

- Chronic history (for at least 3 months) of knee joint pain
- Body mass index (BMI) between 21.5 and 29.5
- Radiographically documented knee osteoarthritis of grades 1–3 (Kellgren-Lawrence (K-L) radiographic classification scale)

Exclusion Criteria:

- Rheumatoid arthritis and other rheumatic diseases
- Varus or valgus more than 10 degrees; lateral subluxation of the patella
- Deformity at the joint levels or adjacent to the knee due to fracture or any other injury
- Complete rupture of the ligament and meniscus leading to laxity or locking
- Serious systemic, oncohematological, autoimmune diseases, history of severe allergy, serious failure of vital organs, inability to walk
- Hyaluronic acid infiltration within the previous six months
- Hemoglobin levels <10 g/dL

Ages Eligible for Study
45–75 years (adult, older adult)
Sexes Eligible for Study
All
Accepts Healthy Volunteers
No
Study Plan
Design Details
Primary purpose: supportive care
Allocation: N/A
Interventional model: single group assignment
Masking: none (open label)

Arms and Interventions

Participant group/arm	Intervention/treatment
Experimental: treatment Patients with moderate to severe osteoarthritis, Kellgren-Lawrence grades 2 and 3 in both knees, accompanied by mild to moderate pain and swelling, are included	Biological: exosome Intra-articular injection is suggested for two times: day 1 and day 90 Other names: EVs

Primary Outcome Measures

Outcome measure	Measure description	Time frame
Western Ontario and McMaster University Osteoarthritis index (WOMAC)	Filling out the WOMAC questionnaire, evaluating the measures related to knee function	1, 3, and 6 months. The second injection is repeated in day 90 after first injection

Sponsor
Isfahan University of Medical Sciences
Investigators

- Principal Investigator: Leila Dehghani, Dr, Isfahan University of Medical Sciences

Recruiting

Clinical Efficacy of Exosome in Degenerative Meniscal Injury (KNEEXO)

ClinicalTrials.gov ID NCT05261360
Sponsor Eskisehir Osmangazi University
Information provided by Ayla Eker Sariboyaci, Eskisehir Osmangazi University (Responsible Party)
Last Update Posted 2022-03-04
Study Overview
Brief Summary
Comparison of intra-articular administration of synovial fluid-derived mesenchymal stem cell-derived exosomes with synovial fluid-derived mesenchymal stem cells on the same patient.
Detailed Description
Mesenchymal stem cell-derived exosomes will be developed and patented as an advanced technology platform as an autologous treatment protocol to repair damaged cartilage tissue. The fact that this treatment is obtained from an autologous source will significantly contribute to the literature in the field of personalized therapy (personalized medicine) and will pave the way for discoveries. Experiences from clinical trials may guide the use of MSC exosomes in other tissue and cell-damaged pathologies and immune pathologies or chronic inflammatory diseases.
This study was supported by a grant (1004, 20AG031) from the Scientific and Technological Research Council of Turkey (TUBITAK).
Official Title
A Phase II Trial to Investigate Clinical Efficacy of Autologous Synovial Fluid Mesenchymal Stem Cell-Derived Exosome Application in Patients with Degenerative Meniscal Injury
Conditions
Knee, injury, meniscus (lateral, medial)
Meniscus tear
Meniscus lesion
Meniscus, degeneration
Intervention/Treatment

- Drug: SF-MSC-EX

- Drug: SF-MSC

Other Study ID Numbers

- 56733164/203

Study Start (Estimated)
2022-03
Primary Completion (Estimated)
2024-03
Study Completion (Estimated)
2025-03
Enrollment (Estimated)
30
Study Type
Interventional
Phase
Phase 2
Study Contact
Name: Ayla Eker Sarıboyacı, AssocProfDr.
Phone Number: +905382696420
Email: aylaekersariboyaci@yahoo.com
This study has 1 location
Turkey
Eskisehir, Turkey, 26040
Recruiting
Eskisehir Osmangazi University
Contact:
Ayla Eker Sariboyaci, AssocProfDr
+905382696420 aylaekersariboyaci@yahoo.com
Principal Investigator:
Ulukan Inan, Prof.Dr.
Eligibility Criteria
Description
Inclusion Criteria:

- Accepting the informed consent form
- Degenerative meniscus damage grade 1, 2, or 3 on MRI in both right and left knees and also the patient not wanting surgical treatment
- Patients with the same degenerative meniscus grade in both knees
- Patients with ongoing pain
- Patients without a history of malignancy
- Absence of signs of unstable meniscus tear such as snagging or locking
- Patients with stage 0, 1, or 2 gonarthrosis according to Kellgren-Lawrence gonarthrosis staging
- Patients without lower extremity malalignment

Exclusion Criteria:

- Patients whose treatment method was explained and who did not accept the method
- Patients outside the working-age range
- Congenital lesion
- Patients requiring surgical treatment (e.g., bucket handle tear and locked knee)
- Active inflammatory or connective tissue disease is thought to affect the patient's pain (e.g., lupus, rheumatoid arthritis, fibromyalgia)
- Local or systemic infection
- Pregnant or breastfeeding women
- Active endocrine disorder that may affect the assessment of the patient's pain (e.g., hypothyroidism, diabetes)
- Active neurological disorder that may affect the assessment of the patient's pain (e.g., peripheral neuropathy, multiple sclerosis)
- Active heart disease
- Presence of a pacemaker
- Conditions where MRI is contraindicated
- Patients with stage 3 or 4 gonarthrosis according to Kellgren-Lawrence gonarthrosis staging
- Patients with lower extremity malalignment
- Patients with signs of unstable meniscus tear such as snagging or locking

Ages Eligible for Study
30–50 years (adult)
Sexes Eligible for Study
All
Accepts Healthy Volunteers
No
Design Details
Primary purpose: treatment
Allocation: randomized
Interventional model: parallel assignment

Interventional model description: The study was planned as three arms. One arm will be the control group, and the other two arms will be the experimental group. The control group defines the group that did not receive treatment. Those in the experimental group, who are the participants other than the control group, will be in both experimental groups. SF-MSC (synovial fluid-derived mesenchymal stem cells) will be applied intra-articularly to the experimental group's right knee, and the experimental group's right knee will be included in the SF-MSC treatment group. SF-MSC-EX (synovial fluid-derived mesenchymal stem cell-derived exosomes) will be applied intra-articularly to the experimental group's left knee, and the experimental group's left knee will be included in the SF-MSC-EX treatment group.

Masking: none (open label)

Arms and Interventions

Participant group/arm	Intervention/treatment
Experimental: SF-MSC-EX treatment group (experimental group's left knees) The left knee will receive 1 million cells/kg SF-MSC-EX (synovial fluid mesenchymal stem cell-derived exosome) by intra-articular injection method	Drug: SF-MSC-EX Intra-articular administration of synovial fluid-derived mesenchymal stem cell-derived exosomes Other names: Intra-articular exosome treatment
Experimental: SF-MSC treatment group (experimental group's right knees) The right knee will receive 1 million cells/kg SF-MSC (synovial fluid-derived mesenchymal stem cell) by intra-articular injection method	Drug: SF-MSC Intra-articular administration of synovial fluid-derived mesenchymal stem cells Other names: Intra-articular stem cell treatment
No intervention: control group Participants who received no treatment were defined as the control group	

Primary Outcome Measures

Outcome measure	Measure description	Time frame
Evaluation of knee functions	The functional evaluation of the participants will be evaluated on the Tegner-Lysholm knee scoring scale. In Tegner-Lysholm knee scoring, examinations for the knee joint (limp, support, pain, instability, locking, swelling, stair-climbing, and squatting) will be evaluated, and a maximum of 100 and a minimum of 0 point will be given. According to the evaluation, <65 points are interpreted as bad, 65–83 points as fair, 84–90 points as good, and >90 points as excellent. Scores will be recorded by being examined before treatment and at the 6th and 12th months after treatment. Knee functions of the control group will be evaluated simultaneously, and the effects of treatments on knee function will be determined	Up to 12th month
Evaluation of physical activity	The physical activity evaluation of the participants will be evaluated with the IPAQ (international physical activity questionnaire) short form. IPAQ short form will be evaluated and recorded before treatment and at the 6th and 12th months after treatment. The control group's physical activity will be evaluated simultaneously, and the effects of treatments on physical activity will be determined	Up to 12th month
Evaluation of pain	Pain assessment of the participants will be evaluated with VAS (visual analog scale). The VAS will be evaluated and recorded before treatment and at the 6th and 12th months after treatment. The physical activity of the control group will be evaluated simultaneously, and the effects of treatments on pain will be determined	Up to 12th month

Outcome measure	Measure description	Time frame
Evaluation of radiological images	Participants will receive knee X-ray imaging and knee magnetic resonance imaging before treatment. The same radiological imaging will be performed at the 6th and 12th months after the treatment. At the same time, the same radiological imaging will be performed on the control group, and the effects of treatments on radiological imaging will be evaluated.	Up to 12th month
Evaluation of cytokine levels and cytokine gene analyzers	Before treatment and at the 6th and 12th months after treatment, cytokine levels (IL-10, IL-6, TNF-α, IL-8, IL-1β, IFN-ɣ, IL-2, IL-4, IL-13, MCP-1, VEGF) and gene analyzes (IL-10, IL-6, TNF-α, IL-8, IL-1β, IFN-ɣ, IL-2, IL-4, IL-13, MCP-1, IL-1ra, MIP-1b, CTGF, TGFβ3, BMP-2, BMP-4, IGF-1, IGF-2, PDGF, EGF, and VEGF genes) will be checked in the samples taken from the synovial fluid and blood. Samples will be taken from the control group along with the treatment group. In this way, the effects of treatments on cytokine levels will be evaluated	Up to 12th month
Evaluation of edema	Edema in both knees will be measured using a tape measure by marking the midpoints of both patellae. Pretreatment measurements will be recorded. Measurements of both knees will be recorded at 6 months and 12 months after treatment. The knees of the patients not receiving treatment will be measured simultaneously, and the changes will be compared.	Up to 12th month
Evaluation of knee joint range of motion	The range of motion of both knees will be measured using the "Baseline Digital Absolute+Axis Goniometer." Knee extension measurements will be made with the patient in the supine position and flexion in the prone position. Pretreatment measurements will be recorded. Post-treatment 6- and 12-month measurements will also be recorded. Measurements of patients not receiving treatment will be recorded simultaneously, and changes will be compared	Up to 12th month
Monitoring of treatment-related complications	Adverse effects and complications will be observed in the treatment group, except for the expected local reactions (redness, swelling, bruising, etc.) after the application	Up to 12th month

Sponsor
Eskisehir Osmangazi University
Collaborators

- The Scientific and Technological Research Council of Turkey

Investigators

- Study Chair: Ayla Eker Sarıboyacı, AssocProfDr., Cell Therapy and Stem Cell Production Application and Research Center (ESTEM)
- Study Director: Onur Uysal, AssocProfDr., Cell Therapy and Stem Cell Production Application and Research Center (ESTEM)
- Principal Investigator: Ulukan İnan, ProfDr., Eskisehir Osmangazi University Faculty of Medicine Department of Orthopedy and Traumatology

Publications

- Tegner Y, Lysholm J. Rating systems in the evaluation of knee ligament injuries. Clin Orthop Relat Res. 1985 Sep;(198):43–9.
- Craig CL, Marshall AL, Sjostrom M, Bauman AE, Booth ML, Ainsworth BE, Pratt M, Ekelund U, Yngve A, Sallis JF, Oja P. International physical activity questionnaire: 12-country reliability and validity. Med Sci Sports Exerc. 2003 Aug;35(8):1381–95. https://doi.org/10.1249/01.MSS.0000078924.61453.FB.
- Pan H, Zhang P, Zhang Z, Yang Q. Arthroscopic partial meniscectomy combined with medical exercise therapy versus isolated medical exercise therapy for degenerative meniscal tear: A meta-analysis of randomized controlled trials. Int J Surg. 2020 Jul;79:222–232. https://doi.org/10.1016/j.ijsu.2020.05.035. Epub 2020 Jun 6.

Recruiting

Intra-articular Injection of UC-MSC Exosome in Knee Osteoarthritis (EXO-OA01)

ClinicalTrials.gov ID NCT06431152

Sponsor Universidad de los Andes, Chile

Information provided by Universidad de los Andes, Chile (Responsible Party)

Last Update Posted 2024-05-29

Study Overview

Brief Summary

The study aims to evaluate the safety of exosomes (sEVs) from allogeneic mesenchymal stromal cells delivered by an intra-articular injection in the knee of patients with mild to moderate symptomatic osteoarthritis. The sEVs will be produced in a GMP facility. The investigators expect to enroll 12 patients in this phase 1 trial, open-label dose-escalation pilot, and the follow-up will be up to 12 months.

Detailed Description

The clinical investigation will represent a phase 1 trial focusing on small extracellular vesicles derived from mesenchymal stem cell (MSC-sEV) in patients with symptomatic Kellgren II–III knee OA. The phase 1 component of the study will be an open-label dose escalation pilot study in which three cohorts of subjects with OA will receive increasing doses of UC-MSC-sEV administered as a single intra-articular (IA) injection. Each cohort will comprise four participants. Eligible study subjects will be enrolled at the "Clinica Universidad de los Andes."

The small extracellular vesicles derived from umbilical cord mesenchymal stem cell (UC-MSC-sEV) will be prepared in the "Clinica Universidad de los Andes" GMP facility. The sEV-based therapeutic for clinical use will be manufactured in compliance with standardized procedures based on Good Manufacture Practice (GMP)) regulations and all quality controls aforementioned. The sEV therapeutic will be transported to the patient administration site under controlled conditions, ensuring maintenance of a temperature range between 2 °C and 8 °C. The sEV injection is expected to be administered within the first 6 h of product manufacture.

The primary study endpoints of this trial will focus on the safety, feasibility, and toxicity of the sEV-based product. The phase I will examine (1) the incidence of immediate post-infiltration adverse reactions in patients; (2) the occurrence of synovitis post-infiltration in patients at 24 and 48 hours, as well as on days 7 and 15; (3) the frequency of post-infiltration pain reported by patients at 24 and 48 h, and on days 7 and 15; and (4) the prevalence of adverse events related to sEV therapy occurring beyond IA infiltration at 24 and 48 h, and on days 7 and 15, as well as at months 2, 4, 6, 8, 10, and 12. The secondary study endpoint will determine the optimal dose for phase II trials. The criteria that will be considered are (1) safety profile at infiltration at 24 and 48 h, and on days 7 and 15, as well as at months 2, 4, 6, 8, 10, and 12; (2) changes in WOMAC scores at months 2, 4, 6, 8, 10, and 12; and (3) alterations in the visual analog scale (VAS) pain scores at months 2, 4, 6, 8, 10, and 12.

Official Title

Administration of sEV Derived from UC-MSC in Patients with Osteoarthritis of the Knee: Safety Determination in a Pilot Dose-Escalation Study

Conditions

Osteoarthritis knee

Intervention/Treatment

- Biological: UC-MSC sEV

Other Study ID Numbers

- EXO-OA01

Study Start (Estimated)
2024-06-01
Primary Completion (Estimated)
2025-06-30
Study Completion (Estimated)
2025-12-31
Enrollment (Estimated)
12
Study Type
Interventional
Phase
Early Phase 1
Study Contact
Name: Jose Matas, MD
Phone Number: +56 2 26183347 ext 3347
Email: jmatas@clinicauandes.cl
Study Contact Backup
Name: Francisco Espinoza, MD
Phone Number: +56 2 26183347 ext 3347

Email: fespinoza@clinicauandes.cl
This study has 1 location
Chile
Las Condes Locations
Santiago, Las Condes, Chile, 2501
Recruiting
Clinica Universidad de los Andes
Contact:
Bernardita Hurtado
226182071 bhurtadodeme@clinicauandes.cl
Contact:
Consuelo Covarrubias
226182071 ccovarrubias@uandes.cl
Eligibility Criteria
Description
Inclusion Criteria:

- Age 30–70 years.
- Kellgren-Lawrence grade II–III knee OA (Rosenberg view X-ray).
- VAS for pain ≥40 mm, without surgical indication in the affected knee.
- In case of bilateral involvement, the most affected knee will be treated. The contralateral knee should be asymptomatic or present a VAS ≤ 20 mm.
- Stable knee with normal physical examination.
- Signed informed consent.

Exclusion Criteria:

- Symptomatic bilateral knee OA
- BMI >30 kg/m^2
- Joint instability at physical examination
- Mechanical meniscal tear on physical examination
- Associated conditions: active local or systemic infection, neoplasia, immunosuppression, pregnancy, anticoagulant therapy, coagulation disorders, inflammatory joint disease (autoimmune, by crystal or other), joint prosthesis, symptomatic spine, or hip disease
- Recent use of intra-articular (last 6 months) or oral (last month) steroid therapy
- Recent use of intra-articular hyaluronic acid therapy (last 6 months)
- Subchondral bone fracture

Ages Eligible for Study
30–70 years (adult, older adult)
Sexes Eligible for Study
All
Accepts Healthy Volunteers
No
Design Details
Primary purpose: treatment

Allocation: randomized
Interventional model: parallel assignment
Masking: none (open label)

Arms and Interventions

Participant group/arm	Intervention/treatment
Experimental: low dose Intra-articular knee injection of exosomes (2 × 10e9 particles/dose) derived from allogeneic mesenchymal stromal cells. Single dose 4 patients	Biological: UC-MSC sEV Small extracellular vesicles derived from allogenic mesenchymal stromal cells, single dose Other names: Cellistem®sEV-OA
Experimental: medial dose Intra-articular knee injection of exosomes (6 × 10e9 particles/dose) derived from allogeneic mesenchymal stromal cells. Single dose 4 patients	Biological: UC-MSC sEV Small extracellular vesicles derived from allogenic mesenchymal stromal cells, single dose Other names: Cellistem®sEV-OA
Experimental: high dose Intra-articular knee injection of exosomes (2 × 10e10 particles/dose) derived from allogeneic mesenchymal stromal cells. Single dose 4 patients	Biological: UC-MSC sEV Small extracellular vesicles derived from allogenic mesenchymal stromal cells, single dose Other names: Cellistem®sEV-OA

Primary Outcome Measures

Outcome measure	Measure description	Time frame
Adverse event	Occurrence of any adverse reactions within 12 months of treatment	12 months

Secondary Outcome Measures

Outcome measure	Measure description	Time frame
Incidence of injection-related pain according to visual analog scale (VAS) (0–100 mm)	Pain measured by visual analog scale (VAS) (0–100 mm) after the first week of treatment	1–2 weeks
Incidence of injection-related synovitis according to the effusion grading scale of the knee joint	Synovitis measured by effusion grading scale (zero to 3+) after the first week of treatment	1–2 weeks
Pain change	Change in visual analog scale (VAS) (0–100 mm) score every 2 months	12 months
Disability change	Change in WOMAC subscale (Western Ontario and McMaster Universities Osteoarthritis IndexWomac) related to function (C) every 2 months. Pain (0–20), stiffness (0–8), functional capacity (0–68)	12 months
Percentage of responders	According to OMERACT-OARSI Criteria Index Response after 52 weeks	52 weeks

Sponsor
Universidad de los Andes, Chile
Not Yet Recruiting

Phase 1b Clinical Trial to Evaluate PEP and EUFLEXXA for Knee Osteoarthritis (KOA)

ClinicalTrials.gov ID NCT06463132

Sponsor Rion Inc.

Information provided by Rion Inc. (Responsible Party)

Last Update Posted 2024-06-17

Study Overview

Brief Summary

Evaluate the safety and exploratory efficacy of single intra-articular injections of PEP reconstituted with 0.9% normal saline at a low dose (one vial PEP) and high dose (two vials PEP), with and without EUFLEXXA, for the treatment of knee osteoarthritis.

Detailed Description

Study plan (with dose escalation): Arm 1 and Arm 2 will run in parallel, such that initially three subjects will be enrolled in Arm 1a (PEP low dose) and three subjects will be enrolled in Arm 2a (PEP-EUFLEXXA low dose). After all six subjects complete the 30-day follow-up and there was not more than 1 AE grade 3 or higher per arm, a further nine subjects will be enrolled in Arm 1b (PEP high dose), and a further nine subjects will be enrolled in Arm 2b (PEP-EUFLEXXA high dose).

Official Title

Phase 1b Open-Label, Multicenter, Randomized Trial to Evaluate the Safety of PEP and EUFLEXXA for the Treatment of Subjects with Knee Osteoarthritis (KOA)

Conditions

Knee osteoarthritis

Intervention/Treatment

- Combination product: PEP/Euflexxa
- Drug: PEP

Other Study ID Numbers

- PRO-00126

Study Start (Estimated)
2024-11-01
Primary Completion (Estimated)
2025-11-01
Study Completion (Estimated)
2025-11-01

Enrollment (Estimated)
24
Study Type
Interventional
Phase
Phase 1
Study Contact
Name: Shariq Khan, M.S.
Phone Number: 847-702-4063
Email: khan@riontx.com
Study Contact Backup
Name: Maureen Merrifield, Ph.D.
Phone Number: 2819146228
Email: merrifield@riontx.com
This study has 1 location
United States
Minnesota Locations
Rochester, Minnesota, United States, 55905
Mayo Clinic in Rochester
Eligibility Criteria
Description
Inclusion Criteria:
Age: adults aged 18–90 years
Type of participant and disease characteristics:

- Diagnosis of unilateral or bilateral symptomatic KOA of at least 6 months duration (meets American College of Rheumatology/Arthritis [ACR] criteria).
- Daily knee pain in the more symptomatic knee of $\geq$ 30 and $\leq$ 80 on a 100-point VAS for greater than 6 months.
- Kellgren-Lawrence grade 2–3 osteoarthritis in the more symptomatic knee based on standard knee radiographs.
- Failed conservative management including at least 2 of the following:
- Lack of improvement with attempted weight loss in the past year if body mass index (BMI) >30 kg/m^2.
- Lack of response to a 4-week trial in the past year of oral acetaminophen or NSAIDs taken as needed.
- Lack of response to a 4-week trial in the past year of topical NSAIDs or capsaicin applied as needed.
- Lack of improvement after injection therapy with cortisone, PRP, or hyaluronic acid.
- Lack of improvement after a 4-week course of physical therapy in the past year.
- Lack of improvement after a 4-week trial of quadriceps strengthening home exercise program in the past year.
- Requesting injection therapy for pain management.

- Contraceptive use by participants and their partners should be consistent with local regulations regarding the methods of contraception for those participating in clinical studies.

A serum pregnancy test (human chorionic gonadotropin [hCG]) should be done for all women of childbearing potential (WOCBP) at screening, and a urine pregnancy test should be done on day 1, prior to injection, with results reviewed before injection to confirm the participant's eligibility. Participants who have positive pregnancy test result will not be permitted to continue in the study.

- Signed informed consent as described in Appendix 1 (Section 10.1) which includes compliance with the requirements and restrictions listed in the informed consent form (ICF) and in this protocol.
- Ability to comply with protocol.

Exclusion Criteria:

- Steroid or viscosupplement injection in the planned treatment knee(s) within the past 3 months
- PRP injection in the planned treatment knee(s) within the past 6 months
- History of documented allergy to intra-articular EUFLEXXA
- History of cancer including melanoma (with the exception of localized skin cancer) in the past 2 years
- HIV positive participants
- BMI >40 kg/m^2
- Arthroscopic debridement in the planned treatment knee(s) in the last 6 months
- Cartilage restoration procedure in the planned treatment knee(s) in the last 5 years
- History of gout or pseudogout
- History of or evidence of active rheumatologic disease, severe peripheral neuropathy, clinically evident cardiac or respiratory disease that interferes with functional status
- Poorly controlled diabetes defined as a glycated hemoglobin (HbA1c) concentration of ≥8.0%
- Currently taking any cancer treatment regimen (including aromatase inhibitors)
- Calcium pyrophosphate deposition disease (CPPD) evident on X-ray
- Systemic (oral, intravenous, or intramuscular) steroids in the last 3 months
- Concurrent participation in another investigational drug or device study or participation in the last 30 days prior to enrollment
- Evidence of recent alcohol or drug abuse, or history of medication misuse or addiction
- Female participants who are pregnant, breastfeeding, or trying to become pregnant
- Women unwilling to use approved contraception method for 3 months after receiving dose of investigational drug
- Unwilling or unable to comply with Telehealth visits (e.g., ability to access Internet, on-camera capabilities, etc.)

Ages Eligible for Study
18–90 years (adult, older adult)
Sexes Eligible for Study
All
Accepts Healthy Volunteers
Yes
Design Details
Primary purpose: treatment
Allocation: randomized
Interventional model: parallel assignment
Interventional model description: Arm 1A, PEP low-dose Arm 1B, PEP high-dose Arm 2A, PEP-EUFLEXXA low-dose Arm 2B, PEP-EUFLEXXA high dose
Masking: none (open label)

Arms and Interventions

Participant group/arm	Intervention/treatment
Experimental: 1A PEP low dose 1A PEP low dose in saline	Drug: PEP PEP (purified exosome product)
Experimental: 1B PEP high dose 1B PEP high dose in saline	Drug: PEP PEP (purified exosome product)
Experimental: 2a PEP-EUFLEXXA low dose 2A PEP-EUFLEXXA low dose	Combination product: PEP/Euflexxa Euflexxa (PMA: P010029)
Experimental: 2b PEP-EUFLEXXA high dose 2B PEP-EUFLEXXA high dose	Combination product: PEP/Euflexxa Euflexxa (PMA: P010029)

Primary Outcome Measures

Outcome measure	Measure description	Time frame
Primary safety follow-up 90 days post-injection occurrence of DLTs	The safety of a single intra-articular injection of PEP, with or without EUFLEXXA, through the initial 90-day treatment period, as assessed by the occurrence of DLTs with severity grading based on the National Cancer Institute-Common Terminology Criteria for Adverse Events (NCI CTCAE)	First 90 days
Long-term safety follow-up occurrence of DLTs from day 91 to day 365	The long-term safety after treatment with a single intra-articular injection of PEP, with or without EUFLEXXA, as assessed from the incidence of DLTs during the day 91 through day 365 follow-up period	Day 365

Secondary Outcome Measures

Outcome measure	Measure description	Time frame
Exploratory endpoints of efficacy-radiographic response	Radiographic response, evaluated pre- and post-injection by an independent, blinded radiologist's assessment: Decrease or lack of progression of cartilage damage (thickness, denudation) and/or bone marrow edema on magnetic resonance imaging (MRI) at 6 or 12 months after injection. Decrease or lack of progression in joint space narrowing on weight-bearing X-ray at 12 months after injection	Day 365
Exploratory endpoints of efficacy-participant-reported responses	Clinical improvement measured using a 100-point pain visual analog scale (VAS) and modified Western Ontario and McMasters University Arthritis Index Questionnaire (WOMAC), which utilizes measures of pain and function and treatment success based on Osteoarthritis Research Society International Outcome Measures in Rheumatology (OARSI OMERACT) responder criteria defined as follows: Absolute change of 20 points or more on the VAS 100-point scale, or improvement of 50% or more in the modified WOMAC pain or function score, or absolute change of 20 points or more in the combined modified WOMAC pain and function score	Day 365

Sponsor
Rion Inc.
Collaborators

- Caidya Clinical Research Organization

Chapter 9
Pulmonary Exosome Trials

Recruiting

Safety and Efficacy of Umbilical Cord Mesenchymal Stem Cell Exosomes in Treating Chronic Cough After COVID-19

ClinicalTrials.gov ID NCT05808400

Sponsor Huazhong University of Science and Technology

Information provided by Jihui Du, Huazhong University of Science and Technology (Responsible Party)

Last Update Posted 2023-04-14

Study Overview

Brief Summary

This clinical trial aims to evaluate the safety and effectiveness of umbilical cord mesenchymal stem cell (UCMSC)-derived extracellular vesicle nebulization inhalation therapy for the treatment of chronic cough after COVID-19 infection. The main objective is to assess whether UCMSC-derived exosome nebulization inhalation therapy alleviates chronic cough after COVID-19.

Participants will be asked to complete a questionnaire to help researchers evaluate their cough severity and to record their scores before nebulization inhalation of UCMSC-derived exosomes. Participants will receive either continuous nebulized inhalation of UCMSC-derived exosomes for 5 days, twice daily, or no treatment. Researchers will compare the experimental and control groups to evaluate the safety and efficacy of UCMSC-derived exosomes for the treatment of chronic cough after COVID-19 infection.

Detailed Description

J. N. Weiss, *Global Exosome Trials*, https://doi.org/10.1007/978-3-031-96420-6_9

1. Background 1.1 Post COVID-19 syndrome, also known as Long COVID, is still causing great trouble to the public despite China having successfully passed the first wave of infection caused by severe acute respiratory syndrome coronavirus 2 (SARS-CoV-2) for over three years, which has resulted in over 5 million deaths globally.

   Long COVID is a multiple-system disease that includes a variety of severe symptoms that persist after infection with COVID-19—(1) heart-related symptoms: chest pain, palpitations; (2) respiratory symptoms: cough, shortness of breath, loss of taste or smell; (3) pancreatic symptoms: diabetes, pancreatic injury; (4) immune system: autoimmunity, mast cell activation syndrome (MCAS); (5) neurological symptoms: cognitive impairment (brain fog), fatigue, sleep disorders, memory loss, tinnitus; (6) vascular symptoms: fatigue, coagulation disorders, deep vein thrombosis, endothelial dysfunction, microvascular disease, and stroke; (7) reproductive symptoms: erectile dysfunction , menstrual disorders, etc., which severely affect the patient's daily life. Long COVID can occur in people of all ages, and the likelihood of developing it is closely related to the severity of acute COVID-19 infection. The main high-risk factors that can trigger Long COVID include (1) type II diabetes, (2) high viral load during COVID-19 infection, (3) previous infection with EB virus, and (4) excessive specific autoantibodies. Treatment strategies for COVID-19 mainly involve using antiviral drugs to block the replication cycle of the virus and various methods to suppress host inflammation to improve symptoms. Currently, the conventional immunotherapy methods used in clinics mainly involve the use of hormones, monoclonal antibody drugs, etc., but they are mainly targeted at more severe inflammatory reactions and suffer from low bioavailability, high cost, and significant side effects, making them unsuitable for the treatment of Long COVID. Therefore, developing new immune-regulating methods with low side effects and costs would be significant for the treatment of Long COVID.

   1.2. Mesenchymal stem cells (MSCs) MSCs have been shown to have comprehensive and powerful immune-regulatory and regenerative functions. MSCs can counteract cell death related to the pathogenesis of chronic obstructive pulmonary disease (COPD), idiopathic pulmonary fibrosis, asthma, acute respiratory distress syndrome (ARDS), and pulmonary hypertension and promote cell regeneration. Exosomes are one of the key paracrine effectors secreted by MSCs, and they are considered powerful candidates for the alternative treatment of various diseases because their biological material is like that of progenitor cells, and they have the ability to maintain healing properties. Under physiological and pathological conditions, exosomes play a critical role in intercellular communication by transporting various biomolecules (such as miRNA and proteins) into target cells.
   1.3. The mechanism of MSC-derived exosomes MSC-derived exosomes inherit immunosuppressive properties from their source cells. Mesenchymal stem cell-derived extracellular vesicles (MSC-EVs) may use multiple mechanisms to balance the function of the immune system. One key mech-

anism is reprogramming and changing the phenotype of various immune cells.

In multiple models, MSC exosomes have therapeutic properties similar to MSCs and are easier to prepare, store, and transport to the bedside, while avoiding some limitations of cell therapy, such as the risk of pulmonary embolism and tumor formation. Exosomes secreted by MSCs can regulate immunity through an interaction with immune cells and inhibit inflammatory reactions through cytokines. Numerous studies have shown that exosomes secreted by MSCs can be used to treat immunodeficiency, inflammation, ARDS, and other lung diseases, so exosomes secreted by MSCs may also be effective in treating COVID-19 infections and pneumonia. The conventional method of stem cell therapy is an intravenous injection, and exosomes are one of the main active components secreted by stem cells with a size of 30–150 nm. After nebulization, exosomes can directly reach the bronchioles and alveoli, which is conducive to maximizing drug absorption.

1.4. Clinical cases of MSC-derived exosomes therapy China has also actively launched relevant clinical studies. A clinical study at Wuxi Fifth People's Hospital in Jiangsu Province confirmed that nebulized umbilical cord mesenchymal stem cell-derived exosomes are safe and feasible for treating COVID-19 pneumonia. Researchers at Ruijin Hospital and Jin Yin-tan Hospital jointly conducted nebulized exosome therapy for COVID-19 using exosomes derived from human allogeneic adipose mesenchymal stem cells (HAMSCs-Exos). Recently, the inhaled anti-COVID-19 drug Exo-CD24, a combination of exosomes and CD24 protein, has shown promising results in phase I clinical trial led by Israeli medical center expert Nadir Arber. Out of 30 critically ill volunteers in the trial, 29 were cured after five days of treatment. Although Exo-CD24 has yet to pass phase III testing, it has already demonstrated enormous potential for the future. The US FDA has approved Direct Biologics to start a phase I/II trial to evaluate ExoFlo™ for treating COVID-19. This marks the first time that extracellular vesicles (EVs) have been approved by the US FDA for treating the disease.

2. Research Purpose The aim of this study is to evaluate the safety and effectiveness of umbilical cord mesenchymal stem cell exosome nebulization inhalation for treating chronic cough in patients after COVID-19 infection through a non-randomized controlled clinical trial.
3. Study Design The study design is a prospective, non-randomized, concurrent controlled trial. Based on the routine treatment regimen for COVID-19 infection according to clinical guidelines, umbilical cord mesenchymal stem cell exosome nebulization inhalation will be used in the experimental group to treat chronic cough in patients after COVID-19 infection. The experimental group (n = 40) and control group (n = 40) will be compared with patients who did not receive exosome nebulization inhalation therapy during the same period. The safety and effectiveness of umbilical cord mesenchymal stem cell exosome nebulization

inhalation for treating chronic cough in patients after COVID-19 infection will be evaluated through cough severity score surveys, symptom improvement time, and adverse event occurrence.

3.1. Study Population A total of 80 participants will be enrolled in the study, with a ratio of 1:1 for the experimental group ($n = 40$) and the control group ($n = 40$). The study population will consist of COVID-19-infected patients who meet the selection criteria and are treated in the COVID-19 rehabilitation outpatient clinic at the Shenzhen Hospital of Southern Medical University.
3.2. Grouping (1) Experimental group: nebulization inhalation of umbilical cord mesenchymal stem cell exosome preparation. Specification: 5 ml, exosome concentration in preparation is 1*10^9 particles/ml.

(2) Control group: Patients during the same period who did not receive treatment with stem cell exosomes.

Official Title

Clinical Study of the Safety and Efficacy of Umbilical Cord Mesenchymal Stem Cell Exosomes in Treating Chronic Cough After COVID-19 Infection

Conditions

Long COVID-19 syndrome

Intervention/Treatment

- Biological: MSC-derived exosomes

Other Study ID Numbers

- KY20230214-V04

Study Start (Actual)
2023-02-15
Primary Completion (Estimated)
2024-02-15
Study Completion (Estimated)
2025-02-15
Enrollment (Estimated)
80
Study Type
Interventional
Phase
Early Phase 1
Study Contact
Name: Jihui Du, PhD
Phone Number: 8613510083963
Email: jihuidu@email.szu.edu.cn
This study has 1 location
China
Guangdong Locations

Shenzhen, Guangdong, China, 518052
Recruiting
Huazhong University of Science and Technology Union Shenzhen Hospital
Contact:
Jihui Du, PhD
8613510083963 jihuidu@email.szu.edu.cn
Eligibility Criteria
Description
Inclusion Criteria:

- Trial participants voluntarily participate in this study and sign an informed consent form.
- At the time of signing the informed consent form, the age of the subject should be ≥18 or ≤80 years old, with no gender restrictions.
- The subject has been diagnosed with COVID-19 (confirmed by positive nucleic acid or antigen test) and has symptoms that have lasted for more than 4 weeks.
- Negative nucleic acid or antigen test at the time of screening.
- The subject has had continuous or intermittent coughing, or loss of taste/smell for ≥4 weeks, which did not occur before the onset of COVID-19 infection.
- No prior treatment with umbilical cord mesenchymal stem cell-derived extracellular vesicles.
- The patient fully understands the purpose and requirements of this clinical study and is willing to complete all trial procedures according to the study requirements.

Exclusion Criteria:

- Age ≤18 or ≥80 years old
- Acute COVID-19 patients
- Suspected or confirmed to have severe, active bacterial, fungal, or other infections that may pose a risk when intervention measures are taken, as determined by the researcher
- Patients with a history of diagnosed bronchial asthma, cough variant asthma, or chronic cough; patients with other pulmonary diseases such as chronic obstructive pulmonary disease, bronchiectasis, tuberculosis, and lung cancer
- Any of the following during the screening period: (1) ALT or AST >3 times the upper limit of normal and (2) eGFR <60 mL/min
- Patients with a history of severe allergies
- Patients with uncontrolled severe cardiovascular, cerebrovascular, liver, kidney, endocrine, blood system diseases, and mental illness
- Patients with active immunosuppression, immunodeficiency, and use of immunosuppressive drugs
- Pregnant and lactating women
- Other factors that the researcher deems unsuitable for participation in the study based on clinical considerations

Ages Eligible for Study
18–80 years (adult, older adult)

Sexes Eligible for Study
All
Accepts Healthy Volunteers
No
Design Details
Primary purpose: treatment
Allocation: non-randomized
Interventional model: parallel assignment
Masking: single (Investigator)

Arms and Interventions

Participant group/arm	Intervention/treatment
Experimental: exosomes treatment group Treated with umbilical cord mesenchymal stem cell-derived extracellular vesicle (EV) preparation (specification: 5 ml, EV concentration of 1*10^9 particles/ml)	Biological: MSC-derived exosomes The total volume of MSC-derived exosomes is 5 ml, and exosome concentration in preparation is 1*10^9 particles/ml
No intervention: non-treatment group No treatment	

Primary Outcome Measures

Outcome measure	Measure description	Time frame
Cough evaluation test	This score is to evaluate the relief of cough symptoms. Higher scores mean worse outcome. Minimum score is 5, and maximum score is 25	6–14 days

Secondary Outcome Measures

Outcome measure	Measure description	Time frame
Improvement or relief time of symptoms	This indicator is used to evaluate how many days it takes to alleviate cough	6th, 15th, 28th day

Other Outcome Measures

Outcome measure	Measure description	Time frame
Pulmonary function tests or lung CT scans	This indicator is used to evaluate lung function	14th day

Sponsor
Huazhong University of Science and Technology
Collaborators

- REGEN-αGEEK (SHENZHEN) MEDICAL TECHNOLOGY CO., LTD.

Investigators

- Principal Investigator: Jihui Du, PhD, Huazhong University of Science and Technology Union Shenzhen Hospital

Publications

- El-Shennawy L, Hoffmann AD, Dashzeveg NK, McAndrews KM, Mehl PJ, Cornish D, Yu Z, Tokars VL, Nicolaescu V, Tomatsidou A, Mao C, Felicelli CJ, Tsai CF, Ostiguin C, Jia Y, Li L, Furlong K, Wysocki J, Luo X, Ruivo CF, Batlle D, Hope TJ, Shen Y, Chae YK, Zhang H, LeBleu VS, Shi T, Swaminathan S, Luo Y, Missiakas D, Randall GC, Demonbreun AR, Ison MG, Kalluri R, Fang D, Liu H. Circulating ACE2-expressing extracellular vesicles block broad strains of SARS-CoV-2. Nat Commun. 2022 Jan 20;13(1):405. https://doi.org/10.1038/s41467-021-27893-2.
- Davis HE, McCorkell L, Vogel JM, Topol EJ. Long COVID: major findings, mechanisms and recommendations. Nat Rev Microbiol. 2023 Mar;21(3):133–146. https://doi.org/10.1038/s41579-022-00846-2. Epub 2023 Jan 13. Erratum In: Nat Rev Microbiol. 2023 Jun;21(6):408. https://doi.org/10.1038/s41579-023-00896-0.
- Davido B, Seang S, Tubiana R, de Truchis P. Post-COVID-19 chronic symptoms: a postinfectious entity? Clin Microbiol Infect. 2020 Nov;26(11):1448–1449. https://doi.org/10.1016/j.cmi.2020.07.028. Epub 2020 Jul 23. No abstract available.
- Su Y, Yuan D, Chen DG, Ng RH, Wang K, Choi J, Li S, Hong S, Zhang R, Xie J, Kornilov SA, Scherler K, Pavlovitch-Bedzyk AJ, Dong S, Lausted C, Lee I, Fallen S, Dai CL, Baloni P, Smith B, Duvvuri VR, Anderson KG, Li J, Yang F, Duncombe CJ, McCulloch DJ, Rostomily C, Troisch P, Zhou J, Mackay S, DeGottardi Q, May DH, Taniguchi R, Gittelman RM, Klinger M, Snyder TM, Roper R, Wojciechowska G, Murray K, Edmark R, Evans S, Jones L, Zhou Y, Rowen L, Liu R, Chour W, Algren HA, Berrington WR, Wallick JA, Cochran RA, Micikas ME; ISB-Swedish COVID-19 Biobanking Unit; Wrin T, Petropoulos CJ, Cole HR, Fischer TD, Wei W, Hoon DSB, Price ND, Subramanian N, Hill JA, Hadlock J, Magis AT, Ribas A, Lanier LL, Boyd SD, Bluestone JA, Chu H, Hood L, Gottardo R, Greenberg PD, Davis MM, Goldman JD, Heath JR. Multiple early factors anticipate post-acute COVID-19 sequelae. Cell. 2022 Mar 3;185(5):881–895.e20. https://doi.org/10.1016/j.cell.2022.01.014. Epub 2022 Jan 25.
- Carrade Holt DD, Wood JA, Granick JL, Walker NJ, Clark KC, Borjesson DL. Equine mesenchymal stem cells inhibit T cell proliferation through different mechanisms depending on tissue source. Stem Cells Dev. 2014 Jun 1;23(11):1258–65. https://doi.org/10.1089/scd.2013.0537. Epub 2014 Mar 4.
- Sauler M, Bazan IS, Lee PJ. Cell Death in the Lung: The Apoptosis-Necroptosis Axis. Annu Rev Physiol. 2019 Feb 10;81:375–402. https://doi.org/10.1146/annurev-physiol-020518-114320. Epub 2018 Nov 28.
- Naji A, Suganuma N, Espagnolle N, Yagyu KI, Baba N, Sensebe L, Deschaseaux F. Rationale for Determining the Functional Potency of Mesenchymal Stem Cells in Preventing Regulated Cell Death for Therapeutic Use. Stem Cells Transl Med. 2017 Mar;6(3):713–719. https://doi.org/10.5966/sctm.2016-0289. Epub 2016 Oct 11.

- Janockova J, Slovinska L, Harvanova D, Spakova T, Rosocha J. New therapeutic approaches of mesenchymal stem cells-derived exosomes. J Biomed Sci. 2021 May 25;28(1):39. https://doi.org/10.1186/s12929-021-00736-4.
- Joo HS, Suh JH, Lee HJ, Bang ES, Lee JM. Current Knowledge and Future Perspectives on Mesenchymal Stem Cell-Derived Exosomes as a New Therapeutic Agent. Int J Mol Sci. 2020 Jan 22;21(3):727. https://doi.org/10.3390/ijms21030727.
- Modani S, Tomar D, Tangirala S, Sriram A, Mehra NK, Kumar R, Khatri DK, Singh PK. An updated review on exosomes: biosynthesis to clinical applications. J Drug Target. 2021 Nov;29(9):925–940. https://doi.org/10.1080/1061186X.2021.1894436. Epub 2021 Mar 12.
- Morrison TJ, Jackson MV, Cunningham EK, Kissenpfennig A, McAuley DF, O'Kane CM, Krasnodembskaya AD. Mesenchymal Stromal Cells Modulate Macrophages in Clinically Relevant Lung Injury Models by Extracellular Vesicle Mitochondrial Transfer. Am J Respir Crit Care Med. 2017 Nov 15;196(10):1275–1286. https://doi.org/10.1164/rccm.201701-0170OC.
- Wu P, Zhang B, Shi H, Qian H, Xu W. MSC-exosome: A novel cell-free therapy for cutaneous regeneration. Cytotherapy. 2018 Mar;20(3):291–301. https://doi.org/10.1016/j.jcyt.2017.11.002. Epub 2018 Feb 9.
- Chu M, Wang H, Bian L, Huang J, Wu D, Zhang R, Fei F, Chen Y, Xia J. Nebulization Therapy with Umbilical Cord Mesenchymal Stem Cell-Derived Exosomes for COVID-19 Pneumonia. Stem Cell Rev Rep. 2022 Aug;18(6):2152–2163. https://doi.org/10.1007/s12015-022-10398-w. Epub 2022 Jun 4.

Recruiting

Safety and Efficacy of EXO-CD24 in Preventing Clinical Deterioration in Patients with Mild-Moderate ARDS

ClinicalTrials.gov ID NCT05947747

Sponsor Nano24med

Information provided by Nano24med (Responsible Party)

Last Update Posted 2023-07-27

Study Overview

Brief Summary

This is phase IIb, randomized, double-blinded, placebo-controlled study to evaluate the safety and efficacy of exosomes overexpressing CD24 of one dose of 10^10 exosome particles, to prevent clinical deterioration in patients with mild-moderate ARDS.

Detailed Description

The study population will include patients with mild-moderate ARDS and laboratory markers predictive of the cytokine storm, who have provided an informed consent.

There will be 90 patients who will be initially screened, randomized, and stratified by center in a 2:1 ratio to receive either 1010 exosome particles (60 patients) or a placebo (30 patients).

The study drug will be delivered using a standard jet nebulizer that produces aerosol particles with a size of 0.4–4.4 μm.

The exosomes will be diluted in 1.5 ml normal saline for inhalation, administered twice a day (bid) for 5 days.

Study treatments will be given as an add-on to the standard of care. Following the 5 days of treatment, patients will remain in follow-up for 23 additional days. In case of hospital discharge before the full follow-up planned, the patient will be required to return to the site for completion of all study assessments.

Official Title

A Phase IIb, Randomized, Double-Blinded, Placebo-Controlled Study to Evaluate the Safety and Efficacy of Exosomes Overexpressing CD24 to Prevent Clinical Deterioration in Patients with Mild-Moderate ARDS

Conditions

ARDS

Intervention/Treatment

- Drug: EXO-CD24
- Other: placebo

Other Study ID Numbers

- SN1

Study Start (Actual)

2023-07-04

Primary Completion (Estimated)

2025-12-20

Study Completion (Estimated)

2025-12-20

Enrollment (Estimated)

90

Study Type

Interventional

Phase

Phase 2

Study Contact

Name: Nimrod Adi, MD

Phone Number: +972-524266719

Email: nimroda@tlvmc.gov.il

Study Contact Backup

Name: Nadir Arber, Prof.

Phone Number: +972-524266595

Email: nadira@tlvmc.gov.il

This study has 1 location

Israel
Tel-Aviv, Israel, 64239
Recruiting
Tel-Aviv Sourasky Medical Center
Contact:
Nadir Arber, Professor
+972-524266595 nadira@tlv.mc.gov.il
Contact:
Nimrod Adi, MD
+972-524266719 nimroda@tlvmc.gov.il
Principal Investigator:
Nimrod Adi, MD
Eligibility Criteria
Description
Inclusion Criteria:

1. Direct and indirect lung injury etiology
2. Age ≥18 years
3. Patients with early acute lung injury (EALI) >2, or patient on HFNC/NIPPV ((1 point for an oxygen requirement >2–6 liters/min or 2 points for >6 liters/min; 1 point each for a respiratory rate ≥30 breaths/min and baseline immune suppression) (immune system compromised by exogenous drug)) (for saturation goal >90%) [1], or ARDS diagnosis (mild/moderate)
4. Willing and able to sign an informed consent, or has a legal guardian who is able to sign

Exclusion Criteria:

1. Any concomitant illness that, based on the judgment of the investigator, might affect the interpretation or the results of the study (immunodeficiency, primary immune deficiency due to virus, hematological malignancy, etc.)
2. Patients with SaO2/FiO2<150
3. Patients with mechanical ventilation (ECMO)
4. Pregnancy (positive urine pregnancy test (women of childbearing potential only)) or breastfeeding
5. Participation in any other interventional study in the last 30 days or within 5 half-lives of receiving an investigational agent

Ages Eligible for Study
18 years and older (adult, older adult)
Sexes Eligible for Study
All
Accepts Healthy Volunteers
No
Design Details
Primary purpose: treatment
Allocation: randomized

Interventional model: parallel assignment

Interventional model description: This is a two-arm study; one arm will receive 10^10 dose of exosomes overexpressing CD24, and the second arm will receive placebo dose.

Masking: single (Participant)

Masking description: the administered dose will be unknown to the patients.

Arms and Interventions

Participant group/Arm	Intervention/treatment
Experimental: group 1, investigational drug EXO-CD24 at a dose of 10^10 60 patients who will receive a 5-day treatment with the investigational drug EXO-CD24 at a dose of 10^10	Drug: EXO-CD24 Twice a day for 5 days, dose 10^10 Other names: Exosomes overexpressing CD24
Placebo comparator: group 2, treatment in a clean sterile saline solution (placebo) 30 patients who will receive a 5-day treatment in a clean sterile saline solution (placebo)	Other: placebo Twice a day for 5 days

Primary Outcome Measures

Outcome measure	Measure description	Time frame
Safety: number of participants with treatment-related adverse Events as assessed by CTCAE v.5 during the 28 days of the study		28 days
Efficacy: the rate of hypoxemic respiratory failure (reported as S/F<150) at day 7		7 days
Efficacy: the rate of hypoxemic respiratory failure (reported as S/F<150) at day 28		28 days

Sponsor

Nano24med

Recruiting

Immune Modulation by Exosomes in COVID-19 (IMECOV19)

ClinicalTrials.gov ID NCT05191381

Sponsor University of Ulm

Information provided by Manfred Weiss, University of Ulm (Responsible Party)

Last Update Posted 2024-01-17

Study Overview

Brief Summary

Following whole blood stimulation with mesenchymal stem cell-derived exosomes, immune phenotype, cytokine release, and mRNA expression patterns from critically ill patients with COVID-19 will be determined.

Detailed Description

Critically ill patients with COVID-19 may develop lung failure and require extracorporal oxygenation due to hyperinflammation and progressive lung fibrosis. The anti-inflammatory and immune modulatory function of mesenchymal stem cells will be investigated by whole blood stimulation experiments using stem cell-derived exosomes. Exosome preparations have been characterized by miRNA and protein expression patterns and suggest their tissue regenerative capacity.

The hypothesis of the present study is that mesenchymal stem cell-derived exosomes attenuate inflammation and support anti-fibrotic pathways.

Official Title

Immune Modulation by Stem Cell-Derived Exosomes in Critically Ill COVID-19

Conditions

COVID-19

Critical illness

Hypercytokinemia

Lung fibrosis

Intervention/Treatment

- Biological: application of exosomes in a whole blood assay

Other Study ID Numbers

- Lung fibrosis in COVID19

Study Start (Actual)

2021-12-22

Primary Completion (Estimated)

2025-07-31

Study Completion (Estimated)

2026-12-31

Enrollment (Estimated)

40

Study Type

Observational [Patient Registry]

Study Contact

Name: Manfred Weiss, MD

Phone Number: +49(0)731500 ext 60226

Email: manfred.weiss@uniklinik-ulm.de

Study Contact Backup

Name: Marion Schneider, PhD

Phone Number: +49(0)731500 ext 60319

Email: marion.schneider@uni-ulm.de

This study has 1 location

Germany

Ulm, Germany, 89070
Recruiting
Ulm University Hospital, Clinic of Anesthesiology and Intensive Care Medicine
Contact:
Manfred Weiss, MD, MBA
+49-(0)731-500-60226 manfred.weiss@uniklinik-ulm.de
Contact:
Marion Schneider, PhD
+49-(0)731-500-60080 marion.schneider@uni-ulm.de
Principal Investigator:
Manfred Weiss, MD
Eligibility Criteria
Description
Inclusion Criteria:

- Critically ill COVID-19 patients with lung dysfunction
- COVID-19 WHO severity degree ≥4, ARDS (WHO Definition March 13. 2020)
- Body weight >50 kg
- Informed consent

Exclusion Criteria:

- Pregnant or breastfeeding women

Study population
Critically ill COVID-19 patients, COVID-19 WHO severity degree ≥4, ARDS (WHO Definition March 13, 2020)
Ages Eligible for Study
18–90 years (adult, older adult)
Sexes Eligible for Study
All
Accepts Healthy Volunteers
Yes
Sampling Method
Probability Sample
Design Details
Observational model: cohort
Time perspective: prospective
Target follow-up duration: 12 months
Biospecimen retention: samples with DNA
Biospecimen description: 4 ml of heparin and 2 ml of EDTA-anti-coagulated blood

Groups and Interventions

Intervention/treatment
Biological: application of exosomes in a whole blood assay Co-incubation of patient-derived whole blood samples with mesenchymal stem cell-derived exosomes and read-out of biomarkers, RNA, and immune phenotypes after 24 h

Primary Outcome Measures

Outcome measure	Measure description	Time frame
Cytokine profile in supernatants	Quantification of pro- and anti-inflammatory biomarkers after 24 h of whole blood culture	24 h, 1 year

Secondary Outcome Measures

Outcome measure	Measure description	Time frame
Immune phenotyping	Immune phenotypes related to type I interferon signaling	1 year
Genetic predisposition to hyperinflammation	Determination of functional single nucleotide polymorphisms of inflammatory genes and receptors	1 year

Sponsor
University of Ulm
Investigators

- Principal investigator: Manfred Weiss, MD, Clinic of Anaesthesiology and Intensive Care Medicine
- Principal investigator: Marion Schneider, PhD, Clinic of Anaesthesiology and Intensive Care Medicine

Publications

- Channappanavar R, Perlman S. Pathogenic human coronavirus infections: causes and consequences of cytokine storm and immunopathology. Semin Immunopathol. 2017 Jul;39(5):529–539. https://doi.org/10.1007/s00281-017-0629-x. Epub 2017 May 2.
- Di Rocco G, Baldari S, Toietta G. Towards Therapeutic Delivery of Extracellular Vesicles: Strategies for In Vivo Tracking and Biodistribution Analysis. Stem Cells Int. 2016;2016:5029619. https://doi.org/10.1155/2016/5029619. Epub 2016 Nov 23.
- Geistlinger J, Du W, Groll J, Liu F, Hoegel J, Foehr KJ, Pasquarelli A, Schneider EM. P2RX7 genotype association in severe sepsis identified by a novel Multi-Individual Array for rapid screening and replication of risk SNPs. Clin Chim Acta. 2012 Jan 18;413(1–2):39–47. https://doi.org/10.1016/j.cca.2011.05.023. Epub 2011 May 25.
- Giamarellos-Bourboulis EJ, Netea MG, Rovina N, Akinosoglou K, Antoniadou A, Antonakos N, Damoraki G, Gkavogianni T, Adami ME, Katsaounou P, Ntaganou M, Kyriakopoulou M, Dimopoulos G, Koutsodimitropoulos I, Velissaris D, Koufargyris P, Karageorgos A, Katrini K, Lekakis V, Lupse M, Kotsaki A, Renieris G, Theodoulou D, Panou V, Koukaki E, Koulouris N, Gogos C, Koutsoukou A. Complex Immune Dysregulation in COVID-19 Patients with Severe Respiratory Failure. Cell Host Microbe. 2020 Jun 10;27(6):992–1000.e3. https://doi.org/10.1016/j.chom.2020.04.009. Epub 2020 Apr 21.

- Gotts JE, Matthay MA. Endogenous and exogenous cell-based pathways for recovery from acute respiratory distress syndrome. Clin Chest Med. 2014 Dec;35(4):797–809. https://doi.org/10.1016/j.ccm.2014.08.015. Epub 2014 Sep 24.
- Haberle H, Magunia H, Lang P, Gloeckner H, Korner A, Koeppen M, Backchoul T, Malek N, Handgretinger R, Rosenberger P, Mirakaj V. Mesenchymal Stem Cell Therapy for Severe COVID-19 ARDS. J Intensive Care Med. 2021 Jun;36(6):681–688. https://doi.org/10.1177/0885066621997365. Epub 2021 Mar 5.
- Lai RC, Arslan F, Lee MM, Sze NS, Choo A, Chen TS, Salto-Tellez M, Timmers L, Lee CN, El Oakley RM, Pasterkamp G, de Kleijn DP, Lim SK. Exosome secreted by MSC reduces myocardial ischemia/reperfusion injury. Stem Cell Res. 2010 May;4(3):214–22. https://doi.org/10.1016/j.scr.2009.12.003. Epub 2010 Jan 4.
- Leng Z, Zhu R, Hou W, Feng Y, Yang Y, Han Q, Shan G, Meng F, Du D, Wang S, Fan J, Wang W, Deng L, Shi H, Li H, Hu Z, Zhang F, Gao J, Liu H, Li X, Zhao Y, Yin K, He X, Gao Z, Wang Y, Yang B, Jin R, Stambler I, Lim LW, Su H, Moskalev A, Cano A, Chakrabarti S, Min KJ, Ellison-Hughes G, Caruso C, Jin K, Zhao RC. Transplantation of ACE2- Mesenchymal Stem Cells Improves the Outcome of Patients with COVID-19 Pneumonia. Aging Dis. 2020 Mar 9;11(2):216–228. https://doi.org/10.14336/AD.2020.0228. eCollection 2020 Apr.
- Mehta P, McAuley DF, Brown M, Sanchez E, Tattersall RS, Manson JJ; HLH Across Speciality Collaboration, UK. COVID-19: consider cytokine storm syndromes and immunosuppression. Lancet. 2020 Mar 28;395(10229):1033–1034. https://doi.org/10.1016/S0140-6736(20)30628-0. Epub 2020 Mar 16. No abstract available.
- Monsel A, Zhu YG, Gudapati V, Lim H, Lee JW. Mesenchymal stem cell derived secretome and extracellular vesicles for acute lung injury and other inflammatory lung diseases. Expert Opin Biol Ther. 2016 Jul;16(7):859–71. https://doi.org/10.1517/14712598.2016.1170804. Epub 2016 Apr 12.
- Shah TG, Predescu D, Predescu S. Mesenchymal stem cells-derived extracellular vesicles in acute respiratory distress syndrome: a review of current literature and potential future treatment options. Clin Transl Med. 2019 Sep 12;8(1):25. https://doi.org/10.1186/s40169-019-0242-9.
- Shi Y, Wang Y, Shao C, Huang J, Gan J, Huang X, Bucci E, Piacentini M, Ippolito G, Melino G. COVID-19 infection: the perspectives on immune responses. Cell Death Differ. 2020 May;27(5):1451–1454. https://doi.org/10.1038/s41418-020-0530-3. Epub 2020 Mar 23. No abstract available.
- Shi L, Huang H, Lu X, Yan X, Jiang X, Xu R, Wang S, Zhang C, Yuan X, Xu Z, Huang L, Fu JL, Li Y, Zhang Y, Yao WQ, Liu T, Song J, Sun L, Yang F, Zhang X, Zhang B, Shi M, Meng F, Song Y, Yu Y, Wen J, Li Q, Mao Q, Maeurer M, Zumla A, Yao C, Xie WF, Wang FS. Effect of human umbilical cord-derived mesenchymal stem cells on lung damage in severe COVID-19 patients: a randomized, double-blind, placebo-controlled phase 2 trial. Signal Transduct Target Ther. 2021 Feb 10;6(1):58. https://doi.org/10.1038/s41392-021-00488-5.
- Shi L, Wang L, Xu R, Zhang C, Xie Y, Liu K, Li T, Hu W, Zhen C, Wang FS. Mesenchymal stem cell therapy for severe COVID-19. Signal Transduct Target Ther. 2021 Sep 8;6(1):339. https://doi.org/10.1038/s41392-021-00754-6.

- Yang X, Yu Y, Xu J, Shu H, Xia J, Liu H, Wu Y, Zhang L, Yu Z, Fang M, Yu T, Wang Y, Pan S, Zou X, Yuan S, Shang Y. Clinical course and outcomes of critically ill patients with SARS-CoV-2 pneumonia in Wuhan, China: a single-centered, retrospective, observational study. Lancet Respir Med. 2020 May;8(5):475–481. https://doi.org/10.1016/S2213-2600(20)30079-5. Epub 2020 Feb 24. Erratum In: Lancet Respir Med. 2020 Apr;8(4):e26. https://doi.org/10.1016/S2213-2600(20)30103-X.
- J. Bindja, M. E. Weiss, M. Schmolz, G. M. Stein, J. Mapes, N. Schneiderhan-Marra, T. O. Joos, E. M. Schneider. Synthetic ligands against TLR2-9 in TruCulture™ - whole blood assays distinguish clinical stages of SIRS (trauma) and sepsis. Trauma, Shock, Inflammation and Sepsis. Trauma, Shock, Inflammation and Sepsis - TSIS 2010; 55 - 63
- Sanders J., Schneider E.M. How severe RNA virus infections such as SARS-CoV-2 disrupt tissue and organ barriers-Reconstitution by mesenchymal stem cell-derived exosomes. Tissue Barriers in Disease, Injury and Regeneration 2021:95–113. https://doi.org/10.1016/B978-0-12-818561-2.00004-7. Epub 2021 Jun 25. PMCID: PMC8225928.

Recruiting

A Clinical Study on Safety and Effectiveness of Mesenchymal Stem Cell Exosomes for the Treatment of COVID-19

ClinicalTrials.gov ID NCT05787288

Sponsor First Affiliated Hospital of Wenzhou Medical University

Information provided by Xiaoying Huang, First Affiliated Hospital of Wenzhou Medical University (Responsible Party)

Last Update Posted 2023-04-07

Study Overview

Brief Summary

This clinical study aims to investigate the safety and efficacy of nebulized inhalation of extracellular vesicles derived from mesenchymal stem cells combined with standard therapy for COVID-19-infected individuals. The primary objective is to determine whether nebulized MSC-secreted extracellular vesicles may be a feasible approach to alleviate COVID-19-induced lung injuries and promote recovery. Participants will be allocated to receive either nebulized MSC-secreted extracellular vesicles twice a day (bid) for 5 days as the test group or nebulized saline solution twice a day for 5 days as the control group. Researchers will compare the test and control groups to evaluate the safety and efficacy of extracellular vesicles in combination with standard therapy.

Detailed Description

1. Background 1.1. New Coronavirus Infection and Current Medical Strategies The 2019 coronavirus disease (COVID-19) caused by severe acute respiratory syndrome coronavirus 2 (SARS-CoV-2) has been raging for over three years, causing more than 5 million deaths worldwide. The World Health Organization has declared COVID-19 pneumonia a global pandemic and a public health emergency. Although diagnostic efficiency and treatment accuracy have improved, the overall treatment effect is still limited. The main causes of death include severe pneumonia, acute respiratory distress syndrome (ARDS), pulmonary edema, or multiple organ failure. Among them, ARDS is the most severe. Pathological studies have shown that the pathogenesis of ARDS is mainly due to the immune response induced by the coronavirus attacking alveolar cells; immune cell infiltration leads to destruction of the pulmonary capillary endothelial structure, causing plasma, plasma proteins, and blood cells to enter the lung interstitium and alveolar cavity, forming pulmonary edema. Due to the destruction of the alveolar epithelial tissue, a large amount of edema fluid enters the alveoli, resulting in limited diffusion function of the alveoli and inability to perform normal respiratory function. At the same time, with the aggravation of tissue damage, cells further release various inflammatory factors to form a so-called cytokine storm, which finally completely destroys most of the pulmonary alveoli and bronchial respiratory structures, causing severe ventilation-perfusion imbalance and ultimately death of the patient.

   In this global emergency event of coronavirus, the main medical strategy to combat COVID-19 is to use antibiotics and antiviral drugs to block the virus replication cycle and suppress host inflammation. This strategy has led to effective supportive and symptomatic treatment in some cases, even yielding promising results, but it is not the ultimate treatment for this infection. For example, immune regulation interventions like tocilizumab (IL-6 receptor blocker), adalimumab (anti-TNF antibody), and eculizumab (anti-C5 antibody) can effectively relieve patient symptoms but cannot cure the disease fundamentally. In fact, there are two major characteristics of COVID-19 pneumonia: first, people with low immunity are more susceptible to COVID-19, and second, the main target organ is the lungs. In fact, respiratory failure has been reported as one of the main causes of death from COVID-19, and autopsies have shown lung damage, significant exudative reactions, and pulmonary embolism in many patients.

   1.2. Mesenchymal Stem Cell Exosomes Mesenchymal stem cells (MSCs) have been shown to have comprehensive and powerful immunomodulatory and regenerative functions. MSCs can combat cell death associated with the pathogenesis of chronic obstructive pulmonary disease (COPD), idiopathic pulmonary fibrosis, asthma, ARDS, and pulmonary hypertension and promote cell regeneration. Exosomes are one of the key paracrine effectors secreted by MSCs and are considered attractive candidates for alternative MSC therapy due to their biocompatibility similar to parent cells and their ability to maintain healing properties. Under physiological and pathological conditions, exosomes play a key role in intercellular communication by transporting various biomolecules such as miRNA and proteins to target cells. Unlike apoptotic bodies and microvesicles derived from the cell surface, exosomes are produced through the endocytic pathway and load the cytoplasmic content of the parent cell. Therefore, they are mini versions of parent cells, mimicking some of their physiological characteristics. Compared to cell counterparts, the nontoxicity, low immunogenicity, high stability, ease of storage, and potential for mass production as ready-made products are several advantages of exosomes, which have led to their expansion in clinical applications as new therapeutic alternatives. In addition, the natural function of exosomes allows them to deliver their membrane and cytoplasmic bioactive components from parent cells to target cells through membrane fusion. There are also other unique characteristics, including the natural ability to cross biological barriers such as the blood-brain barrier (BBB). Furthermore, biocompatibility is another characteristic. Due to their origin from biological sources and inherent targeting ability, exosomes have been used as carriers of drug components in preclinical studies.

1.3. Mechanism of Mesenchymal Stem Cell-Derived Exosome Treatment MSC-derived exosomes inherit immune suppressive properties from their parent cells, and MSC-EVs may use various mechanisms to balance the immune system's function. One key mechanism is reprogramming and altering the phenotype of various immune cells. For example, the ability of MSC-derived exosomes to promote the survival of alveolar macrophages and shift their phenotype from pro-inflammatory (M1) polarization to anti-inflammatory (M2) polarization has been demonstrated in at least two studies. These findings suggest that exosomes can serve as viable alternatives to their parent cells, and this ability has also been reported to alter the Treg/Teff ratio to increase Treg and promote the secretion of anti-inflammatory cytokines.

In multiple models, MSC-EVs have similar therapeutic characteristics to MSCs; are easier to prepare, store, and transport to the bedside; and avoid some limitations of cell therapy, such as the risk of pulmonary embolism and tumor formation. In recent years, MSC-EVs have received widespread attention as biomarkers of pathogenesis and therapeutic drugs for a variety of diseases. In addition, MSC-secreted exosomes can regulate immunity through interaction with immune cells and inhibit inflammatory responses through cytokines. Numerous studies have shown that MSC-secreted exosomes can be used to treat immune deficiencies, inflammation, ARDS, and other pulmonary diseases, so MSC-secreted exosomes may also be effective in treating the lung inflammation caused by COVID-19. Exosomes are one of the main active ingredients secreted by stem cells and are 30–150 nm in size. After nebulization, exosomes can directly reach the bronchioles and alveoli, which is conducive to the maximum absorption of drugs. Multiple clinical trials have shown that intravenous infusion of MSCs and MSC-EVs for the treatment of severe lung damage caused by SARS-CoV-2 is safe and effective, and in the case of lung injury, the nebulization route provides a particularly effective drug delivery method to target lung sites. Therefore, we speculate that nebulized MSC-secreted exosomes may be an effective method for reducing COVID-19 lung damage and promoting recovery.

1.4. Clinical Case Studies of Stem Cell-Derived Exosomes: Recently, the inhaled anti-COVID-19 drug Exo-CD24, led by Israeli medical center expert Nadir Arber, which is a combination of exosomes and CD24 protein, has shown promising results in early clinical trials. The drug was able to cure 29 out of 30 severe patients within 5 days of treatment and has the potential to treat COVID-19 patients within 3–5 days. Although Exo-CD24 has not yet passed phase III testing, it has shown great potential in the future. The US FDA has approved the use of extracellular vesicles (EVs) for the treatment of COVID-19 through a phase I/II trial conducted by Direct Biologics. ExoFlo, the EVs used, restores the health and vitality of patients by reducing sustained inflammation, promoting the revascularization of damaged tissue, and reshaping scar tissue. Domestic clinical studies have also been initiated; clinical research at the Fifth People's Hospital of Wuxi City, Jiangsu Province, has confirmed that nebulized umbilical cord mesenchymal stem cell-derived extracellular vesicles are a safe and viable treatment for COVID-19. The study was published in *Stem Cell Reviews and Reports* in June of this year and included seven patients diagnosed with COVID-19 pneumonia, including two severe cases (patients 2 and 4) and five mild cases (patients 1, 3, 5, 6, and 7). No acute allergic reactions such as throat or tongue swelling, rash, shortness of breath, dizziness, vomiting, or hypotension were observed in any of the patients within two hours after nebulization treatment. There were also no reported adverse events or secondary allergic reactions following treatment. Chest CT scans showed a decrease in lung lobe nodule density and absorption of lung lesions in both severe and mild patients after nebulized treatment with MSC-derived extracellular vesicles. Joint research by Ruijin Hospital and Jinyintan Hospital is being conducted on nebulized COVID-19 treatment using adipose-derived human allogeneic mesenchymal stem cell-derived exosomes (HAMSCs-Exos). Seven critically ill COVID-19 patients were treated with HAMSC-Exos via nebulization inhalation, and all patients tolerated the treatment well without evidence of adverse events or clinical instability during or immediately after nebulization. All patients showed an increase in serum lymphocyte count (median of 1.61 × 10^9/L vs. 1.78×10^9/L), and lung lesions were reduced to varying degrees in all patients after inhaling HAMSC-Exos aerosols, with four patients showing significant improvement. Preliminary results suggest that participants' lung injuries were significantly improved.

However, most clinical trials using stem cell exosomes for COVID-19 infection have the following issues: (a) small sample size, making it difficult to effectively demonstrate the advantages of stem cell exosomes in COVID-19 treatment; (b) lack of a control group; (c) use of traditional two-dimensional production methods, making it difficult to scale up production of large quantities of exosomes for clinical treatment; and (d) lack of in-depth mechanism exploration for relevant phenomena. These problems hinder progress in the use of stem cell exosomes for COVID-19 infection treatment. To address these issues, this project proposes combining nebulized umbilical cord mesenchymal stem cell exosomes with conventional treatment to treat middle to severe COVID-19 patients and evaluate its safety and efficacy.

2. Research Objective: This study aims to evaluate the safety and effectiveness of umbilical cord mesenchymal stem cell-derived exosomes (nebulized) combined with conventional therapy for the treatment of moderate, severe, and critically ill COVID-19 patients through a multicenter, randomized controlled, single-blind clinical trial.
3. Research Design: This study adopts a multicenter, randomized controlled, single-blind trial design. Based on the COVID-19 treatment regimen formulated by clinical guidelines, nebulized umbilical cord mesenchymal stem cell-derived exosomes (experimental group) or medically sterile saline solution (control group) will be administered to treat moderate, severe, and critically ill COVID-19 patients. By comparing the relief of symptoms and the occurrence of adverse events before and after treatment, the safety and effectiveness of umbilical cord mesenchymal stem cell-derived exosomes for the treatment of moderate, severe, and critically ill COVID-19 patients will be evaluated.

Official Title

Clinical Study on the Safety and Efficacy of Mesenchymal Stem Cell Exosomes in the Treatment of Coronavirus Infection

Conditions

COVID-19 pneumonia

Intervention/Treatment

- Biological: extracellular vesicles from mesenchymal stem cells

Other Study ID Numbers

- KY2022-205

Study Start (Actual)

2023-01-23

Primary Completion (Estimated)

2024-01-23

Study Completion (Estimated)

2025-01-23

Enrollment (Estimated)

240

Study Type

Interventional

Phase

Early phase 1

Study Contact

Name: Dan Yao, Master
Phone Number: 0577-55579271
Email: zdyaodan@163.com
Study Contact Backup
Name: Xiaoying Huang, Docter
Phone Number: 0577-55579272
Email: zjwzhxy@126.com
This study has 1 location
China
Zhejiang Locations
Wenzhou, Zhejiang, China, 325000
Recruiting
The First Affiliated Hospital of Wenzhou Medical University
Contact:
Dan Yao The First Affiliated Hospital of Wenzhou Medical University, Master
0577-55579271 zdyaodan@163.com
Eligibility Criteria
Description
Inclusion Criteria:

(a) Voluntary participation of the patient and signing of the informed consent form. (b) The age of the patient at the time of signing the informed consent form should be ≥18 years old and ≤75 years old, regardless of gender. (c) The patient meets the criteria for moderate and severe patients with COVID-19 infection in China's "Diagnosis and Treatment Protocol for Novel Coronavirus Pneumonia (Trial Version 10)," as follows:

1. Moderate: continued fever >3 days and/or cough, dyspnea, or other symptoms, but respiratory rate (RR) <30 breaths/min and oxygen saturation (SpO2) >93% at rest when inhaling air. Characteristic imaging manifestations of COVID-19 pneumonia can be observed (imaging is optional and can be included or excluded).
2. Severe: any one of the following in adults cannot be explained by causes other than COVID-19 infection:
    1. Dyspnea with RR ≥30 breaths/min
    2. SpO2 ≤93% at rest when inhaling air
    3. Ratio of partial pressure of arterial oxygen to fraction of inspired oxygen (PaO2/FiO2) ≤300 mmHg
    4. Disease progression with a significant increase in pulmonary lesions within 24–48 hours
3. Critical: any one of the following conditions:
    1. Respiratory failure requiring mechanical ventilation
    2. Shock
    3. Other organ dysfunction requiring ICU monitoring and treatment.

(d) Positive nucleic acid or antigen test. (e) No prior treatment with umbilical cord mesenchymal stem cell-derived exosomes. (f) The patient has a full understanding of the purpose and requirements of this trial and is willing to complete all trial procedures according to the trial requirements.

Exclusion Criteria:

(a) Female patients of childbearing age who are pregnant, lactating, or planning to conceive within the past year. (b) Severe heart, brain, kidney, and hematopoietic system diseases or other serious illnesses. (c) Neuromuscular diseases causing impaired natural ventilation, including but not limited to spinal cord injury above the level of C5, amyotrophic lateral sclerosis, Guillain-Barre syndrome, and myasthenia gravis. (d) Currently undergoing hemodialysis or peritoneal dialysis. (e) Acute myocardial infarction within 30 days prior to screening. (f) Patients with lung or bone marrow transplantation. (g) History of epilepsy requiring continuous anticonvulsant treatment, or received anticonvulsant treatment within the past 3 years. (h) Active immunosuppression, defined as receiving immunosuppressive drugs or having medical conditions related to immunodeficiency. This includes:

1. HIV (AIDS or CD4 <200 cells/mm3).
2. Chemotherapy within 4 weeks before randomization.
3. Long-term immunosuppressive therapy, including maintenance prednisone therapy (>40 mg/day or equivalent for >1 month).
4. Absolute neutrophil count <500/mm^3. Exceptions are patients who have received short-term systemic (intravenous or oral) steroid treatment for <1 week or topical steroid treatment for skin disorders.

(i) Patients with severe allergic reactions or contraindications to the treatment regimen in this study. (j) Patients with doubts about the treatment plan or obvious mental and psychological disorders. (k) Patients whom the investigator considers unsuitable for participation in this trial (such as factors that may reduce compliance with follow-up or refusal to accept relevant supportive treatment by the patient).

Ages Eligible for Study

18–75 years (adult, older adult)

Sexes Eligible for Study

All

Accepts Healthy Volunteers

No

Design Details

Primary purpose: treatment

Allocation: randomized

Interventional model: parallel assignment

Masking: single (Investigator)

Arms and Interventions

Participant group/arm	Intervention/treatment
Experimental: test group Nebulized mesenchymal stem cell exosome-derived extracellular vesicles twice a day (bid) for 5 days	Biological: extracellular vesicles from mesenchymal stem cells Umbilical cord mesenchymal stem cell-derived extracellular vesicle preparation. Specification: 5 ml, with extracellular vesicle concentration of 1 × 109 particles/ml in the preparation
Sham comparator: control group Nebulized saline solution twice a day (bid) for 5 days	Biological: extracellular vesicles from mesenchymal stem cells Umbilical cord mesenchymal stem cell-derived extracellular vesicle preparation. Specification: 5 ml, with extracellular vesicle concentration of 1 × 109 particles/ml in the preparation

Primary Outcome Measures

Outcome measure	Measure description	Time frame
Symptom remission time after atomizing medication	Symptom remission time after atomizing medication	3 months
Improvement of serum inflammatory markers	Improvement of serum inflammatory markers	3 months
If there is baseline CT, CT review, and comparison	If there is baseline CT, CT review, and comparison	3 months

Secondary Outcome Measures

Outcome measure	Measure description	Time frame
Length of being hospitalized	Length of being hospitalized	3 months
Recovery time (nucleic acid turned negative)	Recovery time (nucleic acid turned negative)	3 months

Sponsor
First Affiliated Hospital of Wenzhou Medical University
Collaborators

- REGEN-αGEEK (SHENZHEN) MEDICAL TECHNOLOGY CO., LTD.

Investigators

- Principal investigator: Xiaoying Huang, Docter, First Affiliated Hospital of Wenzhou Medical University

Publications

- El-Shennawy L, Hoffmann AD, Dashzeveg NK, McAndrews KM, Mehl PJ, Cornish D, Yu Z, Tokars VL, Nicolaescu V, Tomatsidou A, Mao C, Felicelli CJ, Tsai CF, Ostiguin C, Jia Y, Li L, Furlong K, Wysocki J, Luo X, Ruivo CF, Batlle

D, Hope TJ, Shen Y, Chae YK, Zhang H, LeBleu VS, Shi T, Swaminathan S, Luo Y, Missiakas D, Randall GC, Demonbreun AR, Ison MG, Kalluri R, Fang D, Liu H. Circulating ACE2-expressing extracellular vesicles block broad strains of SARS-CoV-2. Nat Commun. 2022 Jan 20;13(1):405. https://doi.org/10.1038/s41467-021-27893-2.

- Huang C, Wang Y, Li X, Ren L, Zhao J, Hu Y, Zhang L, Fan G, Xu J, Gu X, Cheng Z, Yu T, Xia J, Wei Y, Wu W, Xie X, Yin W, Li H, Liu M, Xiao Y, Gao H, Guo L, Xie J, Wang G, Jiang R, Gao Z, Jin Q, Wang J, Cao B. Clinical features of patients infected with 2019 novel coronavirus in Wuhan, China. Lancet. 2020 Feb 15;395(10223):497–506. https://doi.org/10.1016/S0140-6736(20)30183-5. Epub 2020 Jan 24. Erratum In: Lancet. 2020 Feb 15;395(10223):496. https://doi.org/10.1016/S0140-6736(20)30252-X.
- Yildirim F, Karaman I, Kaya A. Current situation in ARDS in the light of recent studies: Classification, epidemiology and pharmacotherapeutics. Tuberk Toraks. 2021 Dec;69(4):535–546. https://doi.org/10.5578/tt.20219611.
- Banerjee A, Pasea L, Harris S, Gonzalez-Izquierdo A, Torralbo A, Shallcross L, Noursadeghi M, Pillay D, Sebire N, Holmes C, Pagel C, Wong WK, Langenberg C, Williams B, Denaxas S, Hemingway H. Estimating excess 1-year mortality associated with the COVID-19 pandemic according to underlying conditions and age: a population-based cohort study. Lancet. 2020 May 30;395(10238):1715–1725. https://doi.org/10.1016/S0140-6736(20)30854-0. Epub 2020 May 12.
- Rubin R. Global Effort to Collect Data on Ventilated Patients With COVID-19. JAMA. 2020 Jun 9;323(22):2233–2234. https://doi.org/10.1001/jama.2020.8341. No abstract available.
- Liang W, Liang H, Ou L, Chen B, Chen A, Li C, Li Y, Guan W, Sang L, Lu J, Xu Y, Chen G, Guo H, Guo J, Chen Z, Zhao Y, Li S, Zhang N, Zhong N, He J; China Medical Treatment Expert Group for COVID-19. Development and Validation of a Clinical Risk Score to Predict the Occurrence of Critical Illness in Hospitalized Patients With COVID-19. JAMA Intern Med. 2020 Aug 1;180(8):1081–1089. https://doi.org/10.1001/jamainternmed.2020.2033.
- Wichmann D, Sperhake JP, Lutgehetmann M, Steurer S, Edler C, Heinemann A, Heinrich F, Mushumba H, Kniep I, Schroder AS, Burdelski C, de Heer G, Nierhaus A, Frings D, Pfefferle S, Becker H, Bredereke-Wiedling H, de Weerth A, Paschen HR, Sheikhzadeh-Eggers S, Stang A, Schmiedel S, Bokemeyer C, Addo MM, Aepfelbacher M, Puschel K, Kluge S. Autopsy Findings and Venous Thromboembolism in Patients With COVID-19: A Prospective Cohort Study. Ann Intern Med. 2020 Aug 18;173(4):268–277. https://doi.org/10.7326/M20-2003. Epub 2020 May 6.
- Carrade Holt DD, Wood JA, Granick JL, Walker NJ, Clark KC, Borjesson DL. Equine mesenchymal stem cells inhibit T cell proliferation through different mechanisms depending on tissue source. Stem Cells Dev. 2014 Jun 1;23(11):1258–65. https://doi.org/10.1089/scd.2013.0537. Epub 2014 Mar 4.
- Sauler M, Bazan IS, Lee PJ. Cell Death in the Lung: The Apoptosis-Necroptosis Axis. Annu Rev Physiol. 2019 Feb 10;81:375–402. https://doi.org/10.1146/annurev-physiol-020518-114320. Epub 2018 Nov 28.

- Naji A, Suganuma N, Espagnolle N, Yagyu KI, Baba N, Sensebe L, Deschaseaux F. Rationale for Determining the Functional Potency of Mesenchymal Stem Cells in Preventing Regulated Cell Death for Therapeutic Use. Stem Cells Transl Med. 2017 Mar;6(3):713–719. https://doi.org/10.5966/sctm.2016-0289. Epub 2016 Oct 11.
- Janockova J, Slovinska L, Harvanova D, Spakova T, Rosocha J. New therapeutic approaches of mesenchymal stem cells-derived exosomes. J Biomed Sci. 2021 May 25;28(1):39. https://doi.org/10.1186/s12929-021-00736-4.
- Yao J, Huang K, Zhu D, Chen T, Jiang Y, Zhang J, Mi L, Xuan H, Hu S, Li J, Zhou Y, Cheng K. A Minimally Invasive Exosome Spray Repairs Heart after Myocardial Infarction. ACS Nano. 2021 Jul 27;15(7):11099–11111. https://doi.org/10.1021/acsnano.1c00628. Epub 2021 Jun 21.
- Noori L, Arabzadeh S, Mohamadi Y, Mojaverrostami S, Mokhtari T, Akbari M, Hassanzadeh G. Intrathecal administration of the extracellular vesicles derived from human Wharton's jelly stem cells inhibit inflammation and attenuate the activity of inflammasome complexes after spinal cord injury in rats. Neurosci Res. 2021 Sep;170:87–98. https://doi.org/10.1016/j.neures.2020.07.011. Epub 2020 Jul 25.
- Park J, Kim S, Lim H, Liu A, Hu S, Lee J, Zhuo H, Hao Q, Matthay MA, Lee JW. Therapeutic effects of human mesenchymal stem cell microvesicles in an ex vivo perfused human lung injured with severe E. coli pneumonia. Thorax. 2019 Jan;74(1):43–50. https://doi.org/10.1136/thoraxjnl-2018-211576. Epub 2018 Aug 3.
- Zhang Y, Chen J, Fu H, Kuang S, He F, Zhang M, Shen Z, Qin W, Lin Z, Huang S. Exosomes derived from 3D-cultured MSCs improve therapeutic effects in periodontitis and experimental colitis and restore the Th17 cell/Treg balance in inflamed periodontium. Int J Oral Sci. 2021 Dec 14;13(1):43. https://doi.org/10.1038/s41368-021-00150-4.
- Joo HS, Suh JH, Lee HJ, Bang ES, Lee JM. Current Knowledge and Future Perspectives on Mesenchymal Stem Cell-Derived Exosomes as a New Therapeutic Agent. Int J Mol Sci. 2020 Jan 22;21(3):727. https://doi.org/10.3390/ijms21030727.
- Modani S, Tomar D, Tangirala S, Sriram A, Mehra NK, Kumar R, Khatri DK, Singh PK. An updated review on exosomes: biosynthesis to clinical applications. J Drug Target. 2021 Nov;29(9):925–940. https://doi.org/10.1080/1061186X.2021.1894436. Epub 2021 Mar 12.
- Morrison TJ, Jackson MV, Cunningham EK, Kissenpfennig A, McAuley DF, O'Kane CM, Krasnodembskaya AD. Mesenchymal Stromal Cells Modulate Macrophages in Clinically Relevant Lung Injury Models by Extracellular Vesicle Mitochondrial Transfer. Am J Respir Crit Care Med. 2017 Nov 15;196(10):1275–1286. https://doi.org/10.1164/rccm.201701-0170OC.
- Wu P, Zhang B, Shi H, Qian H, Xu W. MSC-exosome: A novel cell-free therapy for cutaneous regeneration. Cytotherapy. 2018 Mar;20(3):291–301. https://doi.org/10.1016/j.jcyt.2017.11.002. Epub 2018 Feb 9.
- Chu M, Wang H, Bian L, Huang J, Wu D, Zhang R, Fei F, Chen Y, Xia J. Nebulization Therapy with Umbilical Cord Mesenchymal Stem Cell-Derived Exosomes for COVID-19 Pneumonia. Stem Cell Rev Rep. 2022 Aug;18(6):2152–2163. https://doi.org/10.1007/s12015-022-10398-w. Epub 2022 Jun 4.

- Meng F, Xu R, Wang S, Xu Z, Zhang C, Li Y, Yang T, Shi L, Fu J, Jiang T, Huang L, Zhao P, Yuan X, Fan X, Zhang JY, Song J, Zhang D, Jiao Y, Liu L, Zhou C, Maeurer M, Zumla A, Shi M, Wang FS. Human umbilical cord-derived mesenchymal stem cell therapy in patients with COVID-19: a phase 1 clinical trial. Signal Transduct Target Ther. 2020 Aug 27;5(1):172. https://doi.org/10.1038/s41392-020-00286-5.
- Song NJ, Allen C, Vilgelm AE, Riesenberg BP, Weller KP, Reynolds K, Chakravarthy KB, Kumar A, Khatiwada A, Sun Z, Ma A, Chang Y, Yusuf M, Li A, Zeng C, Evans JP, Bucci D, Gunasena M, Xu M, Liyanage NPM, Bolyard C, Velegraki M, Liu SL, Ma Q, Devenport M, Liu Y, Zheng P, Malvestutto CD, Chung D, Li Z. Treatment with soluble CD24 attenuates COVID-19-associated systemic immunopathology. J Hematol Oncol. 2022 Jan 10;15(1):5. https://doi.org/10.1186/s13045-021-01222-y.

Recruiting

Extracellular Vesicle Treatment for Acute Respiratory Distress Syndrome (ARDS) (EXTINGUISH ARDS)

ClinicalTrials.gov ID NCT05354141

Sponsor Direct Biologics, LLC

Information provided by Direct Biologics, LLC (Responsible Party)

Last Update Posted 2024-11-25

Study Overview

Brief Summary

To evaluate the safety and efficacy of intravenous (IV) administration of bone marrow mesenchymal stem cell-derived extracellular vesicles (EVs), ExoFlo, versus placebo for the treatment of hospitalized patients with moderate-to-severe acute respiratory distress syndrome (ARDS).

Detailed Description

This is a phase III, multicenter, randomized, double-blinded, placebo-controlled trial for the treatment of moderate-to-severe acute respiratory distress syndrome (ARDS).

Official Title

Bone Marrow Mesenchymal Stem Cell-Derived Extracellular Vesicles for Hospitalized Patients with Moderate-to-Severe ARDS: A Phase III Clinical Trial

Conditions

Acute respiratory distress syndrome

ARDS

Intervention/Treatment

- Biological: ExoFlo
- Other: intravenous normal saline

Other Study ID Numbers

- DB-EF-PHASEIII-0001

  Study Start (Actual)
  2022-07-01
  Primary Completion (Estimated)
  2025-03-31
  Study Completion (Estimated)
  2025-08-31
  Enrollment (Estimated)
  970
  Study Type
  Interventional
  Phase
  Phase 3
  Study Contact
  Name: Bill Arana
  Phone Number: 1-800-791-1021
  Email: clinicalaffairs@directbiologics.com
  This study has 38 locations
  United States
  Alabama Locations
  Birmingham, Alabama, United States, 35233
  Recruiting
  Direct Biologics Investigational Site
  Arizona Locations
  Chandler, Arizona, United States, 85224
  Recruiting
  Direct Biologics Investigational Site
  Phoenix, Arizona, United States, 85012
  Recruiting
  Direct Biologics Investigational Site
  Arkansas Locations
  Little Rock, Arkansas, United States, 72205
  Recruiting
  Direct Biologics Investigational Site
  California Locations
  Davis, California, United States, 95817
  Recruiting
  Direct Biologics Investigational Site
  Fullerton, California, United States, 92835
  Recruiting
  Direct Biologics Investigational Site
  Irvine, California, United States, 92627
  Recruiting
  Direct Biologics Investigational Site

Orange, California, United States, 92868
Recruiting
Direct Biologics Investigational Site
Sacramento, California, United States, 95817
Recruiting
Direct Biologics Investigational Site
San Francisco, California, United States, 94143
Recruiting
Direct Biologics Investigational Site
District of Columbia Locations
Washington, District of Columbia, United States, 20010
Recruiting
Direct Biologics Investigational Site
Florida Locations
Jacksonville, Florida, United States, 32224
Recruiting
Direct Biologics Investigational Site
Idaho Locations
Boise, Idaho, United States, 83712
Recruiting
Direct Biologics Investigational Site
Iowa Locations
Iowa City, Iowa, United States, 52242
Recruiting
Direct Biologics Investigational Site
Kansas Locations
Wichita, Kansas, United States, 67214
Recruiting
Direct Biologics Investigational Site
Maryland Locations
Silver Spring, Maryland, United States, 20910
Recruiting
Direct Biologics Investigational Site
Massachusetts Locations
Boston, Massachusetts, United States, 02115
Recruiting
Direct Biologics Investigational Site
Burlington, Massachusetts, United States, 01805
Recruiting
Direct Biologics Investigational Site
Springfield, Massachusetts, United States, 01199
Recruiting
Direct Biologics Investigational Site
Michigan Locations
Ann Arbor, Michigan, United States, 48109

Recruiting
Direct Biologics Investigational Site
Detroit, Michigan, United States, 48202
Recruiting
Direct Biologics Investigational Site
Mississippi Locations
Jackson, Mississippi, United States, 39202
Recruiting
Direct Biologics Investigational Site
New York Locations
Bronx, New York, United States, 10467
Recruiting
Direct Biologics Investigational Site
Flushing, New York, United States, 11368
Recruiting
Direct Biologics Investigational Site
Queens, New York, United States, 11040
Recruiting
Direct Biologics Investigational Site
North Carolina Locations
Durham, North Carolina, United States, 27710
Recruiting
Direct Biologics Investigational Site
Winston-Salem, North Carolina, United States, 27157
Recruiting
Direct Biologics Investigational Site
Ohio Locations
Cincinnati, Ohio, United States, 45219
Recruiting
Direct Biologics Investigational Site
Cleveland, Ohio, United States, 44106
Recruiting
Direct Biologics Investigational Site
Oregon Locations
Portland, Oregon, United States, 97239
Recruiting
Direct Biologics Investigational Site
South Carolina Locations
Charleston, South Carolina, United States, 29425
Recruiting
Direct Biologics Investigational Site
Tennessee Locations
Knoxville, Tennessee, United States, 37996
Recruiting
Direct Biologics Investigational Site

Nashville, Tennessee, United States, 37235
Recruiting
Direct Biologics Investigational Site
Texas Locations
Dallas, Texas, United States, 75246
Recruiting
Direct Biologics Investigational Site
Fort Worth, Texas, United States, 76104
Recruiting
Direct Biologics Investigational Site
Houston, Texas, United States, 77030
Recruiting
Direct Biologics Investigational Site
Utah Locations
Murray, Utah, United States, 84107
Recruiting
Direct Biologics Investigational Site
Salt Lake City, Utah, United States, 84101
Recruiting
Direct Biologics Investigational Site
Eligibility Criteria
Description
Inclusion Criteria:

1. Men and women aged 18–75 years
2. Presence of the following criteria for moderate-to-severe ARDS as defined by the Berlin Criteria within 24 h of the first infusion:
    1. Onset within 7 days of known clinical insult or requiring increasing respiratory rate, increasing oxygen flows, or increased work of breathing
    2. Bilateral lung opacities not fully explained by pleural effusions, atelectasis, or nodules
    3. PaO2/FiO2 (P/F ratio) $\leq$200 mm Hg
    4. Invasive or noninvasive ventilation with a minimum PEEP 5 cm H_2O or a minimum of continuous positive airway pressure (CPAP) 5 cm H_2O, or high flow nasal oxygen at $\geq$30 L/min
    5. Respiratory failure not fully explained by cardiac failure or fluid overload

Exclusion Criteria:

1. Lack of signed and dated informed consent form (either by the individual or by the individual's healthcare proxy).
2. Stated unwillingness to comply with all study procedures and availability for the duration of the study.
3. Vulnerable populations such as pregnant patients, children, and individuals with severe physical or mental disabilities who cannot provide meaningful consent.

4. Active malignancy requiring treatment within the last two years, with the exception of non-melanoma skin cancers.
5. Major physical trauma in the last 2 days, including motor vehicle accidents, assaults, mechanical falls with sequelae of significant bleeding or craniofacial bruising, and surgeries, such that not one or more injury may be undiagnosed at the time of screening.
6. Duration of mechanical ventilation exceeds 3 days or 72 h from diagnosis of ARDS.
7. ALT or AST >8× upper limit of normal (ULN).
8. Documented history of cirrhosis.
9. DNR order, as in electing not to receive chest compressions, cardiac defibrillation, cardiac drugs, or intubation.
10. Moribund-expected survival <24 h.
11. Severe metabolic disturbances at randomization (e.g., ketoacidosis, pH <7.2).
12. Patient currently connected to extracorporeal membrane oxygenation at initiation of screening.
13. If the candidate, either a male or female of reproductive potential, is unwilling to use two methods of highly effective birth control contraception such as condoms with oral contraceptive pill or chooses to remain abstinent if already practicing abstinence during the screening period. The required duration of usage of double method OR maintenance of abstinence must include the time from the beginning of the screening period until day 61, day of withdrawal or early termination.
14. Use of investigational COVID-19 agents or any other investigational agents within 30 days prior to the first dose.

Ages Eligible for Study

18–75 years (adult, older adult)

Sexes Eligible for Study

All

Accepts Healthy Volunteers

No

Design Details

Primary purpose: treatment

Allocation: randomized

Interventional model: parallel assignment

Interventional model description: multicenter, randomized, double-blinded, placebo-controlled trial

Masking: triple (ParticipantCare ProviderInvestigator)

Masking description: double blinded

Arms and Interventions

Participant group/arm	Intervention/treatment
Placebo comparator: placebo Normal saline 100 mL	Other: intravenous normal saline Placebo
Experimental: experimental dose Normal saline 85 mL and ExoFlo 15 mL	Biological: ExoFlo Intravenous administration of bone marrow mesenchymal stem cell-derived extracellular vesicles

Primary Outcome Measures

Outcome measure	Measure description	Time frame
Evaluation of 60-day all-cause mortality	To evaluate the 60-day mortality rate for IMP 15 mL as a treatment for moderate-to-severe ARDS compared to placebo. Reducing the mortality rate for hospitalized patients with moderate-to-severe ARDS is a measure of the treatment effect	60 days

Secondary Outcome Measures

Outcome measure	Measure description	Time frame
Time to death	Reducing the mortality rate for hospitalized patients with moderate-to-severe ARDS is a measure of the treatment effect	60 days
Ventilator-free days (VFDs)	Number of days for which patients are not on mechanical ventilation	Day 29
Oxygen-free days	Number of days for which patients are not on oxygen support	Day 29
ICU-free days	Number of days for which patients are not in the ICU	Day 29
Incidence of treatment-emergent serious adverse events (TESAEs)	Safety comparison performed between IMP 15 mL and placebo arms	61 days

Sponsor
Direct Biologics, LLC
Investigators

- Study Director: Bill Arana, Direct Biologics, LLC

Chapter 10
Rectum/Anus Exosome Trials

Not Yet Recruiting

Human Placenta Mesenchymal Stem Cell-Derived Exosome Injection for Treatment of Complex Anal Fistula

ClinicalTrials.gov ID NCT06568653

Sponsor Tehran University of Medical Sciences

Information provided by Tehran University of Medical Sciences (Responsible Party)

Last Update Posted 2024-08-23

Study Overview

Brief Summary

The goal of this clinical trial is to learn if human placenta mesenchymal stem cell (MSC)-derived exosomes work to treat complex perianal fistula in adults without Crohn's disease. The safety of this treatment will also be learned. The main questions it aims to answer are:

- Does treatment with MSC-derived exosomes lower the number of fistula recurrences in participants?
- Is treatment with MSC-derived exosomes safe? We will compare treatment with MSC-derived exosomes to the routine treatment which is fistulotomy (surgery to close the fistula) alone to see if MSC-derived exosomes work better to treat complex fistula.

Participants will:

- Undergo fistulotomy plus MSC-derived exosome injections or fistulotomy alone.

J. N. Weiss, *Global Exosome Trials*, https://doi.org/10.1007/978-3-031-96420-6_10

- Visit the clinic the week after surgery and then every 4 weeks for checkups and tests.

Official Title
The Efficacy of Human Placenta Mesenchymal Stem Cell-Derived Exosome Injection for Treatment of Complex Anal Fistula in Colorectal Surgery Department of Imam Khomeini Hospital Complex: A Non-randomized Clinical Trial
Conditions
Fistula perianal
Intervention/Treatment

- Procedure: exosome
- Procedure: routine conventional fistulotomy

Other Study ID Numbers

- IR.TUMS.IKHC.REC.1403.113

Study Start (Estimated)
2024-09-15
Primary Completion (Estimated)
2024-11-15
Study Completion (Estimated)
2025-02-15
Enrollment (Estimated)
40
Study Type
Interventional
Phase
Phase 2
No location data
Eligibility Criteria
Description
Inclusion Criteria:

- Participants with complex perianal fistula
- Provided written informed consent

Exclusion Criteria:

- Participants with any inflammatory bowel diseases
- Pregnant or lactating participants
- Participants with contraindications for surgery
- Participants with hepatitis
- Participants with uncontrolled diabetes
- Participants with alcohol or substance abuse

Ages Eligible for Study
18–70 years (adult, older adult)

Sexes Eligible for Study
All
Accepts Healthy Volunteers
No
Study Plan
Design Details
Primary purpose: treatment
Allocation: non-randomized
Interventional model: parallel assignment
Masking: none (open label)

Arms and Interventions

Participant group/arm	Intervention/treatment
Experimental: intervention	Procedure: exosome Human placenta mesenchymal stem cell-derived exosome
Active comparator: control	Procedure: routine conventional fistulotomy Routine conventional fistulotomy

Primary Outcome Measures

Outcome measure	Measure description	Time frame
The number of fistula openings (orifices) will be assessed before and after our intervention	Clinical improvement	3 months

Secondary Outcome Measures

Outcome measure	Measure description	Time frame
QoL questionnaire	Quality of life improvement (before and after intervention) assessed by Persian (Farsi) version of the QoLAF (quality of life in patients with anal fistula) questionnaire	3 months

Sponsor
Tehran University of Medical Sciences
Recruiting

The Role of Mesenchymal Stem Cell and Exosome in Treating Pilonidal Sinus Disease in Children

ClinicalTrials.gov ID NCT06391307

Sponsor Mustafa Azizoğlu

Information provided by Mustafa Azizoğlu, Necmi Kadıoğlu Hospital (Responsible Party)

Last Update Posted 2024-05-14

Study Overview

Brief Summary

Chronic wounds that fail to heal over extended periods pose a significant financial burden on the healthcare system, underscoring the urgent need to enhance clinical treatments. Among the most promising approaches are stem cell-based therapies. Substantial evidence suggests that mesenchymal stem cells (MSCs) can facilitate the healing of chronic wounds in both animal models and preclinical studies, primarily through their paracrine actions. The bioactive factors and cytokines secreted by MSCs can be harvested in the form of conditioned medium. This medium has been processed into a lyophilized powder for clinical use. Patients with chronic wounds will be recruited and divided into two groups: the control group will receive the commonly used fibroblast growth factor, while the experimental group will be treated with the lyophilized powder. The study aims to assess the efficacy and safety of this stem cell and exosome in treating chronic wounds (especially pilonidal sinus).

Detailed Description

Pilonidal sinus disease (PSD) is an infectious or inflammatory condition beneath the skin at the peak of the gluteal cleft in the sacrococcygeal area. It is a chronic condition characterized by discharge, infection, and pain. Although it can occur during adolescence, it is most commonly seen in adult males, leading to a focus on adult treatments in research. Surgical treatment was first implemented by Anderson in 1847. Since then, various surgical and medical treatment options have been explored, yet there is no widely accepted standardized treatment. The ideal treatment should be simple, require a short hospital stay, have low recurrence rates, provide good cosmetic results, be cost-effective, cause minimal pain, and allow a quick return to social life, making the surgical approach contentious.

Maurice and Greenwood first reported the application of liquid phenol in 1964, initially under general anesthesia, later shifting to local anesthesia. Due to high recurrence rates with liquid phenol, Dogru and colleagues introduced the crystallized phenol (CP) procedure, a minimally invasive method now commonly used in adults.

Recent years have shown that stem cells and exosomes promote tissue healing and reduce inflammation. Known for their ability to differentiate into various cell types, stem cells and exosomes play critical roles in intercellular communication, containing a variety of molecules. Their use in surgical fields has become popular as they speed up the postoperative healing process and reduce the risk of complications. Research in the literature supports that stem cells and exosomes accelerate wound healing.

This study is based on two main premises: firstly, to identify the potential healing effects of stem cell and exosome applications in treating pilonidal sinus disease, and secondly, to comparatively assess the impact of these applications on surgical outcomes, specifically regarding surgery duration, complications, and the healing process. Comparing these two groups will help determine the value of stem cell and exosome applications in managing pilonidal sinus disease.

Official Title

The Role of Mesenchymal Stem Cell and Exosome in Treating Pilonidal Sinus Disease in Children: A Prospective Randomized Controlled Trial
Conditions
Pilonidal sinus
Pilonidal disease
Intervention/Treatment

- Other: crystallized phenol
- Biological: crystallized phenol + exosome
- Biological: crystallized phenol + stem cell
- Biological: crystallized phenol + exosome + stem cell

Other Study ID Numbers

- Stem Cell PNS

Study Start (Actual)
2024-05-11
Primary Completion (Estimated)
2024-11-30
Study Completion (Estimated)
2024-12-30
Enrollment (Estimated)
120
Study Type
Interventional
Phase
Not applicable
Study Contact
Name: Mustafa Azizoğlu, MD, PhD
Phone Number: +905447448244
Email: mdmazizoglu@gmail.com
This study has 1 location
Turkey
Istanbul, Turkey, 34430
Recruiting
Mustafa Azizoğlu
Contact:
Mustafa Azizoğlu
+905447448244 mdmazizoglu@gmail.com
Eligibility Criteria
Description
Inclusion Criteria:

- 0–18 years
- Patients with chronic non-healing wound and pilonidal sinus diseases

Exclusion Criteria:

- Patients with epilepsia
- Patients with diabetes
- Patients with hypertension
- Patients with chronic and other diseases

Ages Eligible for Study
1 day to 18 years (child, adult)
Sexes Eligible for Study
All
Accepts Healthy Volunteers
No
Design Details
Primary purpose: treatment
Allocation: randomized
Interventional model: parallel assignment
Masking: none (open label)

Arms and Interventions

Participant group/arm	Intervention/treatment
Active comparator: crystallized phenol In this group, the classic non-operative technique is employed. The pilonidal sinus is debrided under local anesthesia, followed by the injection of crystallized phenol into the wound	Other: crystallized phenol Crystallized phenol + exosome + stem cell Other names: Crystallized phenol will be applied to the wound area
Experimental: crystallized phenol + exosome In this group, the classic non-operative technique is employed. The pilonidal sinus is debrided under local anesthesia, followed by the injection of crystallized phenol + exosome into the wound	Biological: crystallized phenol + exosome Crystallized phenol + exosome will be applied to the wound area
Experimental: crystallized phenol + stem cell In this group, the classic non-operative technique is employed. The pilonidal sinus is debrided under local anesthesia, followed by the injection of crystallized phenol + stem cell into the wound	Biological: crystallized phenol + stem cell Crystallized phenol + stem cell will be applied to the wound area
Experimental: crystallized phenol + exosome + stem cell In this group, the classic non-operative technique is employed. The pilonidal sinus is debrided under local anesthesia, followed by the injection of crystallized phenol + stem cell + exosome into the wound	Biological: crystallized phenol + exosome + stem cell Crystallized phenol + exosome + stem cell will be applied to the wound area

Primary Outcome Measures

Outcome measure	Measure description	Time frame
Wound healing time	In the control group, the healing process generally takes about 2–3 weeks. In the experimental group, a shorter duration is expected. In this study, the wound healing times of both groups will be evaluated and compared	3 weeks
Cosmetic results	In this study, the worst healing wounds will receive a score of 1, and the best-healed wounds, which are closest to normal skin, will receive a score of 10. In short, a low score indicates poor wound healing and poor cosmetic, while a high score indicates that the wound has achieved a good cosmetic appearance	2 months
Skin burn rate	In patients treated with crystallized phenol, skin burns can occur during application. To prevent this, Furacin ointment is applied around the wound. However, we still encounter skin burns. In this study, it is expected that the experimental groups will have a lower burn rate compared to the control group. The burn rate will be evaluated in this study	2 weeks
Average time to full daily activities	It refers to the time when patients return to their routine lives after the procedure	1 week
VAS score	Patient visual analog scale (VAS) scores will be assessed both prior to the procedure and again 10 days and 20 days following the procedure and after recovery	7 weeks
Success rate	The success rate will be calculated after interventions	7 weeks
Recurrence rate	The recurrence rate will be calculated after interventions	7 weeks

Secondary Outcome Measures

Outcome measure	Measure description	Time frame
Bleeding rate	Bleeding during interventions will be calculated	1 week
Infection rate	Infection will be defined during interventions and 10 days after intervention	7 weeks
Total complication rate	Total complications during interventions will be calculated	7 weeks

Sponsor
Mustafa Azizoğlu
Collaborators

- Necmi Kadıoğlu Hospital

Investigators

- Principal Investigator: Mustafa Azizoğlu, MD, Esenyurt State Hospital

Chapter 11
Skin Exosome Trials

Recruiting

MSC EVs in Dystrophic Epidermolysis Bullosa

ClinicalTrials.gov ID NCT04173650

Sponsor Aegle Therapeutics

Information provided by Aegle Therapeutics (Responsible Party)

Last Update Posted 2024-12-30

Study Overview

Brief Summary

Investigational Product: AGLE-102 is an allogeneic-derived extracellular vesicle (EV) product derived from normal donor mesenchymal stem cells (MSCs).

Indication and Rationale: The aim of the study is to assess the safety and efficacy of AGLE-102 in the treatment of lesions in subjects with epidermolysis bullosa (EB).

Study Design: This is a phase 1/2A, non-randomized, multicenter study to assess the effectiveness and safety of AGLE-102 on lesions in subjects with EB.

Detailed Description

Study Design: This trial is a prospective, open-label, randomized, multicenter study, with intra-subject paired-wound control, intended to assess the safety and preliminary efficacy of administering extracellular vesicles (EVs) derived from allogeneic mesenchymal stem cells (MSCs) to 10–50 cm^2 wounds in RDEB subjects with wounds persisting for at least 4 weeks.

After providing written informed consent (assent with parental written consent for pediatric subjects) and undergoing screening evaluations, eligible subjects have a single set of paired wounds identified that are determined by either subject/caregiver reporting, medical history, or other reliable sources to have been present for a minimum of 4 weeks. One of each pair is randomized to treatment with EVs in

J. N. Weiss, *Global Exosome Trials*, https://doi.org/10.1007/978-3-031-96420-6_11

conjunction with standard of care. The other wound of each pair receives standard of care alone, without EV treatment. All wounds in the study continue to receive standard care throughout the study. For the EV-treated wounds, up to six administrations of EVs occur approximately 2 weeks apart over a period of 10 weeks. If the treated wound closes prior to six administrations and remains closed for at least 2 weeks, no additional doses are given. Wound closure is determined by complete re-epithelialization that is not subject to re-injury during dressing changes or as a result of normal daily activities (e.g., wearing clothing, eating, sleeping). This is confirmed by the investigator at least 2 weeks after initial closure. After the initial 10-week treatment period, or from the time of closure of the treated wound if prior to the end of the treatment period, the wounds are followed every 4 weeks for a period of 12 additional weeks, for a total of up to 22 weeks of observation from the start of treatment. Regardless of the closure status of wounds or the timing of the last EV treatment, all subjects must present 10 weeks after the initial treatment to ascertain closure status of both the control and EV-treated wounds. At no time during the study does closure status of the control wound influence the EV treatment or visit schedule.

Study Objectives:
Primary Objectives:

Determine the safety of applying multiple administrations of EVs derived from allogeneic MSCs to 10–50 cm^2 RDEB wounds that have persisted for at least 4 weeks.

Determine if EVs plus standard of care can promote wound healing in RDEB subjects compared to standard of care alone.

Secondary Objectives: Determine if there is clinical benefit of applying EVs to RDEB wounds.

Planned Sample Size: eighth subjects will be treated on the protocol with AGLE-102.

Official Title

A Safety Study of the Administration of Mesenchymal Stem Cell Extracellular Vesicles in the Treatment of Dystrophic Epidermolysis Bullosa Wounds

Conditions

Dystrophic epidermolysis bullosa

Intervention / Treatment

- Drug: AGLE 102

Other Study ID Numbers

- EB IND

Study Start (Actual)

2024-08-13

Primary Completion (Estimated)

2025-03

Study Completion (Estimated)
2025-09
Enrollment (Estimated)
10
Study Type
Interventional
Phase
Phase 1
Phase 2
Study Contact
Name: Mei Chen, Ph.D.
Phone Number: 323-865-0621
Email: chenm@usc.edu
This study has 2 locations
United States
California Locations
Los Angeles, California, United States, 90033
Recruiting
Department of Dermatology USC/Norris Comprehensive Cancer Center University of Southern California
Contact:
Mei Chen, PhD
323-865-0621 chenm@usc.edu
Principal Investigator:
David T Woodley, MD
Pennsylvania Locations
Philadelphia, Pennsylvania, United States, 19104
Recruiting
Children's Hospital of Philadelphia
Contact:
Griffin S Hogrogian, MSEd
215-590-1930 stocktonhg@chop.edu
Principal Investigator:
Marissa Perman, MD
Eligibility Criteria
Description
Inclusion Criteria:

1. The first two subjects must be 18 years or older at the time of signing the informed consent. If approved by the SRC, additional subjects (after the first two subjects) may be 6 years or older at the time of signing the informed consent; otherwise, additional subjects must be 18 years or older until such time it is considered by the SRC as appropriate to lower the age limit to 6 years.
2. Subjects who have a confirmed diagnosis of DEB as determined by electron microscopy, immunomapping, or genetic testing. Subjects with severe DEB

(e.g., RDEB patients with absent Col VII/no anchoring fibrils) and milder forms of DEB (e.g., RDEB patients with reduced Col VII and/or anchoring fibril levels) will be eligible.
3. Subjects who have one or more active wounds (unroofed EB erosions) each between 10 and 50 cm^2 on the arms, legs, or trunk.
4. Females of childbearing potential must have a negative urine or serum pregnancy test at screening and agree to continue use of an acceptable form of birth control throughout the duration of the study. Acceptable forms of birth control include oral, implant, injectable, and transdermal contraceptives, an intrauterine device, or other forms considered acceptable by the investigator.
5. Subjects or guardian of subjects who are under the age of 18 years must be capable of giving signed informed consent, which includes compliance with the requirements and restrictions listed in the informed consent form (ICF) and in this protocol.
6. Subjects must be willing to comply with the protocol requirements.
7. Subjects must be accessible for wound treatments and assessment visits.
8. Subjects must have a negative urine test for drugs of abuse at the screening visit.
9. Female subjects willing to minimize the risk of inducing pregnancy for the duration of the clinical study and follow-up period.
10. A female subject is eligible to participate if she is not pregnant (i.e., has a negative urine pregnancy result at the screening visit and on day 1), and at least one of the following conditions applies:
11. Not a woman of childbearing potential (WOCBP).
12. Or a WOCBP who agrees to follow the contraceptive guidance during the intervention and follow-up period

Exclusion Criteria:

1. The subject has clinical evidence of systemic infection.
2. The subject has a history of bone marrow transplantation.
3. The subject has evidence of autoimmune disease, including insulin-dependent diabetes.
4. The subject has wounds that are considered by the investigator as likely to heal within 1 month after standard therapy.
5. The subject has clinical evidence of an active infection at the wound site.
6. The subject has evidence of significant wound healing before treatment (i.e., $\geq$20% closure of wound during the first month observation period of treatment).
7. The subject has a wound that extends across the fingers, toes, pubic, or perineum region.
8. The subject has a severe medical condition, such as malignancy (including skin cancer), a life expectancy of <2 years, or severe cardiopulmonary disease that restricts ambulation to the clinical facility.
9. The subject has a history of coagulopathy.
10. The subject currently uses systemic steroids or immunosuppressive agents.
11. The subject is allergic to human albumin, streptomycin, or penicillin.
12. The subject is a potential recipient of tissue or organ transplantation.

13. The subject has a current history of alcohol or substance abuse or has a history of alcohol or substance abuse that required treatment within the previous 12 months.
14. The subject has a positive test result for human immunodeficiency virus (HIV) at screening.
15. The subject has a history of poor compliance or unreliability.
16. Females who are pregnant, nursing, or planning a pregnancy during their participation in the study.

Ages Eligible for Study
6 years and older (child, adult, older adult)
Sexes Eligible for Study
All
Accepts Healthy Volunteers
No
Design Details
Primary purpose: treatment
Allocation: N/A
Interventional model: single group assignment

Interventional model description: this trial is a prospective, open-label, randomized, multicenter study, with intra-subject paired-wound control, intended to assess the safety and preliminary efficacy of administering EVs derived from allogeneic MSCs to 10–50 cm^2 wounds in RDEB subjects with wounds persisting for at least 4 weeks.

Masking: none (open label)

Arms and Interventions

Participant group/arm	Intervention/treatment
Experimental: AGLE 102 Treatment arm	Drug: AGLE 102 Exosomes from MSCs up to six administrations

Primary Outcome Measures

Outcome measure	Measure description	Time frame
Treatment-emergent adverse events	Incidence of adverse events after single and repeat administrations of EVs	22 weeks
Wound healing improvement	Change in wound surface area relative to baseline compared with standard of care control	10 weeks

Secondary Outcome Measures

Outcome measure	Measure description	Time frame
Complete wound closure efficacy	Incidence of complete wound closure versus standard of care alone within 10 weeks	10 weeks

(continued)

Outcome measure	Measure description	Time frame
Time from baseline to complete wound closure	Time to wound closure versus standard of care alone	22 weeks
Scar quality improvement	Change from baseline in patient and observer scar assessment scales. The min value is 1 and the max value is 10. The min value is normal skin, and the max value is worst scar imaginable	22 weeks
Pain relief efficacy	Change from baseline in patient-reported measures of pain. Using the Wong-Baker Faces Pain rating scale. The min value is value is 0 and the max value is 10. 0 is no pain, and 10 hurts worst.	22 weeks
Quality of life improvement	Change from baseline in patient-reported quality of life scale. The min value is 1 and the max value is 5. 1 indicates that the wound has minimal impact, and 5 indicates maximum impact	22 weeks

Sponsor
Aegle Therapeutics
Investigators

- Principal Investigator: David T Woodley, MD, University of Southern California Dept of Dermatology

Recruiting

Umbilical Cord Mesenchymal Stem Cell-Derived Exosomes in the Treatment of Melasma

ClinicalTrials.gov ID NCT06677931
Sponsor Fujian Medical University Union Hospital
Information provided by Fujian Medical University Union Hospital (Responsible Party)
Last Update Posted 2024-11-07
Study Overview
Brief Summary
Melasma is a refractory skin disease with a complex pathogenesis and difficult treatment. Research has found that mesenchymal stem cell-derived exosomes have effects such as anti-wrinkle formation, anti-inflammation, antioxidant properties, skin whitening, and promotion of skin regeneration. Recent studies show that there is damage to the basement membrane in melasma skin lesions, and the regenerative repair function of mesenchymal stem cell-derived exosomes can repair the damaged basement membrane in melasma skin lesions, thereby effectively treating melasma. This study aims to observe the therapeutic effect of umbilical cord mesenchymal stem cell-derived exosomes combined with 1565 non-ablative fractional laser treatment for melasma, verify the enhancement effect of 1565 non-ablative fractional

laser, and also explore a new combined treatment method for melasma that is effective, low in side effects, and low in recurrence rate and provides good patient comfort.

Detailed Description

Exosomes are small, uniform lipid bilayer vesicles with a molecular diameter of 30–150 nm, formed by cells and actively secreted into the extracellular space. They contain proteins, peptides, lipids, nucleic acids, growth factors, hormones, and other substances. Exosomes derived from stem cells share similar functions with stem cells, including tissue repair and regeneration, enhancing the survival of transplanted fat, anti-inflammatory, and antioxidant effects. Compared to stem cells, exosomes are more stable, easier to preserve, manage, and control, and their content can be manipulated in terms of type and quantity. They lack live cells and have low immunogenicity. Research has found that stem cell-derived exosomes have various effects in anti-aging and medical aesthetics.

Melasma is an acquired pigmentation disorder predominantly affecting females. Its pathogenesis is complex, and treatment is challenging, making it one of the refractory skin diseases. Current treatment methods have long treatment cycles, high recurrence rates, and poor patient compliance, with treatment outcomes still not ideal. Recent studies show damage to the basement membrane in melasma skin lesions, and the regenerative repair function of stem cell-derived exosomes can repair the damaged basement membrane in these lesions, thus effectively treating melasma.

Due to the skin's barrier function, exosomes from stem cells can hardly penetrate the skin barrier. In recent years, various physicochemical methods such as chemical enhancers, nanotechnology, ultrasound, microneedles, radiofrequency, or thermal ablation have been introduced to facilitate the transdermal delivery of biologics. However, they pose significant issues in terms of skin irritation and damage while aiding in overcoming the skin barrier for effective enhancement. Therefore, finding methods that are minimally irritating to the skin and capable of facilitating the transdermal delivery of biologics remains a challenge in transdermal drug delivery.

This study aims to observe the therapeutic effect of umbilical cord mesenchymal stem cell-derived exosomes combined with 1565 non-ablative fractional laser treatment for melasma, validate the enhancement effect of 1565 non-ablative fractional laser, and explore a new combined treatment method for melasma that is effective, low in side effects, and low in recurrence rate and provides good patient comfort.

Official Title

Safety and Efficacy of Umbilical Cord Mesenchymal Stem Cell-Derived Exosomes in the Treatment of Melasma, a Prospective, Randomized, Controlled Clinical Trial

Conditions

Melasma

Intervention/Treatment

- Procedure: placebo comparator,1565 non-ablative fractional laser combined with normal saline

- Procedure: 1565 non-ablative fractional laser combined with umbilical cord mesenchymal stem cell-derived exosomes

  Other Study ID Numbers

- 2024YF028-01

  Study Start (Actual)
  2024-08-28
  Primary Completion (Estimated)
  2025-04-28
  Study Completion (Estimated)
  2026-08-01
  Enrollment (Estimated)
  60
  Study Type
  Interventional
  Phase
  Not applicable
  Study Contact
  Name: xiaosong chen
  Phone Number: 13365910035 ext 86
  Email: chenxiaosong74@163.com
  Study Contact Backup
  Name: Ting Wang
  Phone Number: 17859556387 ext 86
  Email: wangting1022@fjmu.edu.cn
  This study has 2 locations
  China
  Fujian Locations
  Fuzhou, Fujian, China, 350001
  Recruiting
  Affiliated Union Hospital of Fujian Medical University
  Contact:
  Xiaosong Chen, director
  +86 13365910035 chenxiaosong74@163.com
  Fuzhou Locations
  Fujian, Fuzhou, China, 350001
  Recruiting
  Chenxiaosong
  Contact:
  Xiaosong - Chen, director
  13365910035 chenxiaosong74@163.com
  Eligibility Criteria
  Description
  Inclusion Criteria:

1. Aged 18–60 years with good overall health
2. Diagnosed with melasma according to clinical diagnostic criteria and efficacy standards (revised edition), with facial skin lesions
3. Fully understands and comprehends the content and significance of the study, implementation plan, potential benefits, risks, mitigation measures, participant rights and obligations (including privacy protection and voluntary withdrawal), and willing to sign the informed consent form to participate in the clinical study and can cooperate well
4. Exclusion of inflammatory post-pigmentary disorders, malar melasma, Riehl's melanosis, pigmentary lichenoid dermatosis, and other skin diseases
5. Agrees not to use other cosmetic treatments related to the study during the research period

Exclusion Criteria:

1. Patients who refuse to sign the informed consent form to participate in the trial
2. History of significant organ diseases, autoimmune diseases, or immune dysfunction
3. Abnormal coagulation function, current use of anticoagulants, tendency for thrombosis, or family history of genetic diseases
4. Pregnant or lactating women
5. Patients who have taken oral contraceptives or hormone replacement therapy during the study period or in the past 12 months
6. Patients with a keloid-prone constitution
7. Locally damaged or actively affected by other skin diseases
8. History of severe multiple allergies, genetic allergies, photosensitivity or history of photosensitive drugs such as sulfonamides and tetracyclines, allergy to local anesthetics, lidocaine components, or planned desensitization therapy during the study
9. History of post-inflammatory hyperpigmentation
10. Previously treated for melasma
11. Previous chemical peels, abrasion procedures, or other resurfacing treatments on the face.
12. Chronic skin diseases, especially infectious, allergic, and inflammatory systemic skin diseases such as widespread eczema, pemphigus, and pemphigoid
13. Patients currently participating in other clinical studies
14. Other reasons deemed unsuitable for the clinical study by the investigator

Ages Eligible for Study
18–60 Years (adult)
Sexes Eligible for Study
All
Accepts Healthy Volunteers
Yes
Design Details
Primary purpose: treatment

Allocation: randomized
Interventional model: parallel assignment
Masking: quadruple (ParticipantCare ProviderInvestigatorOutcomes Assessor)

Arms and Interventions

Participant group/arm	Intervention/treatment
Placebo comparator: 1565 non-ablative fractional laser combined with normal Saline 1565 non-ablative fractional laser combined with normal saline	Procedure: placebo comparator,1565 non-ablative fractional laser combined with normal Saline Based on the patient's age, skin color, location of skin lesions, and Fitzpatrick skin type, adjust treatment parameters accordingly. The operator holds the treatment head and vertically applies parallel sweeps closely to the lesion area until the endpoint of slight skin redness is reached. After completion, apply normal saline
Experimental: 1565 non-ablative fractional laser combined with umbilical cord mesenchymal stem cell exosomes 1565 non-ablative fractional laser combined with umbilical cord mesenchymal stem cell exosomes	Procedure: 1565 non-ablative fractional laser combined with umbilical cord mesenchymal stem cell-derived exosomes Based on the patient's age, skin color, location of skin lesions, and Fitzpatrick skin type, adjust treatment parameters accordingly. The operator holds the treatment head and vertically applies parallel sweeps closely to the lesion area until the endpoint of slight skin redness is reached. After completion, apply exosomes

Primary Outcome Measures

Outcome measure	Measure description	Time frame
Melasma area and severity index, MASI	MASI = 0.3 (DMR + HMR) AMR + 0.3 (DF + HF) AF + 0.3 (DML + HML) AML + 0.1 (DC + HC) AC. The total score is 48 points, with lower scores indicating less severity of melasma. MASI is jointly assessed by two physicians from this department, taking the average value. If there is a significant difference in the evaluation results of the two physicians, a third physician from the same department will be consulted, and the average value of the two closest assessments will be taken	1, 2, 3, 4, 5, 6, 7, 8 months after the first treatment

Secondary Outcome Measures

Outcome measure	Measure description	Time frame
Physician's global assessment, PGA	Based on the residual condition of pigmented lesions after treatment, a score of 0–6 is assigned: 0 points for complete clearance (100%) or only minimal residual pigmentation, 1 point for essentially cleared (≥90%), 2 points for marked improvement (75–89%), 3 points for moderate improvement (50–74%), 4 points for slight improvement (25–49%), 5 points for no improvement (<25%), 6 points for worsening compared to before treatment	1, 2, 3, 4, 5, 6, 7, 8 months after the first treatment

(continued)

Outcome measure	Measure description	Time frame
Patient satisfaction evaluation	Patient satisfaction is evaluated using a self-assessment satisfaction scale. It is divided into very satisfied (improvement ≥ 75%), satisfied (improvement 50–75%), average (improvement 25–49%), and dissatisfied (improvement ≤25%). Satisfaction rate = (number of very satisfied cases + number of satisfied cases)/total number of cases × 100%	1, 2, 3, 4, 5, 6, 7, 8 months after the first treatment
Occurrence of adverse reactions	Observation of adverse reactions including erythema, burning, itching, dryness, irritation, hyperpigmentation, edema, scar formation, skin breakdown, and skin infection	1, 2, 3, 4, 5, 6, 7, 8 months after the first treatment

Sponsor
Fujian Medical University Union Hospital
Recruiting

Stem Cell-Derived Exosomes in the Treatment of Melasma and Its Percutaneous Penetration

ClinicalTrials.gov ID NCT06221787

Sponsor Fujian Medical University Union Hospital

Information provided by Chen Xiaosong, Fujian Medical University Union Hospital (Responsible Party)

Last Update Posted 2024-01-30

Study Overview

Brief Summary

Melasma is a refractory skin disease due to its complex pathogenesis and difficult treatment. Studies have found that human umbilical cord mesenchymal stem cell-derived exosomes (hUCMSC-Exos) could serve as a novel cell-free therapeutic strategy in regenerative and aesthetic medicine. It could potentially treat melasma, but the skin barrier is a challenge. This study aims to explore the safety and efficacy of hUCMSC-Exos in the treatment of melasma and means to promote its percutaneous penetration.

Detailed Description

A total of 80 patients with melasma treated in our department were divided into four groups. A 1565 nm non-ablative fractional laser (NAFL) combined with normal saline treatment group was used for Group A. Microneedle, NAFL, and a plasma named Peninsula Blue Aurora Shumin Master (PBASM) combined with hUCMSC-Exos were used for the other treatment groups (B, C, and D, respectively). The treatment was given four times with an interval of 1 month. The degree of pain post-treatment, MASI, improvement rate, physician global assessment score, satisfaction, and complications after treatment were evaluated 6 months later.

Official Title
Stem Cell-Derived Exosomes in the Treatment of Melasma and Its Percutaneous Penetration
Conditions
Melasma
Intervention/Treatment

- Procedure: 1565 nm non-ablative fractional laser combined with normal saline
- Procedure: microneedles combined with hUCMSC-Exos
- Procedure: 1565 nm non-ablative fractional laser combined with hUCMSC-Exos
- Procedure: PBASM combined with hUCMSC-Exos

Other Study ID Numbers

- 2020KY0155

Study Start (Actual)
2022-04-01
Primary Completion (Estimated)
2026-08-01
Study Completion (Estimated)
2026-08-01
Enrollment (Estimated)
80
Study Type
Interventional
Phase
Not applicable
Study Contact
Name: xiaosong chen, director
Phone Number: 13365910035
Email: chenxiaosong74@163.com
This study has 1 location
China
Fujian Locations
Fuzhou, Fujian, China, 350001
Recruiting
Affiliated Union Hospital of Fujian Medical University
Contact:
xiaosong chen, director
+86 13365910035 chenxiaosong74@163.com
Eligibility Criteria
Description
Inclusion Criteria:

- Patients diagnosed with chloasma who meet the clinical diagnostic standards and efficacy standards (revised version) of chloasma and have skin lesions on the face.

It is hoped that exosomes combined with 1565 non-ablative fractional laser, blue aurora, or microneedle can improve facial chloasma.

Fully understand and understand the content and significance of this study, implementation plan, possible benefits, risks and countermeasures, rights and obligations of subjects (including privacy protection, free withdrawal), and willing to participate in this clinical study and able to cooperate well, those who signed the informed consent form.

Exclude post-inflammatory pigmentation, malar brown-green nevus, Riehl's melanosis, pigmented lichen planus, and other skin diseases.

Subjects who agree not to use other cosmetic treatments related to the study during the study period.

Exclusion Criteria:

1. Patients who refuse to sign the informed consent form to participate in the trial
2. Those with a history of important organ diseases, autoimmune diseases, or immune dysfunction
3. Abnormal coagulation function, current use of anticoagulants, thrombophilia, and history of familial genetic diseases
4. Pregnant or lactating women
5. Patients taking oral contraceptives or hormone replacement therapy during the study period or within the past 12 months
6. Patients with scar constitution
7. Active skin infection
8. Those who have a history of multiple severe allergies, hereditary allergies, and photosensitivity or photosensitivity drugs, such as sulfa drugs and tetracyclines, those who are allergic to local anesthetics and lidocaine components, and those who plan to undergo detoxification during the study of allergy healer
9. History of post-inflammatory pigmentation
10. Those who have received treatment for chloasma in the past
11. Those who have undergone chemical peeling, dermabrasion, or other skin resurfacing on their face in the past
12. Patients who are participating in other clinical studies
13. Other reasons that the researcher considers unsuitable for clinical investigators

Ages Eligible for Study

18–60 years (adult)

Sexes Eligible for Study

All

Accepts Healthy Volunteers

Yes

Study Plan

Design Details

Primary purpose: treatment

Allocation: randomized

Interventional model: parallel assignment

Masking: quadruple (ParticipantCare ProviderInvestigatorOutcomes Assessor)

Arms and Interventions

Participant group/arm	Intervention/treatment
Placebo comparator: 1565 nm non-ablative fractional laser combined with normal saline The treatment parameters were adjusted according to each patient's age, skin color, surface area of affected skin, location of melasma, and skin type. After the scanning, infusing with normal saline in the entire face	Procedure: 1565 nm non-ablative fractional laser combined with normal saline After 1565 nm non-ablative fractional laser treatment, patients with melasma were smeared with normal saline and compared with those smeared with exosomes after laser treatment
Experimental: microneedles combined with hUCMSC-Exos The hUCMSC-Exos were applied while rolling a microneedle roller in the entire face	Procedure: microneedles combined with hUCMSC-Exos The hUCMSC-Exos were applied while rolling a microneedle roller and compared with those using 1565 nm non-ablative fractional laser or PBASM combined with hUCMSC-Exos
Experimental: 1565 nm non-ablative fractional laser combined with hUCMSC-Exos The treatment parameters were adjusted according to each patient's age, skin color, surface area of affected skin, location of melasma, and skin type. After the scanning, infusing with hUCMSC-Exos in the entire face	Procedure: 1565 nm non-ablative fractional laser combined with hUCMSC-Exos After 1565 nm non-ablative fractional laser treatment, patients with melasma were smeared with hUCMSC-Exos and compared with those smeared with normal saline after laser treatment. What is more, compared with those using microneedles or PBASM combined with hUCMSC-Exos
Experimental: PBASM combined with hUCMSC-Exos 4–5 levels of intensity were used, rolling each area for 8–10 min before applying the hUCMSC-Exos in the entire face	Procedure: PBASM combined with hUCMSC-Exos A plasma named Peninsula Blue Aurora Shumin Master (PBASM) rolling each area for 8–10 min before applying the hUCMSC-Exos to the entire face. And compared with those using 1565 nm non-ablative fractional laser or microneedles combined with hUCMSC-Exos

Primary Outcome Measures

Outcome measure	Measure Description	Time frame
Melasma area and severity index (MASI)	MASI = 0.3 (DMR+HMR) AMR+0.3 (DF+HF) AF+0.3 (DML+HML) AML+0.1 (DC+HC) AC. A is the area proportion of chloasma, D is the color depth of the spots, H is the color uniformity, F is the forehead, ML is the left cheek, MR is the right cheek, and C is the mandible. Scores for color depth and color uniformity of stains: total score is 4 points each, and the color degree of stains is 0 (no deepening), 1 (slightly deepened), 2 (moderately deepened), 3 (obviously deepened), and 4 points (severely deepened); color uniformity is 0 point (extremely inconsistent), 1 point (slightly consistent), 2 points (moderately consistent), 3 points (obviously consistent), and 4 points (almost completely consistent). Damage area proportion score: total score is 6 points, 0 is normal, 1 is <10%, 2 is 10–29%, 3 is 30–49%, 4 is 50–69%, 5 is 70–89%, and 6 is 90–100%. The total score is 48 points, and the lower the score, the less serious the chloasma	6 months

Sponsor
Fujian Medical University Union Hospital
Investigators

- Study Chair: Xiaosong Chen, Director, Affiliated Union Hospital of Fujian Medical University

Recruiting

Induced Pluripotent Stem Cell-Derived Exosomes for the Treatment of Atopic Dermatitis

ClinicalTrials.gov ID NCT05969717
Sponsor Peking Union Medical College Hospital
Information provided by Peking Union Medical College Hospital (Responsible Party)
Last Update Posted 2023-08-01
Study Overview
Brief Summary
Evaluate the safety, tolerability, and preliminary efficacy of GD-iExo-001 in the treatment of atopic dermatitis
Detailed Description

Atopic dermatitis (AD) is a chronic inflammatory skin disease that is characterized by intense itching and recurrent eczematous lesions. Although it most often starts in infancy and affects two of ten children, it is also highly prevalent in adults. It is the leading non-fatal health burden attributable to skin diseases, inflicts a substantial psychosocial burden on patients and their relatives, and increases the risk of food allergy, asthma, allergic rhinitis, other immune-mediated inflammatory diseases, and mental health disorders. Originally regarded as a childhood disorder mediated by an imbalance toward a T-helper-2 response and exaggerated IgE responses to allergens, it is now recognized as a lifelong disposition with variable clinical manifestations and expressivity, in which defects of the epidermal barrier are central. Present prevention and treatment focus on restoration of epidermal barrier function, which is best achieved through the use of emollients. Topical corticosteroids are still the first-line therapy for acute flares, but they are also used proactively along with topical calcineurin inhibitors to maintain remission.

Exosomes are nano-sized biovesicles released into surrounding body fluids upon fusion of multivesicular bodies and the plasma membrane. They were shown to carry cell-specific cargos of proteins, lipids, and genetic materials and can be selectively taken up by neighboring or distant cells far from their release, reprogramming the recipient cells upon their bioactive compounds. Therefore, the regulated formation of exosomes, specific makeup of their cargo, and cell-targeting specificity are of immense biological interest considering extremely high potential of exosomes as noninvasive diagnostic biomarkers, as well as therapeutic nanocarriers.

Induced pluripotent stem cells (iPSCs) are pluripotent stem cells generated from adult cells by reprogramming. iPSCs have the same properties as embryonic stem cells and therefore self-renew and can differentiate into all cell types of the body except for cells in extra-embryonic tissues such as the placenta. iPSC-derived exosomes contain TGF-β, BDNF, etc., which can inhibit cell apoptosis, inhibit inflammatory response, promote angiogenesis, inhibit fibrosis, and enhance tissue repair potential, with a wide range of potential applications. iPSC-derived exosomes have emerged as an important paracrine factor for iPSCs to repair injured cells through the delivery of bioactive components.

The purpose of this trial is to evaluate the safety, tolerability, and preliminary efficacy of iPSC-derived exosomes in the treatment of atopic dermatitis.

Official Title

Exploratory Clinical Study on Induced Pluripotent Stem Cell-Derived Exosomes (GD-iExo-001) for the Treatment of Atopic Dermatitis

Conditions

Atopic dermatitis

Intervention/Treatment

- Drug: GD-iExo-001
- Other: normal saline

Other Study ID Numbers

- K3016

Study Start (Actual)

2023-04-12

Primary Completion (Estimated)

2025-04-30

Study Completion (Estimated)

2025-06-30

Enrollment (Estimated)

20

Study Type

Interventional

Phase

Early Phase 1

Study Contact

Name: Ju Qiao, PhD

Phone Number: +8615201125788

Email: qiaoqiaoju@aliyun.com

This study has 1 location

China

Beijing Locations

Beijing, Beijing, China, 100730

Recruiting

Chinese Academy of Medical Science & Peking Union Medical College Hospital

Contact:
Ju Qiao, PhD
+8615201125788 qiaoqiaoju@aliyun.com
Eligibility Criteria
Description
Inclusion Criteria:

- Age 18–70 years, body mass index (BMI) between 18 and 35 kg/m^2 (including boundary values)
- Overall good health except AD
- Participants diagnosed with atopic dermatitis (AD) as defined by the Hanifin and Rajka criteria
- Investigator's overall assessment (IGA) score of 2–3
- Participants with a history of subacute or chronic AD symptoms for at least 6 months
- Participants with body surface area (BSA) of AD involvement of ≤5% at screening and baseline
- Participants and their partners agreed to use effective contraception throughout the study period (from screening to 3 months after completion of treatment)
- Participants understood and voluntarily signed the informed consent form

Exclusion Criteria:

- There are obvious active systemic or local infections, including but not limited to the infection of AD secondary infection, local bacterial infection in target lesion, local viral infection in target lesion, and local fungal infection in target lesion. Note: after the infection resolves, the patients can be re-screened.
- Presence of any of the following conditions: HB surface antigen (HBsAg) positive and/or HB e antigen (HBeAg) positive, HB e antibody (HBeAb) and/or hepatitis B core antibody (HBcAb) positive, and hepatitis B virus deoxyribonucleic acid (HBV-DNA) copy number >2000 IU / mL; limited hepatitis C virus (HCV) antibody positive and peripheral blood hepatitis C virus (HCV) RNA positive; positive human immunodeficiency virus (HIV) antibody; positive for syphilis (TPA) test.
- Inoculate live or attenuated vaccine within 4 weeks before screening or during the study period.
- Received allergen-specific immunotherapy within 6 months before screening.
- Use of topical drugs known or may affect AD within 2 weeks before screening (including but not limited to topical glucocorticoids and calcineurin inhibitors, such as tacrolimus and sirolimus).
- Use of immunosuppressants and Janus kinase inhibitors within 4 weeks before screening.
- Use of any biological agent (such as IL-4 receptor inhibitors, IL-13 inhibitors) for 12 weeks before screening or 5 half-lives (whichever is longer).
- Received systemic or local Chinese medicine treatment (including Chinese medicine immersion treatment) within 2 weeks before screening.

- Treated with UV and photochemistry within 4 weeks prior to screening.
- Required systemic treatment of antiviral, antiparasitic, antigenic, or antifungals within 4 weeks prior to screening.
- With significant abnormal findings or laboratory values and clinical significance, such as white blood cell count <3.0e9/L, neutrophils <1 LLN, hemoglobin <90g/L, platelet <100e9/L, serum creatinine >1.5 ULN, ALT or AST 2 ULN, QTcF >450 msec (male), or QTcF >470 msec (female)
- Other combined (or co-occurrence) skin diseases that may affect the study evaluation, such as acne, psoriasis, and lupus erythematosus, or large tattoos, birthmarks, skin scars, skin ulcers, and other conditions that may affect the judgment of the investigator.
- Except for AD, any history of clinical major disease or clinically significant circulatory system abnormality, endocrine system abnormality, neurological or hematological disorders, immune system disease, psychiatric illness, and metabolic instability; clinical significance is defined as the risk of the safety of the subject or aggravating the disease/disease during the study.
- Patients with a history of severe skin allergy and/or allergy to any ingredients of the product.
- History of cancer in the past 5 years (except for surgically removed squamous cell carcinoma, basal cell carcinoma, or skin carcinoma in situ).
- Any major surgery within 8 weeks before screening or subjects expected to undergo surgery during the trial or within 4 weeks after the end of the trial, or 400 mL nonphysiological blood loss (including trauma, blood collection, blood donation within 12 weeks before screening).
- Pregnant women, lactating women, or women who plan to become pregnant during the study (fertile women must have a urine pregnancy test with negative results).
- Subjects who are currently participating in other clinical trials or who have participated in other clinical trials within 90 days.
- The investigator judged any other condition not suitable to participate in this study.

Ages Eligible for Study
18–70 years (adult, older adult)
Sexes Eligible for Study
All
Accepts Healthy Volunteers
No
Design Details
Primary purpose: treatment
Allocation: randomized
Interventional model: parallel assignment
Masking: triple (ParticipantCare ProviderInvestigator)

Arms and Interventions

Participant group/arm	Intervention/treatment
Experimental: GD-iExo-001 treatment Group 1 (low-dose group), 8 patients are treated with 10 μg/mL GD-iExo-001. Group 2 (high-dose group), 8 patients are treated with 50 μg/mL GD-iExo-001. One drop (about 50 μL) of GD-iExo-001 was given to the affected skin area of 2–4 cm^2 for 14 consecutive days, twice per day	Drug: GD-iExo-001 One drop (about 50 μL) of GD-iExo-001 was given to the affected skin area of 2–4 cm^2 for 14 consecutive days, twice per day
Placebo comparator: normal saline control Group 1 (low-dose group), 2 patients are treated with normal saline. Group 2 (high-dose group), 2 patients are treated with normal saline. One drop (about 50 μL) of normal saline was given to the affected skin area of 2–4 cm^2 for 14 consecutive days, twice per day	Other: normal saline One drop (about 50 μL) of normal saline was given to the affected skin area of 2–4 cm^2 for 14 consecutive days, twice per day

Primary Outcome Measures

Outcome measure	Measure description	Time frame
Adverse events as assessed by CTCAE	All potentially treated subjects to assess the safety	42 days from post-administration

Secondary Outcome Measures

Outcome measure	Measure description	Time frame
The proportion of subjects whose IGA score improved by 2 points or more compared with the baseline score		Screening, after the first administration 8 days, 15 days, 21 days, 42 days
The proportion of subjects with an IGA score of 0–1 and an improvement of 2 or more over the baseline score		Screening, after the first administration 8 days, 15 days, 21 days, 42 days
The proportion of subjects whose EASI score improved by more than 50% compared with the baseline period		Screening, after the first administration 8 days, 15 days, 21 days, 42 days
The proportion of subjects whose EASI score improved by more than 75% compared with the baseline period		Screening, after the first administration 8 days, 15 days, 21 days, 42 days
The proportion of subjects whose EASI score improved by more than 90% compared with the baseline period		Screening, after the first administration 8 days, 15 days, 21 days, 42 days
Change in the score of the NRS		Screening, after the first administration 8 days, 15 days, 21 days, 42 days
Change in the score of the DLQI		Screening, after the first administration 8 days, 15 days, 21 days, 42 days

Sponsor
Peking Union Medical College Hospital
Collaborators

- Guidon Pharmaceutics Ltd.

Investigators

- Principal Investigator: Hongzhong Jin, MD, Peking Union Medical College Hospital

Chapter 12
Stroke Exosome Trials

Recruiting

The Effect of GD-iExo-003 in Acute Ischemic Stroke (ExoCURE)

ClinicalTrials.gov ID NCT06138210

Sponsor Xuanwu Hospital, Beijing

Information provided by Junwei Hao, MD, Xuanwu Hospital, Beijing (Responsible Party)

Last Update Posted 2024-05-29

Study Overview

Brief Summary

This is a multicenter, randomized, double-blinded, placebo-controlled, dose-escalation trial. The objective of this study is to evaluate the safety and preliminary efficacy of intravenous exosomes derived from human-induced pluripotent stem cell (GD-iExo-003) in acute ischemic stroke.

Detailed Description

This is a multicenter, randomized, double-blinded, placebo-controlled, dose-escalation trial. This study will consist of two parts, with part 1 being a dose-escalation study and part 2 being an expanded safety study based on part 1 findings.

A traditional 3 + 3 dose escalation design will be implemented in part 1. Cohort 1 receives 2 × 10^9 particles/kg; cohort 2, 4 × 10^9 particles/kg; and cohort 3, 8 × 10^9 particles/kg. If no dose-limiting toxicities (DLTs) are observed for 2 weeks after administration of the first injection, a new cohort will be enrolled at the next planned dose level. If DLTs are observed in one participant in the cohort, another three participants will be treated in the same dose level. Dose escalation will be stopped until DLTs are observed in >33% of the participants.

J. N. Weiss, *Global Exosome Trials*, https://doi.org/10.1007/978-3-031-96420-6_12

In part 2, 20 subjects will be randomized in a 1:1 ratio [exosome (n = 10) or exosome placebo (n = 10)]. The dose level will be determined by Data Safety Monitoring Board based on part 1.

Official Title

The Effect of Exosomes Derived from Human-Induced Pluripotent Stem Cell (GD-iExo-003) in Acute Ischemic Stroke: An Exploratory Study

Conditions

Acute ischemic stroke

Intervention/Treatment

- Drug: exosomes derived from human-induced pluripotent stem cell for injection
- Drug: a placebo of exosomes derived from human-induced pluripotent stem cell for injection

Other Study ID Numbers

- XMEC-2023-004

Study Start (Estimated)
2024-05-27
Primary Completion (Estimated)
2025-08-30
Study Completion (Estimated)
2025-08-30
Enrollment (Estimated)
29
Study Type
Interventional
Phase
Phase 1
Study Contact
Name: Junwei Hao, MD; PhD
Phone Number: 010 8319 8277
Email: haojunwei@vip.163.com
Study Contact Backup
Name: Gaoting Ma, MD
Phone Number: 18301579891
Email: demo_doctor@163.com
This study has 1 location
China
Beijing, China, 100053
Recruiting
Xuanwu Hospital, Capital Medical University
Contact:
Gaoting Ma
18301579891 demo_doctor@163.com
Eligibility Criteria

Description
Inclusion Criteria:

- Clinical diagnosis of acute ischemic stroke
- Age 18–70 years, inclusion of both genders
- Modified Rankin scale score before stroke of 0–1
- NIHSS score 6–20 at inclusion that did not change by ≥4 points from screening to baseline assessment.
- Time of stroke onset is known, and treatment can be started between day 1 and 7 of onset.
- Confirmation of hemispheric cortical infarct with magnetic resonance imaging or computed tomography.
- Subjects who received intravenous thrombolysis or underwent mechanical reperfusion are eligible if they meet all other eligibility criteria.
- Adequate hepatic and renal function: serum aspartate aminotransferase ≤2.5× upper limit of normal, serum alanine aminotransferase ≤2.5× upper limit of normal, blood urea nitrogen ≤1.25× upper limit of normal, and serum creatinine ≤1.25× upper limit of normal.
- Adequate cardiac function.
- Subjects or a legal representative can sign the informed consent and must be willing and able to comply with all aspects of treatment and follow-up schedule.

Exclusion Criteria:

- Presence of intracranial hemorrhage on CT including hemorrhagic stroke, epidural hematoma, subdural hematoma, intraventricular hemorrhage, intraventricular hemorrhage, subarachnoid hemorrhage, or hemorrhagic transformation
- Presence of a lacunar or a brainstem infarct as the etiology of current symptoms.
- Evidence of brain tumor or history of epilepsy or traumatic brain injury.
- Subjects with present malignant disease
- Subjects with severe comorbidities including immunodeficiency or coagulation disorders
- Subjects with Alzheimer's disease, Parkinson's disease, or other degenerative neurological disease
- Ongoing systemic infection, severe local infection, or taking immunosuppressants
- Subjects with negative hepatitis B surface antibody (HBsAg) and positive hepatitis B core antibody (HBcAb), or HBsAg-positive virus carriers, positive hepatitis C antibody, positive syphilis antibody, or HIV
- Allergy to the study products
- Documented allergies
- Participation in any clinical trial in the last 3 months
- Inability or unwillingness to comply with the study schedule
- Pregnancy, childbearing potential (unless it is certain that pregnancy is not possible), or breastfeeding
- Other serious medical or psychiatric illness that is not adequately controlled

- Other circumstances that the investigator considers inappropriate for participation in the trial

  Ages Eligible for Study
  18–70 years (adult, older adult)
  Sexes Eligible for Study
  All
  Accepts Healthy Volunteers
  No
  Design Details
  Primary purpose: treatment
  Allocation: randomized
  Interventional model: sequential assignment
  Masking: quadruple (ParticipantCare ProviderInvestigatorOutcomes Assessor)

Arms and Interventions

Participant group/arm	Intervention/treatment
Experimental: exosome group Patients in this arm will be given exosomes derived from human-induced pluripotent stem cell for injection once a day for 7 days	Drug: exosomes derived from human-induced pluripotent stem cell for injection Exosomes derived from human-induced pluripotent stem cell for injection (3.0 ml, 1 × 10^11 particles/ml) Other names: GD-iExo-003
Placebo comparator: exosome placebo group Patients in this arm will be given a placebo of exosomes derived from human-induced pluripotent stem cell for injection once a day for 7 days	Drug: a placebo of exosomes derived from human-induced pluripotent stem cell for injection Exosomes placebo, 3.0 ml Other names: GD-iExo-003 placebo

Primary Outcome Measures

Outcome measure	Measure description	Time frame
Number of participants who experienced dose-limiting toxicities (DLTs)	DLTs related to exosome are defined as any of the following: (1) Grade 3–4 infusion-related allergic adverse events consisting of perturbation of cardiovascular, respiratory function, or allergic reactions occurring in the first 24 h post-infusion of investigational product. (2) Grade 3–4 adverse events through seven days after administration of the last injection. (3) Neurologic worsening defined as a 4-point increase in NIHSS compared with baseline NIHSS assessed through seven days after administration of the last injection. And (4) rate of intracranial hemorrhage. Adverse event is graded in Common Terminology Criteria for Adverse Events Version 5.0 (CTCAE 5.0)	14±2 days

Secondary Outcome Measures

Outcome measure	Measure description	Time frame
Incidence of severe adverse events	The proportion of patients who experienced severe adverse events	90±7 days
Favorable functional outcome	Rate of favorable functional outcome defined as a modified Rankin scale (mRS, scores range from 0 to 6, with 0–2 indicating favorable outcome and 3–6 indicating unfavorable outcome including 6 as death) score of 0–2)	90±7 days
Functional outcome	The range of mRS scores by shift analysis	90±7 days
NIHSS score change	The change of the National Institutes of Health Stroke Scale (NIHSS) score from day 7 to baseline	7 days
NIHSS score change	The change of the National Institutes of Health Stroke Scale (NIHSS) score from day 14 to baseline	14±2 days
Quality of life (EQ-5D-5L)	The value of EQ-5D-5L score	90±7 days
Barthel index (BI)	The value of BI	90±7 days

Other Outcome Measures

Outcome measure	Measure description	Time frame
Change of infarct volume	The infarct volume is measured by CT or MRI from the baseline to 14 days	14±2 days
Blood marker changes from baseline to discharge	A number of blood markers will be examined including C-reactive protein, glial fibrillary acidic protein, IL-1β, IL-6, IL-8, IL-10, and tumor necrosis factor-alpha	At discharge, an average of 14 days

Sponsor
Xuanwu Hospital, Beijing
Collaborators

- Guidon Pharmaceutics Ltd.

Investigators

- Principal Investigator: Junwei Hao, MD; PhD, Xuanwu Hospital, Beijing

Active, Not Recruiting

Extracellular Vesicles as Stroke Biomarkers (EXO4STROKE)

ClinicalTrials.gov ID NCT05370105
Sponsor Fondazione Don Carlo Gnocchi Onlus

Information provided by Fondazione Don Carlo Gnocchi Onlus (Responsible Party)

Last Update Posted 2024-01-03

Study Overview

Brief Summary

The combination of rehabilitation protocols and regenerative therapies offers the outstanding opportunity to promote and enhance the endogenous regenerative and repair processes occurring in tissues damaged or lost due to injury, disease, or age. Still, one of the main hurdles in the clinical approach to regenerative rehabilitation is the lack of easily accessible and sensitive biomarkers for the evaluation of rehabilitation and therapy efficacy. Extracellular vesicles (EVs) are nanoscaled vesicles that mediate intercellular communication among organs. EVs were shown to be involved in the onset, progression, and resolution of many disorders, being also used as a valuable tool in the regenerative medicine field. However, the initial enthusiastic approach to EVs has been hindered in its transfer to clinics because of technological obstacles related to their dimensions and limited availability. The present project proposes the application of a surface plasmon resonance imaging (SPRi)-based biosensor for the detection and characterization of blood EVs from stroke patients, before and after rehabilitation. After the successful SPRi detection of EVs of different cellular origin (brain and non-brain cells), the quantification of specific surface molecules related to pathological or regeneration processes will be accomplished. If successful, the project will (1) demonstrate the ability of the SPRi biosensor to reveal differences in the relative amount of specific cell-derived EV subpopulations and in their cargo during disease progression and rehabilitation-induced recovery, (2) provide support for using the proposed SPRi-based biosensor for the detection and characterization of circulating EVs in order to evaluate the efficacy of rehabilitation protocols and regenerative therapies, (3) and identify new biomarkers for the profiling of stroke patients to personalize the rehabilitation therapies.

Detailed Description

OBJECTIVE: The aim of the project will be the evaluation of the prognostic power of circulating extracellular vesicles (EVs) in the serum of stroke patients. The characterization by SPRi of different families of EVs will allow to evaluate the activation status of the processes of neuroinflammation, neuronal regeneration, angiogenesis, and cellular damage to provide a picture of the mechanisms of response to the damage taking place in the patient. These data will be correlated with emerging prognostic markers derived from the literature and with the outcome of the rehabilitation evaluated with specific functional and neurological scales that allow accurate profiling of the patient and the evaluation of functional recovery, according to what recently validated in the "Minimum rehabilitation evaluation protocol of the person with Cerebral Stroke Version 2020—PMIC 2020" by the Italian Society of Physical and Rehabilitative Medicine (SIMFER) (https://springerhealthcare.it/mr/numero/volume-34-n- 2-June-2020).

The PMIC 2020 aims to provide each physiatrist (rehabilitation team) with a uniform tool for the assessment of the person with stroke in the different phases of the disease, from acute hospital to territorial rehabilitation.

Specific objectives will be:

(i) optimization of the SPRi method for the identification of different families of EVs in the serum of healthy subjects, ii) evaluation of the feasibility of the SPRi-based method for the characterization of EVs from the serum of stroke patients, and iii) preliminary study of the correlation between SPRi data, soluble markers of inflammation and regeneration, patient profiling, and rehabilitation outcome at discharge.

IMPACT: The personalization of the rehabilitation plan in relation to the injury suffered and the patient's active response would lead to an increased probability of functional recovery, with benefits in terms of quality of life for the patient and family members, and a reduction in the management costs of the for the National Health System.

SAMPLE COLLECTION: 80 post-stroke patients will be asked to undergo three samples of biological material (10 ml of blood, two 5 ml tubes suitable for serum isolation), the first collection on the second day of hospitalization (t0) at IRCCS S. Maria Nascente (Milan) or IRCCS Don Gnocchi (Florence) of Fondazione Don Gnocchi and a second withdrawal at discharge (t1), or approximately 2 months after the first withdrawal. Where possible, a third sampling (t2 – follow-up) will be performed 6 months after the event at the IRCCS S. Maria Nascente or at the IRCCS in Florence. A total of 20 healthy subjects will be asked to undergo a single sample of biological material (10 ml of blood, two 5 ml tubes suitable for serum isolation).

EV ISOLATION: The blood sample will be processed for serum separation. The samples will be coded, sterile aliquoted, and stored at −80 °C at the Laboratory of Nanomedicine and Clinical Biophotonics of IRCCS S. Maria Nascente (Milan) until used.

EVs will be isolated from serum by size exclusion chromatography (qEV; Izon). The actual isolation will be verified with standard techniques, including Western blot for specific protein markers (CD63, Flotillin 1), nanoparticle tracking analysis, or transmission electron microscopy.

SPRi BIOSENSOR: The functionalization of the SPRi chip will be optimized for known markers of apoptotic bodies (Annexin V; index of extent of brain damage) and of EVs from neurons (Ephrin), microglia (IB4 or CD11b), astrocytes (GLAST), and endothelial cells (CD31). The chip will be also functionalized for the recognition of the Klotho protein (Sahu et al. 2018).

Immobilized EVs will be tested also for the presence on the surface of receptors related to neuronal regeneration (TGFbR1/2), microglial activation (TSPO), and angiogenesis (VEGFR-2).

RAMAN ANALYSIS: EVs isolated from patient serum will also be analyzed by Raman spectroscopy according to a protocol already optimized for patients with

Parkinson's disease (Gualerzi et al. 2019). Raman analysis will provide information on the biochemical characteristics of the EVs, which can be correlated with the molecular data obtained in SPRi.

ELISA: Known markers of inflammation and neuronal activation will be quantified in serum by ELISA assays—inflammatory cytokines (IL6 and TNFa), adipokines (leptin), soluble adhesion molecules (sICAM, sFAS), and growth factors (BDNF).

Correlation between SPRi data, soluble inflammatory, and neurotrophic factors will be performed to identify new rehabilitation markers for stroke patients

Official Title

Characterization of Circulating Extracellular Vesicles/Exosomes as New Predictive Biomarkers in Stroke Patients

Conditions

Stroke

Rehabilitation

Intervention/Treatment

- Other: blood withdrawal

Other Study ID Numbers

- EXO4STROKE

Study Start (Actual)

2018-06-25

Primary Completion (Actual)

2022-09-30

Study Completion (Estimated)

2023-12-31

Enrollment (Estimated)

100

Study Type

Observational

This study has 2 locations

Italy

Florence, Italy

IRCCS Don Gnocchi, Fondazione Don Carlo Gnocchi ONLUS

Milano, Italy, 20148

IRCCS S. Maria Nascente, Fondazione Don Carlo Gnocchi ONLUS

Eligibility Criteria

Description

Inclusion Criteria:

- Diagnosis of ischemic or hemorrhagic stroke related to intensive post-stroke rehabilitation hospitalization
- Within 15 days of the ictal event

Exclusion Criteria:

- Previous head injuries/traumas
- Oncological diseases
- Diseases of the immune and hematological system
- Neurodegenerative diseases

Study Population

Patients hospitalized at Fondazione Don Gnocchi after stroke injury and undergoing an intensive rehabilitation program.

Ages Eligible for Study

35–75 years (adult, older adult)

Sexes Eligible for Study

All

Accepts Healthy Volunteers

Yes

Sampling Method

Probability Sample

Study Plan

Design Details

Observational model: case-control

Time perspective: prospective

Biospecimen retention: samples with DNA

Biospecimen description: Serum samples used for extracellular vesicles isolation. DNA content will not be considered.

Groups and Interventions

Groups/cohorts	Intervention/treatment
Stroke patients 80 post-stroke patients will be asked to undergo three samples of biological material (10 ml of blood): the first collection on the second day of hospitalization at IRCCS S. Maria Nascente (Milano) or at IRCCS Don Gnocchi (Florence) of Fondazione Don Gnocchi (t0) and a second withdrawal at discharge (t1), or approximately 2 months after the first withdrawal. Where possible, a third sampling (t2 – follow-up) will be performed 6 months after the event	Other: blood withdrawal 10 ml of blood, two 5 ml tubes suitable for serum isolation. Given the nature and objectives of the study, there are no risks and/or inconveniences of particular importance for the patient since the blood samples will be performed according to the common procedure used in all analysis laboratories. At the end of the collection, in the area where the blood sample was taken, a small bruise may form which will disappear in the following hours; in any case during the collection, particular attention will be paid to the subjects being treated with antiplatelet and anticoagulants The study does not include the execution of interventional treatments or therapies

(continued)

Groups/cohorts	Intervention/treatment
Healthy controls The healthy controls will be volunteers recruited at Fondazione Don Gnocchi, who are not affected by neurodegenerative and cardiovascular diseases and who have not taken anti-inflammatory drugs in the week prior to recruitment	Other: blood withdrawal 10 ml of blood, two 5 ml tubes suitable for serum isolation. Given the nature and objectives of the study, there are no risks and/or inconveniences of particular importance for the patient since the blood samples will be performed according to the common procedure used in all analysis laboratories. At the end of the collection, in the area where the blood sample was taken, a small bruise may form which will disappear in the following hours; in any case during the collection, particular attention will be paid to the subjects being treated with antiplatelet and anticoagulants The study does not include the execution of interventional treatments or therapies

Primary Outcome Measures

Outcome measure	Measure description	Time frame
Change in modified Barthel index after rehabilitation	modified Barthel index (Shah et al. 1989)	01/11/2020–30/03/2022

Secondary Outcome Measures

Outcome measure	Measure description	Time frame
Extracellular vesicle characterization by SPRi	EVs will be isolated from serum, characterized by standard procedures, and injected on the SPRi biosensor for the differential quantification of multiple EV subfamilies. Secondary antigens will be evaluated on the surface of immobilized EVs Changes in biomarker expression will be assessed after rehabilitation	25/06/2018–30/09/2022
Change in numeric rating scale (NRS) PAIN or PAINAD for non-verbal patient after rehabilitation	Numeric rating scale (NRS) PAIN or PAINAD for non-verbal patient, validated in the literature and already proposed in the PMIC 2020 by SIMFER, will be used for accurate patient profiling and assessment of functional recovery	25/06/2018–30/09/2022
Change in anamnestic and current modified Rankin scale after rehabilitation	Anamnestic and current modified Rankin scale, validated in the literature and already proposed in the PMIC 2020 by SIMFER, will be used for accurate patient profiling and assessment of functional recovery	25/06/2018–30/09/2022
Change in NIH-STROKE scale after rehabilitation	NIHSS scale (Brott et al. 1989), validated in the literature and already proposed in the PMIC 2020 by SIMFER, will be used for accurate patient profiling and assessment of functional recovery	25/06/2018–30/09/2022

(continued)

Outcome measure	Measure description	Time frame
Change in Fugl-Meyer Assessment (FMA) scale after rehabilitation	Fugl-Meyer Assessment (FMA) scale (Fugl-Meyer et al. 1975; Cecchi et al. 2020), validated in the literature and already proposed in the PMIC 2020 by SIMFER, will be used for accurate patient profiling and assessment of functional recovery	25/06/2018–30/09/2022
Change in Trunk control test after rehabilitation	Trunk control test (Franchignoni et al. 1997), validated in the literature and already proposed in the PMIC 2020 by SIMFER, will be used for accurate patient profiling and assessment of functional recovery	25/06/2018–30/09/2022
Change in short physical performance battery (SPPB) after rehabilitation	SPPB (Guralnik et al. 1994), validated in the literature and already proposed in the PMIC 2020 by SIMFER, will be used for accurate patient profiling and assessment of functional recovery	25/06/2018–30/09/2022
Change in functional ambulation classification	Functional ambulation classification (Jan Mehrholz et al. 2007), validated in the literature and already proposed in the PMIC 2020 by SIMFER, will be used for accurate patient profiling and assessment of functional recovery	25/06/2018–30/09/2022
Change in Addenbrooke's cognitive examination scale after rehabilitation	Addenbrooke's cognitive examination (Mathuranath et al. 2000), validated in the literature and already proposed in the PMIC 2020 by SIMFER, will be used for accurate patient profiling and assessment of functional recovery	25/06/2018–30/09/2022
Change in hospital anxiety and depression scale (HADS) after rehabilitation	HADS, validated in the literature and already proposed in the PMIC 2020 by SIMFER, will be used for accurate patient profiling and assessment of functional recovery	25/06/2018–30/09/2022
Change in cumulative illness rating scale (CIRS) after rehabilitation	CIRS (Linn et al. 1968), validated in the literature and already proposed in the PMIC 2020 by SIMFER, will be used for accurate patient profiling and assessment of functional recovery	25/06/2018–30/09/2022

Sponsor
Fondazione Don Carlo Gnocchi Onlus
Investigators

- Principal Investigator: Alice Gualerzi, PhD, Fondazione Don Carlo Gnocchi, Laboratory of Nanomedicine and Clinical Biophotonics

Publications

- Picciolini S, Gualerzi A, Vanna R, Sguassero A, Gramatica F, Bedoni M, Masserini M, Morasso C. Detection and Characterization of Different Brain-Derived Subpopulations of Plasma Exosomes by Surface Plasmon Resonance

Imaging. Anal Chem. 2018 Aug 7;90(15):8873–8880. doi: 10.1021/acs.analchem.8b00941. Epub 2018 Jul 17.

- Gualerzi A, Picciolini S, Carlomagno C, Terenzi F, Ramat S, Sorbi S, Bedoni M. Raman profiling of circulating extracellular vesicles for the stratification of Parkinson's patients. Nanomedicine. 2019 Nov;22:102097. doi: 10.1016/j.nano.2019.102097. Epub 2019 Oct 21.
- Picciolini S, Gualerzi A, Carlomagno C, Cabinio M, Sorrentino S, Baglio F, Bedoni M. An SPRi-based biosensor pilot study: Analysis of multiple circulating extracellular vesicles and hippocampal volume in Alzheimer's disease. J Pharm Biomed Anal. 2021 Jan 5;192:113649. doi: 10.1016/j.jpba.2020.113649. Epub 2020 Sep 23.
- Gualerzi A, Picciolini S, Carlomagno C, Roda F, Bedoni M. Biophotonics for diagnostic detection of extracellular vesicles. Adv Drug Deliv Rev. 2021 Jul;174:229-249. doi: 10.1016/j.addr.2021.04.014. Epub 2021 Apr 19.
- Gualerzi A, Picciolini S, Roda F, Bedoni M. Extracellular Vesicles in Regeneration and Rehabilitation Recovery after Stroke. Biology (Basel). 2021 Aug 30;10(9):843. doi: 10.3390/biology10090843.

Recruiting

The Role of Acupuncture-Induced Exosome in Treating Post-Stroke Dementia

ClinicalTrials.gov ID NCT05326724

Sponsor China Medical University Hospital

Information provided by China Medical University Hospital (Responsible Party)

Last Update Posted 2022-04-13

Study Overview

Brief Summary

Stroke is the main cause of disability and the second main cause of dementia. Approximately 21.5% of patients develop dementia within 4 years after stroke. The main clinical manifestation of dementia is memory and cognitive impairment. At present, acetylcholinesterase inhibitors and NMDA glutamate receptor antagonists are used for dementia treatment, but those drugs have limited efficacy. Exosome is an extracellular vesicle from the endosomal, size ranging from ~40 to 160 nm (average ~100 nm). It contains many cells including DNA, RNA, fat, and metabolites, as well as cytoplasm and cell surface proteins that play a role in regulating intercellular communication. Some studies believe that exosomes in the circulation are an ideal marker to reflect the pathological progress and recovery of stroke and play a key role in the reorganization of tissues and the progress of neurodegeneration after stroke. Our previous studies have known that acupuncture can increase the long-term potentiation of hippocampal CA1 in rats with ischemic stroke and improve learning-memory and neurological function. Therefore, the purpose of this study is to explore the role of acupuncture-induced exosome in the treatment of post-stroke dementia.

Official Title
The Role of Acupuncture-Induced Exosome in Treating Post-Stroke Dementia
Conditions
Exosome
Post-stroke dementia
Acupuncture
Intervention/Treatment

- Device: acupuncture

Other Study ID Numbers

- CMUH111-REC2-024

Study Start (Estimated)
2022-08-01
Primary Completion (Estimated)
2025-07-31
Study Completion (Estimated)
2025-07-31
Enrollment (Estimated)
30
Study Type
Interventional
Phase
Not applicable
Study Contact
Name: Ching-Liang Hsieh, Ph.D
Phone Number: +886-4-22053366 ext 3127
Email: clhsieh@mail.cmuh.org.tw
This study has 1 location
Taiwan
North District Locations
Taichung, North District, Taiwan, 40447
Recruiting
China Medical University Hospital
Contact:
Ching-Liang Hsieh, PhD
+886-4-22053366 ext 3127 clhsieh@mail.cmuh.org.tw
Eligibility Criteria
Description
Inclusion Criteria:

1. History of stroke
2. MMSE score between 16 and 26

Exclusion Criteria:

1. Those with serious diseases, such as heart failure, chronic failure, or cancer patients
2. Intolerance to acupuncture treatment
3. Allergy to acupuncture needles
4. Refusal to sign the informed consent form

Ages Eligible for Study
50–75 years (adult, older adult)
Sexes Eligible for Study
All
Accepts Healthy Volunteers
No
Study Plan
Design Details
Primary purpose: treatment
Allocation: N/A
Interventional model: single group assignment
Masking: none (open label)

Arms and Interventions

Participant group/arm	Intervention/treatment
Experimental: acupuncture	Device: acupuncture The stainless steel needles are used to insert into the three points of Sishencong, the Baihui, and the Dazhui, once a week, once for 20 min, for 12 consecutive weeks

Primary Outcome Measures

Outcome measure	Measure description	Time frame
Concentration of exosome		12 weeks
Alzheimer's disease assessment scale-cognitive subscale scale	Higher scores indicate greater cognitive impairment	12 weeks
Behavioral and psychological symptoms of dementia scale	The greater cognitive impairment or dementia severity is associated with higher rates of some BPSD (behavioral and psychological symptoms of dementia)	12 weeks

Sponsor
China Medical University Hospital
Recruiting

Extracellular Vesicle Surface Markers in Acute Cerebrovascular Syndromes (ElViS-ACS)

ClinicalTrials.gov ID NCT06319742

Sponsor Ospedale Civico, Lugano

Information provided by Dr. med. Carlo Cereda, Ospedale Civico, Lugano (Responsible Party)

Last Update Posted 2024-04-18

Study Overview

Brief Summary

Clinical implication of eventual blood biomarkers for stroke diagnosis and prognosis would be limited, mainly because clinical evaluation and scales (providing stroke severity) or neuroimaging (providing accurate size of the lesion) are more reliable predictors for clinical outcome prediction. In clinical practice, it would be more useful to find a biomarker that can help orient the physician in conditions in which the clinical picture and imaging provide limited support.

Transient ischemic attacks (TIAs) represent a classical example for which a biomarker would be of interest to confirm and distinguish a brain ischemic process from a stroke mimic. Diagnostic biomarkers of TIA have been investigated, but none of the potential candidates have reached enough accuracy for TIA diagnosis. Our group has found that extracellular vesicles (EVs) could be useful as biomarkers for detecting brain ischemia in patients with TIA because the EV surface antigen profile appears to be different in patients with transient symptoms, adjudicated to be very likely caused by brain ischemia, compared to patients whose symptoms were less likely due to brain ischemia. Our study has raised interest in the scientific community recognizing the promising role of blood-derived EV analysis in expanding the possibilities to correctly diagnose and classify TIA and stroke events and discriminate them from TIA or stroke mimics, with important future implications in management and therapy of the patients with acute ischemic cerebrovascular syndrome. The validity of our approach needs to be tested in a larger, prospective, multicenter study.

Detailed Description

Characterization of extracellular vesicles

Extracellular vesicles (EVs) will be characterized in pre-cleared serum samples (see transfer and managements of blood samples). EVs will be characterized by nanoparticle tracking analysis, western blot, bead-based flow cytometry (direct and inverse approach), and ELISA.

We will evaluate diameter and concentration of serum nanoparticles (NPs) by nanoparticle tracking analysis (NTA) using NanoSight LM10 (Malvern Instruments, United Kingdom) equipped with a 405 nm laser and Nanoparticle Tracking Analysis NTA 2.3 analytic software. A camera will record Brownian movement of EVs, and the size and number of EVs per mL will be calculated by Stokes-Einstein equation. Three videos of 60 s will be recorded for each analysis.

Western blot analysis will be performed on protein lysate after EV immunocapture (using beads covered with antibodies against EV-specific tetraspanins, CD9, CD63, and CD81). Blots of representative samples will be incubated with primary antibodies against specific markers expressed on the surface or within EVs (TSG101, syntenin-1, CD81, Alix) and potential contaminants (GRP94, apolipoprotein A1, apolipoprotein B48).

EV profiling will be performed using a standardized multiplex bead-based flow cytometric assay, using MACSPlex Human Exosome Kit (Miltenyi Biotec; Bergisch Gladbach, Germany), as previously described. The detection of 37 different surface antigens commonly expressed on EV membrane (including markers from activated platelets, endothelium, and inflammatory cells) will be simultaneously performed. Background will be subtracted from the MFI value of each marker and then normalized by using the mean fluorescence intensity levels (MFI) of CD9, CD63, and CD81. Levels of expression will be reported as normalized MFI (nMFI; %) for each EV-surface antigen (median value and interquartile range).

After an initial screening by multiplexed assay, single candidate EV biomarkers will be confirmed by either reverse flow cytometry and ELISA techniques.

The reverse flow cytometric assay will be performed by isolating EVs by capture beads coated with antibodies against CD9-CD63-CD81 (EpCam; JSR Micro) and then incubating with fluorochrome-conjugated antibodies against single EV surface antigens, associated with patient diagnosis during the initial screening by MACSPlex assay. Beads incubated with isotype-matched antibodies and beads incubated in absence of vesicles will serve as controls. Candidate EV biomarkers will be confirmed also by ELISA technique, using specific antibodies as per the manufacturer's instructions.

Official Title

Extracellular Vesicle Surface Markers in Acute Cerebrovascular Syndromes

Conditions

Stroke, TIA, stroke mimics, stroke biomarkers

Intervention/Treatment

- Diagnostic test: extracellular vesicle (EV) analysis

Other Study ID Numbers

- NSISTRCR_2201

Study Start (Actual)

2022-11-18

Primary Completion (Estimated)

2025-12-31

Study Completion (Estimated)

2026-01-31

Enrollment (Estimated)

200

Study Type

Observational

Study Contact
Name: Carlo Walter Cereda, PI
Phone Number: +41918116691
Email: carlo.cereda@eoc.ch
Study Contact Backup
Name: Giovanni Bianco
Phone Number: +41918117073
Email: giovanni.bianco@eoc.ch
This study has 1 location
Switzerland
Ticino Locations
Lugano, Ticino, Switzerland, CH-6900
Recruiting
Neurocenter of Southern Switzerland, Ospedale Civico
Contact:
Carlo Cereda, MD
+41 91 811 6691 carlo.cereda@eoc.ch
Principal Investigator:
Carlo Cereda
Eligibility Criteria
Description
Inclusion Criteria:
Affected by:

1. Suspect ischemic minor stroke (acute loss of focal cerebral function of presumed vascular etiology and NIHSS ≤327, 28) within 48 h of symptom onset or II TIA (defined as the acute onset of focal neurological symptoms lasting <24 h and presumed to be caused by brain ischemia at the time of referral) 19 III. Symptoms mimicking I or II with high suspicion of a non-ischemic condition being the cause of the event
2. Age ≥18 years
3. If cerebral magnetic resonance imaging will be performed within 48–72 h from admission
4. If baseline CT/MRI is without hemorrhage
5. If informed consent obtained

Exclusion Criteria:

1. Ocular TIA (amaurosis fugax)
2. Contraindications for MRI
3. Pregnancy
4. Concomitant acute/chronic inflammatory disease (e.g., infections, autoimmune disease)
5. Concomitant hematological diseases
6. Central nervous system infection within 30 days
7. Serious head trauma within 30 days

8. Major surgery within 90 days

Study Population

We will enroll all patients admitted to the stroke units because of symptoms suggesting a cerebrovascular syndrome.

Ages Eligible for Study

18 years and older (adult, older adult)

Sexes Eligible for Study

All

Accepts Healthy Volunteers

No

Sampling Method

Probability Sample

Design Details

Observational model: cohort

Time perspective: prospective

Groups and Interventions

Groups/cohorts	Intervention/treatment
Stroke	Diagnostic test: extracellular vesicle (EV) analysis The patients undergo a blood sample for EV analyses: EVs will be characterized by nanoparticle tracking analysis, western blot, bead-based flow cytometry (direct and inverse approach), and ELISA We will evaluate diameter and concentration of serum nanoparticles (NPs) by nanoparticle tracking analysis (NTA) using NanoSight LM10. Western blot analysis will be performed on protein lysate after EV immuno-capture (using beads covered with antibodies against EV-specific tetraspanins, CD9, CD63, and CD81). EV profiling will be performed using a standardized multiplex bead-based flow cytometric assay, using MACSPlex Human Exosome Kit (Miltenyi Biotec; Bergisch Gladbach, Germany), as previously described. The detection of 37 different surface antigens commonly expressed on EV membrane (including markers from activated platelets, endothelium, and inflammatory cells) will be simultaneously performed
TIA	Diagnostic test: extracellular vesicle (EV) analysis The patients undergo a blood sample for EV analyses: EVs will be characterized by nanoparticle tracking analysis, western blot, bead-based flow cytometry (direct and inverse approach), and ELISA We will evaluate the diameter and concentration of serum nanoparticles (NPs) by nanoparticle tracking analysis (NTA) using NanoSight LM10. Western blot analysis will be performed on protein lysate after EV immuno-capture (using beads covered with antibodies against EV-specific tetraspanins, CD9, CD63, and CD81). EV profiling will be performed using a standardized multiplex bead-based flow cytometric assay, using MACSPlex Human Exosome Kit (Miltenyi Biotec; Bergisch Gladbach, Germany), as previously described. The detection of 37 different surface antigens commonly expressed on EV membrane (including markers from activated platelets, endothelium, and inflammatory cells) will be simultaneously performed

(continued)

Groups/cohorts	Intervention/treatment
Stroke mimic	Diagnostic test: extracellular vesicle (EV) analysis The patients undergo a blood sample for EV analyses: EVs will be characterized by nanoparticle tracking analysis, western blot, bead-based flow cytometry (direct and inverse approach), and ELISA We will evaluate the diameter and concentration of serum nanoparticles (NPs) by nanoparticle tracking analysis (NTA) using NanoSight LM10. Western blot analysis will be performed on protein lysate after EV immuno-capture (using beads covered with antibodies against EV-specific tetraspanins, CD9, CD63, and CD81). EV profiling will be performed using a standardized multiplex bead-based flow cytometric assay, using MACSPlex Human Exosome Kit (Miltenyi Biotec; Bergisch Gladbach, Germany), as previously described. The detection of 37 different surface antigens commonly expressed on EV membrane (including markers from activated platelets, endothelium, and inflammatory cells) will be simultaneously performed

Primary Outcome Measures

Outcome measure	Measure description	Time frame
TIA differentiation from TIA mimics	Determine the performance of EV profiling (analysis of antigens expressed on vesicle surface), added to a structured clinical (PREDISC score) and imaging evaluation (brain MRI), to discriminate TIAs from TIA mimics (non-ischemic events)	72 h from symptom onset

Secondary Outcome Measures

Outcome measure	Measure description	Time frame
TIA differentiation from stroke	Determine the performance of EV profiling to differentiate between TIAs (with negative MRI for acute lesion) and acute ischemic strokes (AIS, MRI confirmed)	Acute phase, 3 and 12 months
Stroke etiology	Determine the performance of EV profiling to categorize pre-specified causes of ischemic events	Acute phase, 3 and 12 months

Sponsor
Ospedale Civico, Lugano

Index

A
Active immunosuppression, 310
Acupuncture, 258, 259, 360–362
Acupuncture-induced exosome, 187, 188
Acute exercise, 218, 219
Acute ischemic stroke, 349–351
Acute myeloid leukemia, 32–37
Acute myocardial infarction, 310
Acute/chronic pancreatitis, 118
Acute respiratory distress syndrome (ARDS), 305
Acute type A aortic dissection (ATAAD), 237–239
Adjuvant chemotherapy (ACT), 76
Advanced adenomas (AAs), 104
Advanced adenomas and colorectal cancer (AACRC), 104–113
Adverse events (AEs), 35
Aegle therapeutics, 334
Aging, 181, 182
AGLE-102, 329
Allogeneic mesenchymal stromal cells, 279
Alternating current electric (ACE), 114
Alzheimer's disease (AD), 140
Amyotrophic lateral sclerosis, 175–181
Anastomotic leakage, 8, 9
Androgenetic alopecia, 212, 216
Anemia, 32
Anemia recovery, 36
Anlotinib, 125–128
Antiaging, 181–184
Anti-infective agents, 37
Anti-inflammatory therapies, 254
Applied behavioral analysis (ABA), 186
Artificial tear replacement, 254
Atopic dermatitis (AD), 343–348
Autism, 184–187
Autism Diagnostic Observation Schedule (ADOS), 187
Autism spectrum disorder (ASD), 184, 186
Autologous adipose tissue-derived stem cells (ADSCs), 195–197, 200
Autologous platelet-rich plasma, 184

B
B cell non-Hodgkin lymphoma (B-NHL), 47
BENEV exosome regenerative complex+ for self-perceived thinning hair, 204, 205
BENEV Exosome Regenerative Complex+ post SylFirmX® RF microneedling procedure, 204
Beta-catenin, 12
β-hCG pregnancy test, 152
Bioinformatics methods, 80
Biomarkers, 42
Bipolar disorder (BD), 241–243
Blood biomarkers, 363
Blood microvesicles and exosomes in patients with graft occlusion after aortocoronary bypass surgery (MVBYPASS), 137–139
Blood transfusion, 37
Blood-brain barrier (BBB), 306
Brain metastases, 4
Breastmilk, 202
Bronchopulmonary dysplasia (BPD), 229, 232

J. N. Weiss, *Global Exosome Trials*, https://doi.org/10.1007/978-3-031-96420-6

C

CA9, 42
Cancer, 3–6
Cancer cell-derived exosomes, 101
Carbohydrate antigen 19-9 (CA19-9), 16
Carbon footprint, 42
Cardiac function, 32
Cardiac remodeling, 133
Cardiovascular magnetic resonance (CMR), 133
Cardiovascular surgery, delirium, 140–142
Case group, 51
CD9, 42
CD9+, 44
CD9+/VGEFR2+ exosomes, 45
CD20, 47
Cellular metabolism, 13
Cerebrospinal fluid, 3, 5, 6
cf-miRNA, 104
Chemoradiation therapy, 25
Chemotherapy, 152
Chemotherapy-induced myelosuppression, 32–37
Childhood Autism Rating Scale (CARS), 184, 187
Chloasma, 340–342
CHOP chemotherapy (R-CHOP), 46
Chronic cough, after COVID-19, 289, 292
Chronic dry eye, 254–255
Chronic kidney disease (CKD), 168
Chronic obstructive pulmonary disease (COPD), 290
Chronic wounds, 324
Clear cell renal cell carcinoma, 42–46
Clinical diagnostic value, 166–169
Cognitive delay, 229, 232
Colon carcinogenesis, 12
Colonoscopy, 11
Colorectal cancer (CRC), 104, 108
Column extraction method, 264
Complete remission (CR), 32
Computed tomography (CT), 4
Control group, 51, 52
Controlled ankle movement (CAM), 154
Conventional immunotherapy, 290
Coronary artery bypass graft (CABG) surgery, 137
Coronary artery disease (CAD), 137
COVID-19
  chronic cough after, 289, 292
  extracellular vesicles for, 307
  extracorporal oxygenation, 300
  lung failure, 300
  lungs and, 305
  nebulized exosome therapy for, 291
  nebulized MSC-secreted extracellular vesicles, 304
  people with low immunity, 305
  rehabilitation outpatient clinic, 292
  stem cell exosomes for, 307
  treatment strategies for, 290
Crystallized phenol (CP) procedure, 324
CtDNA/exosome evaluation, 7
Curcumin, 12
Cytarabine, 33
Cytology, 99

D

Data-independent acquisition (DIA) proteomics, 80
Daunorubicin, 33
Decompensated liver cirrhosis, 143–147
Delirium, 140–142
Dementia, 188–190, 192, 360–362
DEtection of colorectal NEoplasias in blood (DENEB), 108, 109
Diabetic foot ulcers (DFU), 149–155
Diabetic nephropathy, 165, 167
Diabetic retinopathy (DR), 264–267
  exosomes, 267
  treatment, 266
Dietary protein, 155–162
Diffuse large B cell lymphomas (DLBCL), 46, 47
Disease-free survival (DFS), 69
Dose-limiting toxicities (DLTs), 36, 175, 176, 179, 349, 352
Dry eye disease (DED), 250
Dry eye syndrome (DES), 258
  acupuncture, 258
  Chinese herbal tea bag TBDESJS, 258, 259
  limbal stem cells derived exosomes (LSC-Exo), 255
Dual-energy X-ray absorptiometry (DXA), 174
Ductal adenocarcinoma, 120

E

Early Onset Colorectal Cancer Detection (ENCODE), 90–96
Early-staged lung cancer, 55–58
Electrocardiogram (ECG), 135
Electron microscopy technique, 42, 44, 45
ELISA assays, 356

Endocrine malignancy, 96
Epidermal growth factor receptor (EGFR) mutations, 70–73
Epidermolysis bullosa (EB), 329, 330, 332
Epilepsy, 190–194
Erectile dysfunction (ED), 195–200
Esophagus cancer group, 83
Exo-CD24, 291, 307
ExoFlo, 307
ExoLuminate study, 113–119
Exo-PRECISE, 122–124
ExoReBLy, 46–49
Exosomal expression, 27
Exosomal microRNAs (exo-miRNA), 59, 104
Exosomes, 1, 3, 6–8, 12, 175, 176, 178, 179, 181, 182, 186, 188, 190, 196, 197, 200, 202, 205, 209, 213, 215–218, 220, 221, 224, 225, 228, 229, 231, 237, 239, 241, 242, 244–246, 271, 290, 291, 300, 305, 324, 333–344, 360–362, 364, 366, 367
  as correlative biomarker in clinical outcomes, 25
  diabetic retinopathy (DR), 266
  dry eye, 255
  as predictive biomarkers, 73–75
  in rectal cancer, 24–27
  intraperitoneal administration of, 9
  molecular profiling of, 55–58
  non-Hodgkin B-cell lymphomas, 46–49
  rectal cancer patients, preventing early leakage in, 8–12
  safety of, 279
Exosome microRNA expression, 155–162
Exosome RNA, 66–70
Exosome testing, 86–89
Exosome therapy, 184
Exosome-based liquid biopsies, for upper gastrointestinal cancers diagnosis, 80–83
Exosome-based liquid biopsy for the differential diagnosis of primary liver cancer (ELUCIDATE), 58–64
Exosome-based miRNA, 16
Exosome-Based Nanoplatform for Ldlr mRNA Delivery in FH (ENDFH), 220
Exosome-based OCS scores, 52–55
Exosome-mediated intercellular signaling, 119–122
Exosome-mediated single-cell transcriptomics, 49–52
Exosomes in Melanoma Patients (EXOMEL1), 37–39
Exosomes in Monitoring Patients with Sarcoma (EXOSARC), 28–31
ExoVerita™ assay, 114
Extracellular Vesicle Treatment for Acute Respiratory Distress Syndrome (ARDS) (EXTINGUISH ARDS), 314–320
Extracellular vesicles (EVs), 128–131, 228, 229, 231, 232, 291, 307, 354–356, 358, 363, 364, 366, 367
Extracorporal oxygenation, 300
Extremely low birth weight (ELBW) infants, 228, 229, 231

F

Familial hypercholesterolemia (FH), 220, 221
Fat mass, 174
Fat-free mass, 174
Febrile neutropenia, 36
Fecal immunochemical testing (FIT), 104
Fistulotomy, 321
Flow cytometry, 45
Follicular thyroid cancer, 96–100

G

Galectin-3, 100–103
Gastric cardia cancer, 49–52
Glial tumor exosomes (ExoGLIE), 39–42
Gliomas, 39
Good manufacture practice (GMP), 279

H

Hair, 204–218
Healthy, 178, 183, 186, 189, 192, 199, 203–206, 208, 214, 218–220, 223, 227, 230, 235, 239, 242, 243, 246
Hepatocellular carcinoma (HCC), 58, 61
HOMA index, 160
Homozygous familial hypercholesterolemia (HoFH), 220, 221
Host inflammation, 305
Human allogeneic mesenchymal stem cell-derived exosomes (HAMSCs-Exos), 291, 307
Human papillomavirus (HPV), 87
  HPV-OPSCC, 87
  HPV-positive cancer, 89
Human papillomavirus-positive oropharyngeal squamous cell carcinoma, 86–89
Human placenta mesenchymal stem cell (hPMSC), 8

Human placenta mesenchymal stem cell-derived exosomes, 8
Human umbilical cord mesenchymal stem cell-derived exosomes (hUCMSC-Exos), 339, 340, 342
Hypercholesterolemia, 220–222, 224, 225
Hyperinflammation, 300

I

Idarubicin, 33
Immune checkpoint inhibitors, 73
Immune modulation, 13
Induced pluripotent stem cell (iPSC), 191, 193, 344
Induced Pluripotent Stem Cell-Derived Exosomes, 343–348
Insulin, 169–174
- resistance, 155–162, 170
- sensitivity, 173

International Index of Erectile Function (IIEF) score, 195–198, 200, 201
Intraductal papillary mucinous neoplasm (IPMN), 120
Intrahepatic cholangiocarcinoma (ICC), 58, 61, 62
Intrahepatic triglyceride, 174
Intraventricular hemorrhage (IVH), 228

J

Jaundice, neonatal, 202–204

L

Limbal stem cells derived exosomes (LSC-Exo), 254
Liquid biopsy, 90
Liquid CDx test, 39
Liquid phenol, 324
Liver cirrhosis (LC), 143
Liver fibrosis, 143
lncRNA-ELNAT1, 86
Local immunosuppressive treatments, 254
Long COVID, 290
- heart-related symptoms, 290
- high-risk factors, 290
- immune system, 290
- neurological symptoms, 290
- pancreatic symptoms, 290
- reproductive symptoms, 290
- respiratory symptoms, 290
- vascular symptoms, 290

Low anterior resection (LAR), 9
Low-risk adenoma, 108
Lung adenocarcinoma, 70–73
Lung cancer
- with brain metastasis, 5
- with leptomeningeal metastasis, 5
- metastasis, 6

M

Machine learning, 104, 258
Magnetic resonance (MRI) images, 4
Major depressive disorder (MDD), 241, 243
Malondialdehyde, 161
Matrix metalloproteinase (MMP), 271
Maximum population concentration ratio (MCC) method, 248
Maximum tolerated dose (MTD), 36
Melanoma, 37
Melasma, 334–343
Meningeal metastases, 4
Mental developmental index (MDI) score, 229, 232
Mesenchymal stem cell exosomes, 274, 290, 291
- clinical case studies of, 307
- mechanism of, 306, 307

Mesenchymal stem cell-derived exosomes (MSC-Exo), 143–147, 250, 321–327
Mesenchymal stem cell-derived extracellular vesicles (MSC-EVs), 290
Mesenchymal stem cell-derived small extracellular vesicles (MSC-sEVs), 279
Mesenchymal stem cells (MSCs), 181, 191, 221, 228, 229, 231, 237, 239, 290, 305, 324
- clinical cases of, 291, 292
- mechanism of, 290, 291

Metabolic bone disease of prematurity (MBDP), 244, 245
Metabolically healthy and lean (MHL), 170
Metabolically unhealthy (MUO), 170
Metabolism, 225–228
Metastatic/locally advanced sarcoma, 31
MicroRNA (miRNA), 16, 104, 156, 247
MicroRNA biomarkers, 234
Microvesicles (MVs), 137, 181
MIRACLE Study, 133–137
miRTarBase, 165
Molecular residual disease (MRD), 75–80
Monoclonal anti-CD20 antibody, 46

mRNA therapy, 220
Multicenter cohort study, 83–86
Multidimensional statistical methods, 258
Multiple organ dysfunction syndrome (MODS), 237–240

N

Nanoparticle tracking analysis (NTA), 363
Nanoparticles (NPs), 363, 366, 367
Nanosomes, 101
Nebulized MSC-secreted extracellular vesicles, 304
Necrotizing enterocolitis (NEC), 229
Neoadjuvant chemoradiation therapy, 9, 25, 31
Neoadjuvant treatment (NT), 128
Neonatal abstinence syndrome (NAS), 234
Neonatal jaundice, 202–204
Neonatal opioid withdrawal syndrome, 234
Neurodevelopmental disorders, 228–233
Neuro-muscular diseases, 310
Newborn jaundice, 202
Next-generation sequencing (NGS), 41, 69
NF-κB pathways, 12
Nonablative fractional laser (NAFL), 339
Noncancer group, 83
Non-coding RNAs (ncRNAs), 271
Non-disease controls, 108
Non-Hodgkin B-cell lymphomas, 46–49
Non-small cell lung cancer (NSCLC), 4, 56, 125–128
Non-small cell lung cancer with central nervous system metastasis, 3–6

O

Obesity, 156
Ocular myasthenia gravis (OMG), 247, 248
Ocular Surface Index Score (OSDI), 255
Opioid withdrawal, 234–236
Oral glucose tolerance test (OGTT), 164, 167
Oropharyngeal squamous cell carcinoma (OPSCC), 87
Oropharynx, 87
Osteoarthritis (OA), 271
Ovarian cancer recurrence, 52–55
Oxidative stress, 156

P

Padded three-layer, 154
Pancreatic cancer
  ExoLuminate study, early detection of, 113–119
  exosome-mediated intercellular signaling, interrogation with, 119–122
  tumor exosome liquid biopsy strategy, 64–66
Pancreatic cancer detection consortium (PCDC), 16–24
Pancreatic cancer ductal adenocarcinoma, 20
PANcreatic cancer Exosome Early detectiON (PANXEON), 20
Pancreatic cyst, 118
Pancreatic ductal adenocarcinoma (PDAC), 16, 114
Pancreatic neuroendocrine tumors, 120
Pancreaticoduodenectomy, 120
Pancreatitis, 65
Parallel reaction monitoring (PRM) technology, 80
PASS software Test, 53
Pathological neonatal jaundice, 202
PD-1, 73
PD-L1 (programmed death-ligand 1), 37, 39, 73
PEP-TISSEEL, 154
Periventricular leukomalacia (PVL), 228
Phase 2a Multi-Center Prospective, Randomized Trial, 149–155
Phospholipid, 13
Photo-biomodulation (PBM), 184
Pilonidal sinus disease (PSD), 324
Plant exosomes, 12–16
Plasma Exosome RNA to Diagnose Prostate Cancer (exo-PRECISE), 122–124
Plasma exosomes, 70–73
Plasma proteins, 83
Platelet-rich plasma (PRP), 184
Pluripotent stem cell-derived mesenchymal stem cell exosome (PSC-MSC-Exo) eye drops, 250
Post COVID-19 syndrome, 290
Post-stroke dementia, 188, 361
Prematurity, 244–246
Primary high-grade osteosarcoma, 66–70
Primary liver cancers (PLCs), 58
Programmed cell death ligand 1 (PD-L1), 37, 39, 47, 73
Progression-free survival (PFS), 69
Progressive disease (PD), 127
Progressive lung fibrosis, 300
Proteomics, 49–52
Pulmonary vein, 56

Q
Quantitative reverse transcriptase polymerase chain reaction (qRT-PCR), 20

R
Radiation, 25
Raman analysis, 355
Real-time fluorescence quantification (RT-qPCR), 163, 248
RECC-EV, 128–131
Receiver operating characteristic (ROC) analysis, 241
Rectal cancer
  exosomes in, 24–27
  liquid biopsy, neoadjuvant treatment response assessment in, 128–131
Refractory focal epilepsy, 190, 191
Regenerative Injection of Stem Cells or Stem Cell-Derived Exosomes for Erectile Dysfunction (RISE), 195
Regenerative therapies, 354
Rehabilitation protocols, 354
Renal cell carcinoma, 73–75
Resistance exercise (RE), 225
Retinopathy of prematurity (ROP), 229
Reverse flow cytometric assay, 364
Reverse transcription quantitative polymerase chain reaction (RT-qPCR), 45, 46
Rituximab, 46

S
Sarcomas, 28
Schirmer's test, 258
Sclerosis, 175–181
Sequential organ failure assessment (SOFA) scores, 237–239
Serious adverse events (SAEs), 35
Serum exosomes, 202
Serum pregnancy test, 285
Severe acute respiratory syndrome coronavirus 2 (SARS-CoV-2), 290, 305
Sham comparator, 154
Single-vesicle membrane protein detection techniques, 80
Sjögren's syndrome (SJS), 258
Skin aging, 182
Small extracellular vesicles (SEV), 169–174
Spearman's ρ test, 124
Stable disease (SD), 127
Stage II–III colorectal cancer, 75–80
Statistical analysis, 165
ST-elevation myocardial infarction (STEMI), 133, 134, 136
Stem cells, 324, 335
Stem cell exosomes for COVID-19, 307
Stem cell-derived exosomes, 195
STONEES criteria, 152
Stroke, 187, 188, 349–362, 364, 366, 367
Surface plasmon resonance imaging (SPRi)-based biosensor, 354, 355
Surgical brain surgery, 4
Synovial fluid-derived mesenchymal stem cells (SF-MSC), 276
Synovial fluid-derived mesenchymal stem cells-derived exosomes (SF-MSC-EX), 276

T
TBDESJS, 258, 259
3M Cavilon®, 154
3-Minute Diagnostic Interview for Confusion Assessment Method (3D-CAM) diagnostic algorithm, 142
Thyroglobulin, urinary exosomal biomarkers of, 100–103
Thyroid cancer, 97
Thyroid follicular neoplasm, 96–100
TISSEEL, 154
Tissue factor (TF), 138
Topical PEP-TISSEEL, 149–155
Total mesorectum excision (TME), 128
Training-Induced Muscle Exosome Release (TIMER), 225
Transient ischemic attacks (TIAs), 363, 367
Tumor exosome liquid biopsy strategy, 64–66
Tumor-draining vein, 55–58
Tumorgenesis, 28
Type 2 diabetic kidney disease, 166–169
Type 2 diabetic nephropathy, 162–166

U
Umbilical cord mesenchymal stem cell (UCMSC), 289
Umbilical cord mesenchymal stem cell exosome nebulization inhalation, 291
Umbilical cord-derived mesenchymal stem cells exosomes (UCMSC-Exo), 32–37, 335
Upper gastrointestinal cancers, exosome-based liquid biopsies for, 80–83
Urinary exosomal protein biomarkers, 96–100

Urinary exosomal thyroglobulin (UExTg), 97
Urinary exosome
  from clear cell renal cell carcinoma, 42–46
  lncRNAs, 83–86
  in type 2 diabetic kidney disease, 166–169
  in type 2 diabetic nephropathy, 162–166
Urine pregnancy test, 285

V
Virus replication cycle, 305

W
Western blot analysis, 364
Women of childbearing potential (WOCBP), 285
Wound closure, 330

MIX
Papier aus verantwortungsvollen Quellen
Paper from responsible sources
FSC® C105338

If you have any concerns about our products,
you can contact us on
ProductSafety@springernature.com

In case Publisher is established outside the EU,
the EU authorized representative is:
Springer Nature Customer Service Center GmbH
Europaplatz 3, 69115 Heidelberg, Germany

Printed by Libri Plureos GmbH
in Hamburg, Germany